OXFORD HANDBOOK OF

Emergencies in Cardiology

Published and forthcoming titles in the Emergencies in . . . series:

Emergencies in Paediatrics and Neonatology
Stuart Crisp

Emergencies in Adult Nursing
Edited by Philip Downing

Emergencies in Anaesthesia
Edited by Keith Allman, Andrew McIndoe, and Iain H. Wilson

Emergencies in Children's and Young People's Nursing
Edited by E.A. Glasper, Gill McEwing, and Jim Richardson

Emergencies in Clinical Surgery
Edited by Chris Callaghan, Chris Watson and Andrew Bradley

Emergencies in Critical Care, 2e
Edited by Martin Beed, Richard Sherman, and Ravi Mahajan

Emergencies in Gastroenterology and Hepatology
Marcus Harbord and Daniel Marks

Emergencies in Mental Health Nursing
Edited by Patrick Callaghan

Emergencies in Obstetrics and Gynaecology
Edited by S. Arulkumaran

Emergencies in Oncology
Edited by Martin Scott-Brown, Roy A.J. Spence, and Patrick G. Johnston

Emergencies in Paediatrics and Neonatology, 2e
Edited by Stuart Crisp and Jo Rainbow

Emergencies in Palliative and Supportive Care
Edited by David Currow and Katherine Clark

Emergencies in Primary Care
Chantal Simon, Karen O'Reilly, John Buckmaster, and Robin Proctor

Emergencies in Psychiatry, 2e
Basant Puri and Ian Treasaden

Emergencies in Respiratory Medicine
Edited by Robert Parker, Catherine Thomas, and Lesley Bennett

Emergencies in Sports Medicine
Edited by Julian Redhead and Jonathan Gordon

Head, Neck and Dental Emergencies
Edited by Mike Perry

Medical Emergencies in Dentistry
Nigel Robb and Jason Leitch

OXFORD HANDBOOK OF

Emergencies in Cardiology

THIRD EDITION

EDITED BY

Robin P. Choudhury
Professor of Cardiovascular Medicine, University of Oxford. UK; Honorary Consultant Cardiologist, Oxford University Hospitals, UK

Thomas J. Cahill
Consultant Structural & Interventional Cardiologist, Oxford University Hospitals, UK

Andrew R.J. Mitchell
Consultant Cardiologist, Jersey General Hospital, Jersey & Honorary Consultant Cardiologist, Oxford University Hospitals, UK

OXFORD
UNIVERSITY PRESS

OXFORD
UNIVERSITY PRESS

Great Clarendon Street, Oxford, OX2 6DP,
United Kingdom

Oxford University Press is a department of the University of Oxford. It furthers the University's objective of excellence in research, scholarship, and education by publishing worldwide. Oxford is a registered trade mark of Oxford University Press in the UK and in certain other countries.

First Edition published in 2006
Second Edition published in 2010
Third Edition published in 2026

Published in the United States of America by Oxford University Press
198 Madison Avenue, New York, NY 10016, United States of America.

British Library Cataloguing in Publication Data
Data available

Library of Congress Control Number: 2025951458

ISBN 978–0–19–891484–6

DOI: 10.1093/med/9780198914846.001.0001

Printed in India by
Replika Press Pvt. Ltd.

MIX
Paper | Supporting responsible forestry
FSC www.fsc.org
FSC™ C016779

Preface for 3rd edition

Acute cardiology problems often require rapid and appropriate diagnosis and treatment. With the increasing complexity and rapidly evolving nature of available therapies, knowing which to use—and in what situation—can be challenging.

This book provides an easily accessible guide to diagnosing and managing acute cardiovascular problems. It is designed for busy medical and cardiology teams, offering expert advice in a clear, concise format. The familiar *Oxford Handbook* style, with bullet-point information for speed and clarity, is combined with an integral cross-referencing system that enables rapid access to essential information.

This third edition includes updated sections throughout and introduces chapters to guide safe emergency management in conditions with which the on-call doctor may be unfamiliar: pregnancy/maternal cardiology, adult congenital heart disease, drug-related cardiac conditions, hypertensive emergencies, transplantation, inherited cardiac conditions, emergency imaging, digital technologies, and end of life and palliation.

The first section of the book is symptom based and aims to help clinicians reach a diagnosis quickly, with suggestions regarding key points in the history, physical findings, investigations, and extensive cross-referencing to specific cardiac conditions later in the book.

The second section, 'Specific conditions', describes the presentation, investigation, and management of all common—and some uncommon—acute cardiac problems. The chapter authors use their specialist expertise to guide management in all areas, including complex issues such as arrhythmias (and implantable defibrillators), cardiac problems in pregnancy, perioperative cardiac issues, adults with congenital heart disease, and cardiac trauma.

The final section addresses 'Practical issues', with clear descriptions of how to perform common cardiac procedures. It also includes a chapter on the art of ECG recognition, with a library of example ECGs to support pattern recognition.

We hope that you enjoy the new edition of the book and find it valuable in enhancing the care of your patients. We welcome further suggestions for changes and additions in future editions RPC, TJC & ARJM 2026.

Contents

Contributors

Thomas J. Cahill
Consultant Cardiologist (Structural Intervention), Oxford University Hospitals, UK

Jason Chai
British Heart Foundation Clinical Research Fellow, University of Oxford, UK

Charles Chan
Consultant in Cardiothoracic Anaesthesia, Oxford University Hospitals, UK

Robin P. Choudhury
Professor of Cardiovascular Medicine, University of Oxford, UK; Honorary Consultant Cardiologist, Oxford University Hospitals, UK

Giovanni Luigi De Maria
Consultant Cardiologist (Intervention), Oxford University Hospitals, UK; Honorary Senior Clinical Lecturer, University of Oxford, UK

James Gamble
Consultant Cardiologist (Heart Failure), Oxford University Hospitals, UK

Michael Gatzoulis
Consultant Cardiologist, Royal Brompton; Professor of Cardiology (Congenital Heart Disease), National Heart and Lung Institute, Imperial College London, UK

Victoria Hedges
Consultant in Palliative Medicine, Oxford University Hospitals, UK

John A Henry
NIHR Academic Clinical Fellow in Cardiology, Oxford University Hospitals, UK

Aaron Henry
Academic Clinical Fellow, John Radcliffe Hospital, Oxford, UK

Andrew Johnson
Consultant in Cardiothoracic Intensive Care and Anaesthesia, Oxford University Hospitals, UK

Sujatha Kesavan
Registrar in Cardiology, Oxford University Hospitals, UK

Antonios Kouriolous
Consultant Cardiac Surgeon, Oxford University Hospitals, UK

Andrew Lewis
British Heart Foundation Intermediate Clinical Research Fellow, University of Oxford, UK; Honorary Consultant Cardiologist, Oxford University Hospitals, UK

Robert Lewis
Respiratory and Sleep Physician, Department of Respiratory Medicine, Middlemore Hospital, Auckland, New Zealand

Joanna Lim
Consultant Cardiologist (Adult Congenital Heart Disease), Oxford University Hospitals, UK

Andrew R.J. Mitchell
Consultant Cardiologist, Jersey General Hospital, Jersey; Honorary Consultant Cardiologist, Oxford University Hospitals, UK

Jim Newton
Consultant Cardiologist (Echocardiography and Valvular Heart Disease), Oxford University Hospitals, UK

Elizabeth Orchard
Consultant Cardiologist (Adult Congenital Heart Disease), Oxford University Hospitals, UK

Julian Ormerod
Consultant Cardiologist (Inherited Cardiac Conditions), Oxford University Hospitals, UK

Jennifer J. Rayner
Senior Clinical Research Fellow and Honorary Consultant Cardiologist, Oxford University Hospitals, UK

Nik Sabharwal
Consultant Cardiologist (Cardiac Imaging), Oxford University Hospitals, UK

Rod Stables
Professor of Cardiology and Consultant Cardiologist, Liverpool Heart and Chest Centre, UK

William D Watson
Clinical Lecturer in Cardiology, University of Cambridge and Royal Papworth Hospital, UK

Rohan Wijesurendra
Senior Clinical Research Fellow, University of Oxford, UK; Honorary Consultant Cardiologist (Electrophysiology), Oxford University Hospitals, UK

Emergency symbols

A true life-threatening emergency. Memorizing these conditions may help. Call immediately for help. Try to remain calm and quickly assess ABC. Once the problem has been dealt with remember to reassess—other problems may have been forgotten or missed in the heat of the moment.

These people need to be assessed very quickly, because they can rapidly deteriorate. Consider senior help/advice as you assess the person.

These conditions require careful assessment and correction but are unlikely to become life-threatening emergencies.

These sections cover management guidelines or advice on clinical dilemmas. The timing of clinical intervention is under the control of you, their caring clinician.

Symbols and Abbreviations

➲	cross reference
⚠	warning
►	important
►►	don't delay
∴	therefore
↑	increased
↓	decreased
→	leading to
Δ	differential diagnosis
1°	primary
2°	secondary
>	greater than
<	less than
~	approximately
_	website
∴	therefore
3D	three-dimensional
ACEi	ACE inhibitor
ACHD	adult congenital heart disease
ACR	acute cellular rejection
ACS	acute coronary syndrome
AED	automated external defibrillator
AI	artificial intelligence
ALS	advanced life support
AMI	acute myocardial infarction
AMR	antibody-mediated rejection
ANA	antinuclear antibodies
ANCA	antineutrophil cytoplasmic antibodies
AP	atriopulmonary
ApoAI	apolipoprotein AI
ApoB	apolipoprotein B
AR	aortic regurgitation
ARB	angiotensin receptor blocker
ARF	acute rheumatic fever
ARNI	angiotensin receptor–neprilysin inhibitor
AS	aortic stenosis
ASD	atrial septal defect
ASI	Aortic Size Index
AST	aspartate aminotransferase
ATG	anti-thymocyte globulin
ATP	antitachycardia pacing
AV	aortic valve
AVNRT	atrioventricular nodal re-entrant tachycardia
AVRT	atrioventricular re-entrant tachycardia
BD	twice daily
BiVAD	biventricular assist device assist device
BMI	body mass index
BMV	balloon mitral valvuloplasty
BNP	B-type natriuretic peptide
bpm	beats per minute
BrS	Brugada syndrome
CABG	coronary artery bypass graft
CAD	coronary artery disease
CAV	cardiac allograft vasculopathy
CCS	chronic cardiac syndrome
ccTGA	congenitally corrected transposition of the great arteries
CHB	complete heart block
CHD	congenital heart disease
CK	creatine kinase
cm	centimetre
CMR	cardiovascular magnetic resonance
CMV	*cytomegalovirus*
CNI	calcineurin inhibitor
CO	cardiac output
COX	cyclooxygenase
CPAP	continuous positive airway pressure
CpcPH	combined post- and pre-capillary pulmonary hypertension
CPR	cardiopulmonary resuscitation
CRDS	calcium release deficiency syndrome
CRS	cytokine release syndrome
CRT	cardiac resynchronization therapy
CPVT	catecholaminergic polymorphic ventricular tachycardia
CSCI	continuous subcutaneous infusion
CSF	cerebrospinal fluid

CT	computed tomography
CTPA	computed tomography pulmonary angiography
CXR	chest X-ray
DAPT	dual antiplatelet therapy
DCCV	direct current cardioversion
DCM	dilated cardiomyopathy
DIC	disseminated intravascular coagulation
DKA	diabetic ketoacidosis
DOAC	direct oral anticoagulant
dsDNA	double-stranded DNA
DVT	deep vein thrombosis
EBV	*Epstein Barr virus*
ECG	electrocardiogram
ECMO	extra-corporeal membrane oxygenation
EF	ejection fraction
eGFR	estimated glomerular filtration rate
EMI	electromagnetic interference
ERS	early repolarization syndrome
$ETCO_2$	end-tidal carbon dioxide
FALD	Fontan-associated liver disease
FBC	full blood count
FEV1	forced expiratory volume in 1 second
Fr	French
FVC	forced vital capacity
GA	general anaesthetic
GP	General Practitioner
GP	glycoprotein
GTN	glyceryl trinitrate
HBV	hepatitis B virus
HCM	hypertrophic cardiomyopathy
Hct	haematocrit
HCV	hepatitis C virus
HDL	high-density lipoprotein
HDU	High-dependency Unit
HF	heart failure
HFpEF	heart failure with preserved ejection fraction
HR	heart rate
HTAD	heritable thoracic aortic disease
IABP	intra-aortic balloon pump
ICD	implantable cardioverter defibrillator
IE	infective endocarditis
IHD	ischaemic heart disease
IJ	internal jugular
IM	intramuscular
IO	intraosseous
IpcPH	isolated post-capillary pulmonary hypertension
ITU	Intensive Therapy Unit
IV	intravenous
IVC	inferior vena cava
JLN	Jervell and Lange–Nielsen syndrome
JVP	jugular venous pressure
LA	left atrial
LAD	left anterior descending
LBBB	left bundle branch block
LCA	left coronary artery
LCX	circumflex (artery)
LDA	low-dose aspirin
LDH	lactate dehydrogenase
LDL	low-density lipoprotein
LFT	liver function test
Lp(a)	lipoprotein (a)
LMWH	low-molecular-weight heparin
LQTS	long QT syndrome
LV	left ventricle/ventricular
LVAD	left ventricular assist device
LVESD	left ventricular end-systolic diameter
LVH	left ventricular hypertrophy
LVOTO	left ventricular outflow tract obstruction
MAP	mean arterial pressure
METS	metabolic equivalents
MI	myocardial infarction
MINOCA	myocardial infarction with non-obstructed coronary arteries
MR	mitral regurgitation
MRA	mineralocorticoid receptor antagonist
MRI	magnetic resonance imaging
MS	mitral stenosis
MVO_2	myocardial oxygen consumption
MVR	mitral valve replacement
MVT	mechanical valve thrombosis
NIV	non-invasive ventilation
NCS	non-cardiac surgery
NSTEMI	non-ST-segment elevation myocardial infarction

NSVT	non-sustained ventricular tachycardia
NYHA	New York Heart Association
OAC	oral anticoagulation
PA	pulmonary artery
PAC	pulmonary artery catheterization
PAH	pulmonary arterial hypertension
PAWP	pulmonary artery wedge pressure
PCC	prothrombin complex concentrate
PCI	percutaneous coronary intervention
PDA	patent ductus arteriosus
PDE3	phosphodiesterase 3
PE	pulmonary embolism
PEA	pulseless electrical activity
PESI	Pulmonary Embolism Severity Index
PET	positron emission tomography
PFO	patent foramen ovale
PH	pulmonary hypertension
PJP	*pneumocystis jirovecii pneumonia*
PLE	protein-losing enteropathy
PND	paroxysmal nocturnal dyspnoea
PO	*per os* (by mouth)
POCUS	point of care ultrasound
PPCI	primary percutaneous coronary intervention
PS	pulmonary stenosis
P-SCAD	pregnancy-related spontaneous coronary artery dissection
PTLD	post-transplant lymphoproliferative disorder
pVA-ECMO	peripheral veno-arterial extracorporeal membrane oxygenation
PVD	peripheral vascular disease
PVR	pulmonary valve replacement
PVR	pulmonary vascular resistance
PVT	portal vein thrombosis
QDS	four times per day
RA	right atrial
RBBB	right bundle branch block
RCA	right coronary artery
ROSC	return of spontaneous circulation
RRT	renal replacement therapy
rtPA	recombinant tissue plasminogen activator
RV	right ventricle/ventricular
RVAD	right ventricular assist device
RVOT	right ventricular outflow tract
RVOTO	right ventricular outflow tract obstruction
SAM	systolic anterior motion
SBP	systolic blood pressure
SCAI	Society for Cardiovascular Angiography and Interventions
SCD	sudden cardiac death
siRNA	small interfering RNA
SIRS	systemic inflammatory response syndrome
SL	sublingual
SOB	shortness of breath
SOP	standard operating procedure
SPECT	single photon emission computed tomography
STEMI	ST-segment elevation myocardial infarction
SVD	structural valve degeneration
SVR	systemic vascular resistance
SVT	supraventricular tachycardia
TAVI	transcatheter aortic valve implantation
TCPC	total cavopulmonary connection
TCS	temporary circulatory support
TDS	three times daily
TEER	transcatheter edge-to-edge repair
TEVAR	thoracic endovascular repair
TFT	thyroid function test
TMVR	transcatheter mitral valve replacement
TNK	tenecteplase
TOE	transoesophageal echocardiogram
TOF	Tetralogy of Fallot
TR	tricuspid regurgitation
TTE	transthoracic echocardiogram
TTR	transthyretin
TV	tricuspid valve
U&Es	urea and electrolytes
UFH	unfractionated heparin
URTI	upper respiratory tract infection
US	ultrasound
V-A	veno-arterial
VAD	ventricular assist device
VF	ventricular fibrillation

VKA	vitamin K antagonist
VQ	ventilation/perfusion
VR	virtual reality
VSD	ventricular septal defect
VT	ventricular tachycardia/ tachyarrhythmia
VTE	venous thromboembolism
VV	veno-venous
WCC	white cell count
WPW	Wolff–Parkinson–White
WU	Wood units

Part 1

Presentations

Chapter 1

Cardiac arrest

Adult basic life support

Adult basic life support follows stepwise assessment to recognize cardiac arrest and begin CPR. Effective teamwork and communication while maintaining safety are important in this resuscitative response (Fig 1.1).

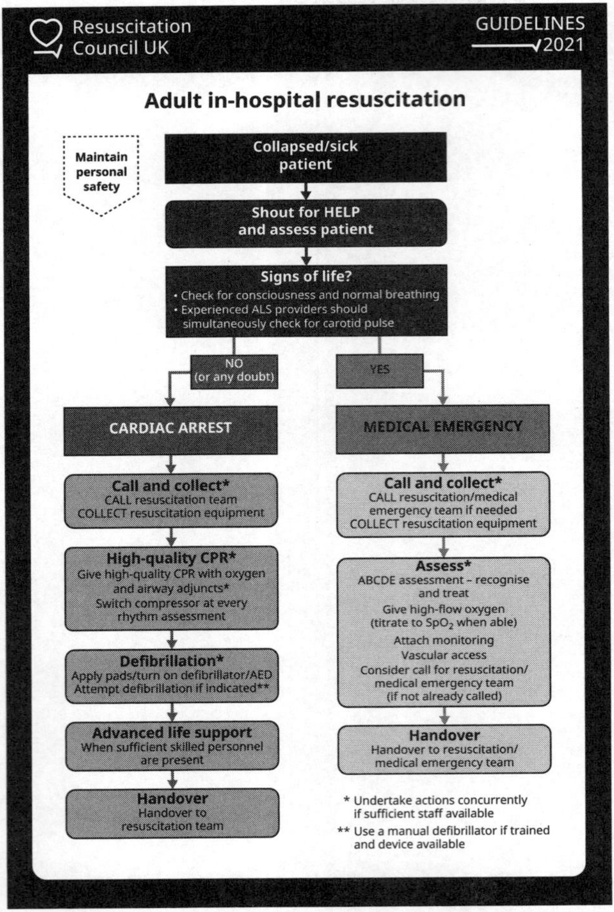

Fig. 1.1 Adult in-hospital resuscitation.

Patient assessment and recognition of cardiac arrest

- Ensure safety of rescuer and patient
- Check for responsiveness by gently shaking and asking loudly ***'are you all right?'***
- If patient is unresponsive, call for help and assess airway
- Open the airway. With two fingertips under the point of chin, tilt head up. If this fails, place fingers behind the angles of lower jaw and apply steady pressure upwards and forwards. Remove any visible airway obstruction
- LOOK, LISTEN, and FEEL for signs of life. Put your ear by patient's mouth while observing for chest/abdominal movements and feeling for a carotid pulse. Take no more than 10 seconds
- Start CPR if no signs of life
- Slow laboured breathing (agonal breathing) should be considered a sign of cardiac arrest
- A short period of seizure-like movement can occur at the start of cardiac arrest. Assess the person after seizure has stopped. If unresponsive with absent or abnormal breathing, start CPR

Call and Collect

- CALL resuscitation team
- COLLECT resuscitation equipment
- If you are a lone bystander and you have to leave the patient to ring for help, CALL and COLLECT first then start CPR

Chest compression

- Start chest compression as early as possible
- Locate the middle of lower half of the sternum. Place the heel of one hand there with the other hand on top of the first. Interlock the fingers of both hands and lift them to ensure that pressure is not applied over patients ribs. Do not apply pressure over bottom tip of sternum or upper abdomen
- Compress to a depth of at least 5 cm but not more than 6 cm
- Compress at rate of 100–120 per minute with as few interruptions as possible
- Allow for chest to completely recoil after each compression
- The pressure should be firm, controlled, and applied vertically. Do not lean on the chest. Erratic or violent action is dangerous
- Perform chest compressions on a firm surface whenever feasible

Breathing

- Give 30 chest compressions before 2 rescue breaths
- Alternate between providing 30 compressions and 2 rescue breaths.
- Add supplemental O_2 as soon as it is available
- Once airway is secure, give uninterrupted compressions at 100 per minute and simultaneously ventilate at 10 per minute

Application of defibrillation pads or AED

- Analyse rhythm as soon as possible
- Do not interrupt chest compression until you are ready to assess rhythm

- Do not delay defibrillation to provide additional CPR once defibrillator read
- Immediately resume CPR after rhythm check and/or defibrillation

Foreign body airway obstruction

- Suspect choking if someone is suddenly unable to speak or talk, especially after eating
- Encourage the person to COUGH
- If the cough becomes ineffective, give 5 BACK BLOWS. Lean the person forward and apply blows between the shoulder blades using the heel of one hand
- If back blows are ineffective, give 5 ABDOMINAL THRUSTS. Stand behind the person and put both your arms around the abdomen. Lean the person forwards, clench your fist and place it between the umbilicus and the rib cage. Grasp your fist with the hand and pull sharply inwards and upwards
- If choking has not been relived after 5 abdominal thrusts, continue alternating 5 back blows with 5 abdominal thrusts until it is relieved
- If the person becomes unresponsive, start CPR

Suspected cervical spine injury

- Despite risk of spinal cord damage, untreated cardiorespiratory arrest will kill the patient
- Minimize potential secondary injury with in-line immobilization of the cervical spine
- Use jaw thrust and/or an oral airway adjunct to open the airway rather than tilting the neck
- Avoid placing patient in lateral recovery position

Safety

- Make sure you, the patient, and the team are safe
- Separate guidelines have been developed for resuscitation of those suspected or confirmed SARS-CoV-2 infection

Further reading

- Resuscitation Council UK Guidelines 2025

Adult advanced life support

Adult advanced life support follows basic life support to provide time-critical diagnostics and intervention. Effective teamwork and communication while maintaining safety continue to be important in this resuscitative response (Fig 1.2).

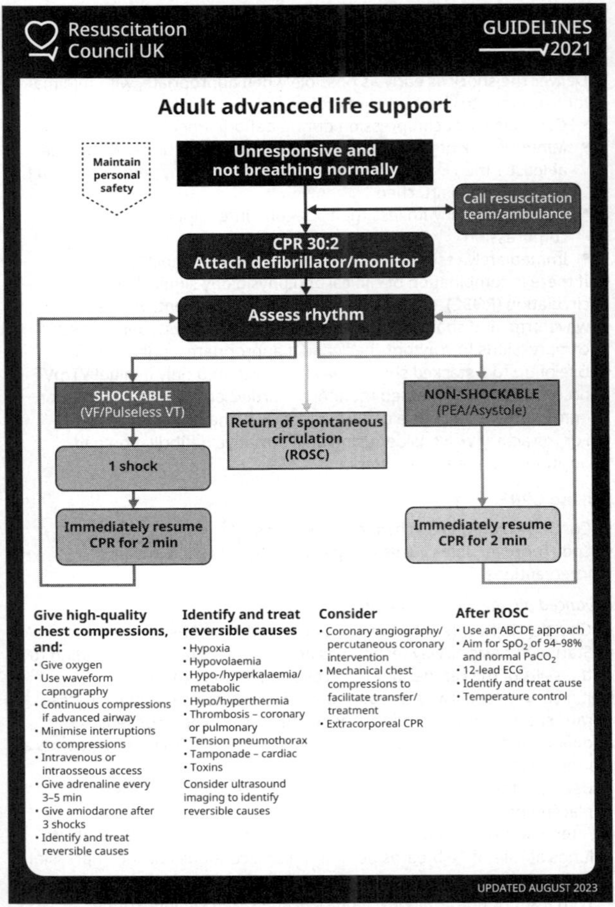

Fig. 1.2 Adult advanced life support.

Assess rhythm

- Attach AED or defibrillator pad to assess rhythm
- SHOCKABLE rhythms are VT and VF
- NON-SHOCKABLE rhythms are asystole and PEA

Defibrillation

- Continue CPR while defibrillator retrieved and pads applied
- Anterolateral pad placement is the first position of choice. In patients with an implantable device, place pad more than 8 cm away from device or use an alternative pad position
- Deliver the shock as early as possible when appropriate, with minimal interruptions to chest compression
    - Continue chest compression during defibrillator charging
    - Minimize risk of fire by placing any oxygen mask or nasal cannula at least 1 metre away from the patient's chest. Any ventilator circuit should remain attached
    - Deliver a shock with less than 5 second interruption in chest compression
    - Immediately resume chest compressions after shock delivered
- If there is combination of clinical and physiology signs of spontaneous circulation (ROSC), e.g. waking, purposeful movement, arterial waveform, and sharp rise in end-tidal CO_2, consider stopping chest compressions for rhythm check and if appropriate a pulse check
- Use of up to 3 stacked shocks may be considered only if initial VT/pVT occurs during a witnessed monitored cardiac arrest with defibrillator immediately available, e.g. during cardiac catheterization
- For refractory VF, consider using an alternative defibrillation pad position, e.g. anterior–posterior

During CPR

- Continue high-quality chest compressions
- Look for reversible causes and perform the following advance interventions

Advanced airway and ventilation

- Give the highest feasible inspired oxygen during CPR
- Start with basic airway techniques and progress stepwise according to the skills of the rescuer until effective ventilation is achieved
- If an advanced airway is required, only a rescuer with a 'high success rate' should perform endotracheal intubation. Expert consensus defines 'high success rate' is defined as over 95% within two attempts at intubation
- Use waveform capnography to confirm correct advance airway placement
- After insertion of endotracheal tube or supra-glottic airway, ventilate lungs at rate of 10 breaths per minute and continue chest compression without pause
- With a supra-glottic airway, if gas leakage results in inadequate ventilation, pause compression for ventilation using compression: ventilation ratio 30:2

Vascular access and drugs

- Establish intravenous access
- Consider intraossesous access if attempt at intravenous access unsuccessful or not feasible

Adrenaline

- Give adrenaline 1 mg IV/IO as soon as possible for adults in cardiac arrest with a non-shockable rhythm
- Give adrenaline 1 mg IV/IO after the third shock for adults in cardiac arrest with a shockable rhythm
- Repeat adrenaline 1 mg IV/IO every 3–5 minutes while ALS continues

Anti-arrhythmic drugs

- Give amiodarone 300 mg IV/IO for adult in cardiac arrest in VT/VF after 3 shocks have been given
- Give a further dose of amiodarone 150 mg IV/IO for adult patients in cardiac arrest who are in VF/pVT after 5 shocks have been given
- Lidocaine 100 mg IV/IO may be used as an alternative of amiodarone. An additional bolus of lidocaine 50 mg can be given after 5 defibrillation attempts

Thrombolytic drugs

- Consider thrombolysis when pulmonary embolus is suspected or confirmed as cause of cardiac arrest
- Consider CPR 60–90 mins after administration of thrombolysis

Fluid

- Give IV/IO fluids only where cardiac arrest is suspected or caused by hypovolaemia

Others

- Consider 10% calcium chloride 10 mL slow IV if PEA is thought to be due to hyperkalaemia, hypocalcemia, calcium-channel blocker overdose, or magnesium overdose
- Consider magnesium sulphate 8 mmol (4 mL 50% solution) for refractory VT if patient is thought to be has hypomagnesaemia, digoxin toxicity, or torsade de pointes
- Consider sodium bicarbonate 50 mmol (50 mL 8.4% solution) in patient thought to have hyperkalaemia or tricyclic antidepressant overdose. Note sodium bicarbonate raises PCO_2 and requires increase in minute ventilation

Reversible causes

- Look for reversible causes: 4Hs and 4Ts
  - Hypoxia
  - Hypovolaemia
  - Hyper/hypokalemia
  - Hypothermia
  - Tamponade
  - Tension pneumothorax
  - Toxins
  - Thrombosis (ACS/PE)

- Only skilled operators should use intra-arrest point of care ultrasound (POCUS). POCUS must not cause additional or prolonged interruptions in chest compressions
- POCUS may be useful to diagnose treatable cause of cardiac arrest such as cardiac tamponade and pneumothorax. Right ventricular dilatation in isolation during cardiac arrest should not be used to diagnose pulmonary embolism. Do not use POCUS to assess myocardial contractility as sole indicator for terminating CPR

Waveform capnography during ALS

- Use waveform capnography to confirm correct endotracheal tube placement during CPR
- Use waveform capnography to monitor the quality of CPR
- The trend or value of $ETCO_2$ should not be used solely to interrupt chest compression or decide whether a resuscitative attempt should be stopped

Mechanical chest compression devices

- Consider mechanical chest compressions only if high-quality manual chest compression is not practical or compromises provider safety

Periarrest arrhythmias

Patient assessment

- Define nature of the arrhythmia
- Look for life-threatening features in the unstable patient
  - SHOCK—appreciated as hypotension and symptoms of increased sympathetic activity and reduced cerebral blood flow
  - SYNCOPE—as consequence of reduced cerebral blood flow
  - SEVERE HEART FAILURE—manifest as pulmonary oedema and/or raised jugular venous pressure
  - MYOCARDIAL ISCHAEMIA—may present with angina and/or isolated finings on the 12-lead ECG

Tachyarrhythmia

- Electrical cardioversion is preferred for tachyarrhythmia in unstable patients with life-threatening signs
- To convert atrial/ventricular tachyarrhythmia, shock must be synchronized to occur with the R wave of the electrocardiogram
- Conscious patients require sedation/anaesthesia before synchronized cardioversion
- If cardioversion fails to restore sinus rhythm and patient remains unstable, give amiodarone 300 mg over 10–20mins (or procainamide 10–15 mg/kg over 20 mins) and reattempt cardioversion. Loading amiodarone can be followed by infusion 900 mg over 24 hrs
- If patient with tachyarrhythmia is stable and not deteriorating, pharmacological therapy is preferred

Atrial fibrillation

- Initial synchronized shock at maximum output rather than an escalating approach is reasonable (ALS 2021)

Atrial flutter or paroxysmal supra-ventricular tachycardia

- Give initial synchronized shock of 70–120 J
- Give subsequent shocks using stepwise increase in energy

Ventricular tachycardia with pulse

- Give initial synchronized shock of 120–150 J
- Give subsequent shocks using stepwise increase in energy

Bradyarrhythmia

- If bradycardia is accompanied by life-threatening signs, Give atropine 500 mcg (IV/IO) and repeat every 3–5 mins if necessary to total 3 mg
- Consider second-line agents if atropine is ineffective. Examples include isoprenaline (5 mcg/min as starting dose) and adrenaline (2–10 mcg/min as starting dose)
- For bradycardia caused by (i) inferior myocardial infarction, (ii) cardiac transplant, or (iii) spinal cord injury, consider aminophylline (100–200 mg slow IV bolus)
- Avoid atropine in patients with cardiac transplants as it can cause high degree AV block or sinus arrest, use aminophylline
- Consider glucagon if β blockers or calcium-channel blockers are potential causes of bradycardia

- Consider pacing in patients who are unstable and refractory to drug therapy. If transcutaneous pacing is ineffective, consider transvenous pacing
- If atropine is ineffective and transcutaneous pacing is not immediately available, fist pacing can be attempted while waiting for pacing equipment
- Assess risk of asystole if no immediate adverse signs: (i) recent asystole, (ii) Mobitz type II AV block, (iii) ventricular pauses for 3 seconds, (iv) complete heart block with broad QRS complex
- Indications for pacing referral (i) second-degree AV block, (ii) complete heart block, and (iii) symptomatic sinus node disease

Chapter 2

Cardiogenic shock

Introduction

Cardiogenic shock represents the most severe presentation of cardiac dysfunction. It is a medical emergency with a high mortality. Despite modern management approximately 40–50% of patients with cardiogenic shock die in hospital. Improved survival is now being demonstrated with earlier diagnosis, structured multidisciplinary team management, involvement of specialist centres, and selective use of mechanical circulatory support.

Definition

Cardiogenic shock is traditionally defined as a clinical syndrome characterized by low cardiac output and end-organ hypoperfusion. It is perhaps better thought of as a global circulatory disorder initiated by a decreased cardiac output. Patients may present with peripheral vasodilation, rather than conventional vasoconstriction, in the context of out-of-hospital cardiac arrest, post-cardiotomy, or concurrent infection. Extreme hypoperfusion may present as multiple organ dysfunction syndrome and if untreated will result in death.

As cardiac output is difficult to measure, a low cardiac output is inferred from refractory hypotension in the presence of pathology known to cause decreased cardiac output.

Clinical criteria used to diagnose cardiogenic shock include:

- SBP < 90 mmHg for > 30 mins, or inotropes/vasopressors to maintain SBP > 90 mmHg
- End-organ hypoperfusion (urine output < 30 mL/hr, cool extremities, altered mental state, lactate > 2 mmol/L)

Classification

There are a number of different classification schemes of cardiogenic shock, but most current guidelines utilize the SCAI SHOCK classification (Fig. 2.1). This has 5 stages from A to E, with each further stage associated with worse prognosis across all aetiologies of cardiogenic shock. This simple classification facilitates the standardized assessment and communication of shock severity, and identification of patients who require escalating support.

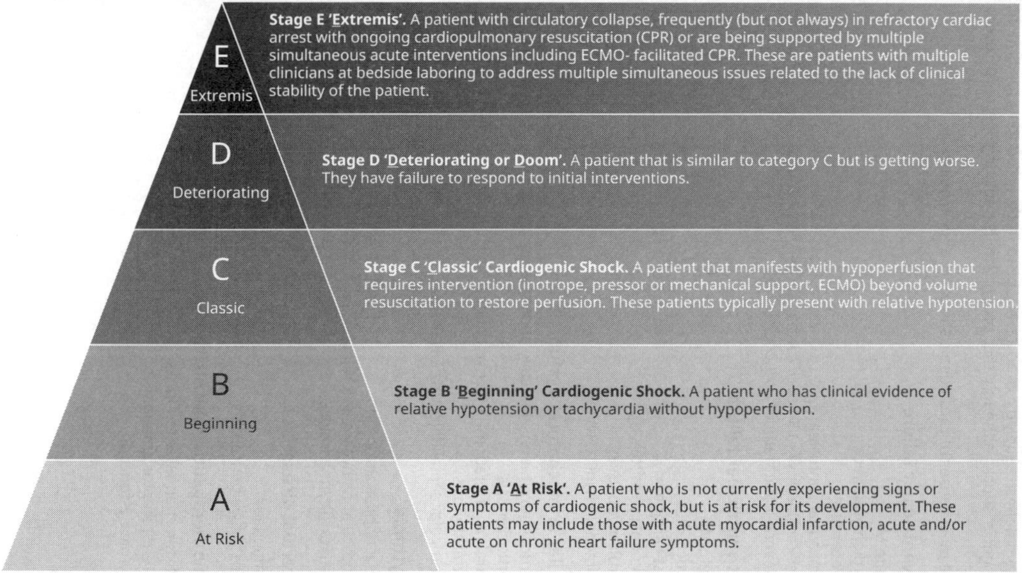

Fig. 2.1 SCAI SHOCK classification.

Incidence and aetiology

Cardiogenic shock accounts for 2–5% of acute heart failure presentations. The commonest aetiology is acute MI, historically accounting for 80% of cardiogenic shock, although this proportion is reducing in more recent series.

The main causes of cardiogenic shock are shown below.

Left ventricular failure

- Acute MI
- Cardiomyopathies
- Myocarditis
- Myocardial contusion
- Post-cardiotomy—0.5–1% of cardiac surgery procedures
- Left ventricular outflow tract obstruction

Right ventricular failure

- Acute MI
- Myocarditis
- Post-cardiotomy
- Pulmonary embolism
- Cardiomyopathies
- Pulmonary hypertension

Valvular or mechanical dysfunction

- Aortic regurgitation—infective endocarditis
- Aortic stenosis
- Mitral regurgitation—infective endocarditis, ischaemia/infarction
- Mitral stenosis
- Ventricular septal defect/free wall rupture

Arrhythmia

- Atrial fibrillation/flutter
- Ventricular tachycardia/fibrillation
- Bradycardia/heart block

Pericardial disease

- Tamponade
- Constrictive pericarditis

Chemotherapeutic/toxic/metabolic

- Calcium channel antagonists
- Adrenoreceptor antagonists
- Thyroid dysfunction

Pathophysiology

An initial cardiac insult decreases cardiac output resulting in central haemodynamic alterations, microcirculatory dysfunction, systemic inflammation, and multiple organ dysfunction syndrome. Upstream precipitating factors may be non-cardiovascular: e.g. infection may result in an acute decompensation of heart failure leading to cardiogenic shock.

Cardiac dysfunction

- The mechanism of cardiac dysfunction is variable
- Classically, acute LV dysfunction and cardiogenic shock arises from extensive loss of contractile myocardium (e.g. acute MI)
- Altered ventricular loading conditions may also lead to severe LV and/or RV dysfunction (e.g. acute valve dysfunction)
- RV dysfunction may result from primary contractile failure or as a result of preload/afterload mismatching

Haemodynamic changes

- Decreased stroke volume
- Decreased cardiac output
- Increased uni-/bi-ventricular end-diastolic pressure
- Decreased blood pressure
- Compensatory vasoconstriction

Microcirculatory changes

- Microcirculatory dysfunction occurs early
- May precede central haemodynamic perturbation
- Cellular hypoxia occurs, contributing to organ dysfunction

Systemic inflammation

- A systemic inflammatory response is common, with circulating proinflammatory cytokines
- This results in vasodilation, which is exacerbated by production of vasodilatory metabolites as a result of tissue hypoxia
- Overt infection may also be present contributing to systemic inflammation and vasodilation

End-organ effects

- A combination of low arterial pressure and high venous pressure contribute to reduced organ perfusion
- Hypoperfusion is compounded by microcirculatory dysfunction
- This drives injury and dysfunction of multiple organs, including the heart, lungs, kidneys, and brain
- Bacterial translocation from the gut occurs due to breakdown of the intestinal barrier, further driving inflammation and vasodilation

Management

Immediate initial assessment of ABC (Airway, Breathing, and Circulation).

Airway

- If there is airway compromise, including from decreased conscious state, call critical care/anaesthesia immediately

Breathing

- Supplemental oxygen to maintain $SpO_2 > 90\%$
- Consider CPAP if pulmonary oedema present—as well as the gas exchange benefit of positive alveolar pressure and increase in functional residual capacity, positive intrathoracic pressure results in LV afterload reduction
- Caution—CPAP may also increase RV afterload which can result in haemodynamic deterioration

Circulation

- Assessment of the circulation includes basic haemodynamic assessment—heart rate and rhythm, blood pressure; and assessment of distal perfusion—hands/feet cool and dusky, or warm and well-perfused
- 12-lead ECG—if evidence of STEMI, emergency coronary angiography and primary percutaneous coronary intervention is indicated

Investigations

- Arterial blood gas
- Bloods—FBC, U&Es, LFTs, Mg, PO_4, Ca, troponin, BNP, coagulation screen; consider TFTs and procalcitonin
- 12-lead ECG—as above
- Transthoracic echocardiography—essential for making the diagnosis and establishing the aetiology of shock
- Consider lung ultrasound at the time of echo to assess pulmonary congestion, consolidation, pleural collections/pneumothorax
- Coronary angiography—emergently if STEMI, consider urgently in other cases of acute coronary syndrome

Next steps

- Use the SCAI SHOCK pyramid (Fig. 2.1) to classify severity and phenotype of shock
- Call the 'shock team' (if applicable) and/or involve critical care early, as there is high risk of deterioration, and immediately if the patient is in SCAI class C or worse
- Consider evidence of fluid balance and distribution—pulmonary/peripheral oedema, and vascular tone (vasoconstricted/vasodilated
- Patient stabilization may need to occur concurrently with initial investigations
- Emergency coronary revascularization for patients presenting with STEMI has been clearly demonstrated to improve outcome and should not be delayed

Initial management

- If SBP < 90 mmHg, it is reasonable to give a fluid challenge (e.g. 250 mL crystalloid) unless overt pulmonary oedema is present
- If echocardiography is immediately available, assessment of preload can be used to guide further fluid challenges
- In order to achieve clinical stability, it may be necessary to deliver inotropic and vasoconstrictive drugs peripherally whilst obtaining central venous access
- 1mg adrenaline diluted in 50 mL 0.9% saline may be infused into a large peripheral vein as a temporizing measure
- If vasodilation is suspected, metaraminol is a useful vasoconstrictor that can be administered peripherally—dilute 10 mg in 50 mL 0.9% saline and titrate to effect

Intensive care management

- Intubation and ventilation—may be necessary where cardiac output is critically low and/or tissue hypoperfusion is severe
- Invasive monitoring—vital in guiding haemodynamic management—initially arterial line, central line
- Inotropic support—patients very commonly need inotropic/vasopressor support, which can be guided by the clinical phenotype of shock. See options in Table 2.1
- Consider pulmonary artery catheterization (PAC)—see Box 2.1
- Renal replacement therapy (RRT) is often required for acute kidney injury. If required fluid removal can also be achieved via RRT. There is emerging interest in pro-inflammatory cytokine removal, either using haemofiltration or specific cytokine adsorbers

Table 2.1 Inotropes and vasopressors in common clinical use

Drug	Mechanism	Typical doses	Notes
Adrenaline	α1, β1/2/3 adrenoreceptors Positive inotropy, lusitropy, chronotropy, and vasoconstriction	0.01–0.5 mcg/kg/min	Dose-dependent action on all adrenoreceptors Ideally given centrally
Dobutamine	β1(+β2) adrenoreceptors Positive inotropy, lusitropy, chronotropy, and vasodilation	1–10 mcg/kg/min	Useful in bradycardic and vasoconstricted pts, otherwise tachycardia and vasodilation often limit its use
Dopamine	β1(±α1) adrenoreceptors; D1/2 dopaminergic receptors Splanchnic vasodilation, positive inotropy, lusitropy. Chronotropy, and vasoconstriction in higher doses	5–10 mcg/kg/min as an inotrope	Less tachycardia than dobutamine In low dose (0–5 μg/kg/min) mediates splanchnic vasodilatation (but no evidence this improves outcomes)

(Continued)

Table 2.1 (*Contd.*)

Drug	Mechanism	Typical doses	Notes
Levosimendan	Calcium sensitizer and inhibition of PDE3 Positive inotropy, lusitropy, and vasodilation	0.1mcg/kg/min for 24 hrs	Calcium sensitizer—less increase in MVO_2 c/f catecholamines Metabolites with long duration of action
Milrinone	PDE3 inhibition Positive inotropy, lusitropy, and vasodilation	0.1–0.5 mcg/kg/min	Tends not to increase heart rate Causes dose-dependent vasodilation Accumulates in renal dysfunction
Noradrenaline	α1(±β1) adrenoreceptors Vasoconstriction	0.01–1.0 mcg/kg/min	Predominant effect is vasocontriction CO may also increase through venoconstrictive preload augmentation
Vasopressin	V1 vasopressin receptor Vasoconstriction	0.1,–2.4 IU/hr	Adrenoreceptor independent effect which is useful when adrenoreceptors are downregulated

Abbreviations: CO—cardiac output; PDE3—phosphodiesterase 3

Box 2.1 Pulmonary artery (PA) catheterization

- PA catheterization (PAC; using a balloon-tipped Swan–Ganz catheter) is the gold standard for continuous cardiac output monitoring
- It allows direct measurement of RA pressure, RV pressure, PA pressure, PA wedge pressure (estimating LA pressure), and mixed venous oxygen saturations
- Derived measurements from PAC include cardiac output, cardiac index, and systemic/pulmonary vascular resistance
- PAC has *not* been demonstrated to improve patient outcome but may be valuable in guiding management in selected patients in experienced centres
- It carries small risks of arrhythmia, bleeding, infection, myocardial or pulmonary artery injury

Advanced management

There is evidence that standardized management led by a multidisciplinary team can improve outcomes in cardiogenic shock. This is particularly useful in considering appropriateness of short term mechanical circulatory support (MCS). The aim of MCS is to provide short-term haemodynamic assistance for an initial period ranging from hours to weeks. It can provide a bridge to a clinical decision or diagnosis, to recovery, or to a more durable form of support (left ventricular assist device or cardiac transplantation).

Patient selection for MCS

There are currently no universally accepted guidelines on patient selection. In the UK, several factors are associated with adverse outcome (despite MCS) and function as exclusion criteria for its use:

- Unwitnessed cardiac arrest
- Initial rhythm asystole
- No bystander CPR
- CPR > 60 minutes
- Frailty
- Perceived difficulties with cannulation
- Terminal illness
- Non-cardiac cause of cardiac arrest
- Lactate > 15 mmol/L
- PaO_2 < 6 kPa
- $ETCO_2$ < 1.3 kPa

Options for MCS in cardiogenic shock

See Chapter 21. Table 2.2 provides a summary of available devices.

Box 2.2 References

- ESC HFA position statement on the management of cardiogenic shock. *European Journal of Heart Failure* 2020; 22(8): 1315–41
- SCAI clinical expert consensus statement on the classification of cardiogenic shock. *Catheterisation and Cardiovascular Interventions.* 2019; 94: 29–37
- Tehrani et al. Standardized management of cardiogenic shock. *JACC: Heart Failure*. 2020 ;8:879–91

Table 2.2 Options for MCS in cardiogenic shock

	IABP	Impella	pVA-ECMO
Action	Diastolic augmentation and LV afterload reduction	Expels blood from ventricle to aorta (or PA if Impella RP)	RA drainage through extracorporeal pump and oxygenator with arterial return
Access	7–8 Fr	12–14 Fr (CP device) 22 Fr (RP/5.5 device)	19–25 Fr venous 15–19 Fr arterial
Flow	Pulsatile flow	Continuous flow via axial pump CO up to 5.5 L/min depending on device	Continuous flow via centrifugal pump CO < 7L/min
Duration	Usually < 1 week	10 days	< 30 days
LV unloading	+	++	-
Rhythm dependent	Yes	No	No
Pros	Insertion at bedside or in cath lab No extracorporeal blood Increased coronary and cerebral blood flow	Relative ease of insertion in cath lab No extracorporeal blood	Rapid insertion—no cath lab Full circulatory support Rapid improvement in oxygenation
Cons	Limb ischaemia Haemolysis Platelets ↓ Bleeding	Limb ischaemia Haemolysis Platelets ↓ Bleeding	Limb ischaemia Haemolysis Platelets ↓ Bleeding LV overloading
Contraindications	> Moderate AR Severe PVD Aortic dissection	Severe AS Prosthetic AV LV thrombus VSD PVD Inability to anticoagulate	Severe AR Aortic dissection Inability to anticoagulate

Abbreviations: AR—aortic regurgitation; AS—aortic stenosis; AV—aortic valve; Fr—French; IABP—intra-aortic balloon pump; pVA-ECMO—peripheral veno-arterial extracorporeal membrane oxygenation; LV—left ventricle; PA—pulmonary artery; CO—cardiac output; PVD—peripheral vascular disease; VSD—ventricular septal defect

Chest pain

Diagnosing chest pain

Aspects to ask about, with more likely diagnoses, include:

- *Nature* of the pain: what is its quality, distribution, and severity?
  - Retrosternal, heavy/crushing/squeezing pain/ache—ACS/AMI
  - Abrupt onset, 'tearing' pain—aortic dissection
  - Sharp, lateral chest wall, easy to localize—?pleuritic/muscular
- Associated features:
  - Diaphoresis (sweating), breathlessness—ACS, PE?
  - (Pre)syncope—PE, ACS?
  - Cough, sputum, haemoptysis—chest infection, PE?
  - Superficial tenderness—musculoskeletal?
- *Pattern* of occurrence—exacerbating and relieving factors:
  - Relationship to exertion—CAD, esp. if predictable
  - With emotional stress—can be CAD
  - After extreme physical or emotional stressors—Takotsubo?
  - Eating—?gastrointestinal source, but can be CAD
  - Respiration—pleuritic/pericarditic pain
- *Change*:
  - In frequency or intensity of chest pain
  - With posture—pericarditic pain might ease leaning forward
- *Previous history*:
  - Of cardiac, respiratory, or upper gastrointestinal pathology?
- *Background risk*:
  - Pulmonary embolism (cancer, immobility, surgery, prior PE)
  - CAD risk (smoking, diabetes, hyperlipidaemia, hypertension)
  - Aortic dissection (hypertension, Marfan, bicuspid AoV)

Causes of chest pain

Cardiovascular

- Angina/MI, see ➲ p.47
- Pulmonary embolism, see ➲ p.208
- Aortic dissection, see ➲ p.179
- Pericarditis, see ➲ p.198
- Myocarditis, see ➲ p.90.

Non-cardiovascular

- Pneumonia
- Pneumothorax
- Chest wall pain
- Muscular
- Oesophageal reflux
- Oesophageal rupture
- Nerve root pain
- Herpes zoster

Patterns of presentation

Acute coronary syndromes and Angina pectoris (➲ p.47)

Typically 'tight', 'heavy', 'band-like', or 'compressing' in quality with retrosternal location ± radiation to (left) arm or throat and occasionally to the back or epigastrium. The severity is highly variable. Angina may not necessarily indicate coronary artery disease—aortic stenosis, LVOTO, and anaemia are all possible causes.

- Chronic stable angina is provoked by physical exertion, cold (leading to peripheral vasoconstriction), and emotional stress, and is relieved by rest. Sublingual GTN, where effective, will work within a couple of minutes
- Unstable angina (see ➲ p.62) occurs at rest or on minimal exertion and is more likely to be severe and sustained. Stuttering or rapidly increasing symptoms leading up to the acute presentation may occur and are termed crescendo angina
- Acute MI often presents as severe sustained, ischaemic-type pain. There may be associated 'autonomic' features, e.g. sweating and nausea ± vomiting
- Sharp stabbing pains, pains that are well localized, e.g. left submammary, of fleeting duration e.g. < 30 sec, or of flitting location are unlikely to reflect myocardial ischaemia

Thoracic aortic dissection (➲ p.179)

Typically has abrupt, even instantaneous, onset. A tearing sensation from anterior to posterior in the chest may be described and the pain is severe and often terrifying. Other features may supervene, according to compromised vascular territories, e.g. angina, neurological symptoms due to coronary, carotid, or spinal artery involvement. The usual cause is hypertension, which may be previously undiagnosed. Marfan syndrome is an important predisposition.

Pulmonary embolism (➲ p.208)

May present with pleuritic chest pain (sharp, localized, worse with inspiration) ± associated breathlessness/haemoptysis. Large pulmonary emboli may diminish cardiac output to the extent that syncope occurs. Ask about risk factors such as prolonged immobility (travel, surgery—esp. orthopaedic), malignancy, postpartum, previous DVT/PE, personal or familial tendency to thrombosis, smoking, and oral contraceptive use.

Pericarditis (➲ p.198)

A gnawing, sore, retrosternal pain, often relieved by leaning forward (probably separates the inflamed pericardial layers). May also cause pleuritic pain. There may be associated 'viral-type' symptoms or features of the underlying disease. Breathlessness may indicate the accumulation of pericardial fluid, or tamponade.

Oesophageal pain

Can mimic angina to the extent that it may be associated with physical exertion and relieved by nitrates. Association with acid reflux, exacerbation when supine, with food or alcohol, and relief from antacids points towards oesophageal pain, but the distinction can be difficult and investigation is often required. Remember that meals can also provoke angina.

Associated physical signs

Unstable angina and acute myocardial infarction

(Also see ➲ p.47, p.62.)

- Since things can change quickly it is important to document normal and negative findings clearly, so that new problems will be immediately apparent
- Note pulse (either tachycardia or bradycardia occur) and BP
- Pay attention for any signs of heart failure
- Record the heart sounds including any added sounds (e.g. pericardial rubs) and the nature or absence of murmurs
- A rapid survey for neurological deficits is appropriate (as anticoagulation or thrombolysis may be indicated), with more detailed examination reserved for those where relevant abnormalities are identified

Pulmonary embolism

(Also see ➲ p.208.)

- Sinus tachycardia
- Hypotension
- Cyanosis
- Tachypnoea
- Low grade fever
- Palpable RV
- Loud pulmonary component of S_2 (loud P_2)
- Pleural rub
- Signs of DVT

Pericarditis

(Also see ➲ p.198.)

- Pericardial friction rub
- Check the pulse character
- Measure the BP yourself (pulsus paradoxus if systolic pressure difference through respiratory cycle >10 mmHg)
- Look for other signs of tamponade, e.g. hypotension, Kussmaul's sign (JVP rises on inspiration), and quiet or absent heart sounds

Investigations

Investigations will reflect the possible diagnoses and complications based on the history and physical examination. They will also be directed towards risk factors and secondary prevention measures, e.g. cholesterol measurement and treatment in ischaemic heart disease. More detailed consideration of the investigation and management is given in the chapters that deal with each condition.

Unstable angina/acute myocardial infarction

(Also see ➲ p.47, p.62.)

- FBC and U&E
- Glucose
- Total cholesterol and HDL cholesterol
- Troponin
- ECG
- Invasive X-ray coronary arteriography
- *Selected patients*: echocardiogram, CT coronary angiogram, chest X-ray

Pulmonary embolism

(Also see ➲ p.208.)

- FBC
- D-dimer
- Arterial blood gases
- ECG
- CXR
- Echocardiogram
- CT pulmonary angiogram
- *Selected patients*: ventilation perfusion (VQ) scan, pulmonary angiogram, Doppler ultrasound leg veins, thrombophilia screen

Aortic dissection

(Also see ➲ p.179.)

- FBC and U&E
- Group and save blood/cross match
- ECG
- CXR
- Contrast CT - thoracic and abdominal aortogram
- Echocardiogram
- *Selected patients*: TTE and/or TOE, MRI

Pericarditis

(Also see ➲ p.198.)

- FBC and U&E
- CRP
- Troponin
- ECG
- *Selected patients*: ANA, dsDNA, viral titres, pericardial fluid microscopy and culture, echocardiogram

Shortness of breath

Diagnosing breathlessness

- ▶ Lots of things can make people *feel* short of breath. Ask about speed of onset, associated symptoms, previous cardiac and respiratory history, current medication, allergies, cardiac risk factors, smoking history. Obtain additional information from relatives, GP, notes.
- ▶ Read the ambulance sheet—it is a vital source of information

Speed of onset

- Sudden —acute PE, arrhythmia, acute valve disease, pneumothorax, airway obstruction, anaphylaxis
- Minutes —angina/MI, pulmonary oedema, asthma
- Hours/days —pneumonia, exacerbation of COPD, congestive cardiac failure, pleural effusion
- Weeks/months —constrictive/restrictive cardiomyopathy, pulmonary fibrosis, pneumonitis, chronic PE
- Intermittent —asthma, LV failure, arrhythmias

Associated symptoms

- Chest pain —ischaemic (angina, MI)
  —pericarditic (pericarditis)
  —pleural (pneumonia, PE)
  —musculoskeletal (chest wall pain)
- Palpitation —AF is the commonest clinical arrhythmia
- Wheeze —asthma/COPD, anaphylactoid
- Orthopnoea, paroxysmal nocturnal dyspnoea
  —cardiac failure, effusions
- Sweats/weight loss —malignancy, infection
- Cough/sputum —pneumonia
- Haemoptysis —pink froth suggests pulmonary oedema
- Hyper-anxious —thyrotoxicosis, anxiety. Breathlessness that *only* occurs at rest is unlikely to be pathological

Associated signs

- Clammy, pale —left ventricular failure, MI
- Cardiac murmur —valve disease, but beware incidental murmur
- Crackles —early/coarse (pulmonary oedema, pneumonia) —late/fine (fibrosis)
- Clubbing —malignancy, cyanotic congenital heart disease
  —endocarditis, bronchiectasis
  —pulmonary hypertension
- Cyanosis —severe hypoxaemia
- Displaced apex —left ventricular dilatation
- RV heave —elevated right heart pressures
- Elevated JVP —right heart failure, fluid overload
  —pericardial tamponade/constriction
  —large PE
- Stridor —upper airway obstruction
- Peripheral oedema —right heart failure
- CO_2 retention flap —Type 2 failure (see Box 4.1)

Box 4.1 Causes of breathlessness

Cardiovascular

- LV failure ± pulmonary oedema ➲ p.74
- Angina/MI ➲ p.48
- Severe ± acute ± decompensated valve disease ➲ p.92
- Arrhythmias (especially AF) ➲ p.143
- Constrictive pericarditis/cardiac tamponade ➲ p.201
- Restrictive/dilated cardiomyopathy ➲ p.344
- Pulmonary embolus ➲ p.208
- Pulmonary hypertension ➲ p.213

Non-cardiovascular

- Pneumonia
- Asthma
- COPD
- Pneumothorax
- Pleural effusion
- Upper airway obstruction
- Bronchial carcinoma
- Lymphangitis carcinomatosis
- SVC obstruction
- Pneumonitis/pulmonary fibrosis
- Anaemia
- Thyrotoxicosis
- Metabolic, e.g. acidosis
- Chest wall pain—pleuritic/musculoskeletal
- Skeletal abnormalities
- Neuromuscular—diaphragmatic weakness
- Central nervous system disorder—meningitis, pontine infarction, haemorrhage
- Anxiety/psychogenic

Box 4.2 Respiratory failure

- Diagnosed if the PaO_2 < 8 kPa
- Subdivided according to the $PaCO_2$:
  - Type 1: $PaCO_2$ < 6.5 kPa. Seen in virtually all acute disease of the lung, e.g. pulmonary oedema, pneumonia, asthma
  - Type 2: $PaCO_2$ > 6.5 kPa. The problem is hypoventilation. Neuromuscular disorders, severe pneumonia, drug overdose

Investigations

- ECG—ischaemic changes, arrhythmias
- CXR
- Pulse oximetry
- Arterial blood gases
- FBC—anaemia, white cell count
- Cardiac enzymes—troponin, CK
- Further investigations according to differential diagnosis:
  - B-type natriuretic peptide—if low then cardiac failure unlikely
  - D-dimers—unlikely PE if negative
  - CRP
  - Renal function and electrolytes
  - Blood cultures if pyrexial
  - Peak expiratory flow rate
  - Spirometry ± lung function testing—including gas transfer
  - Echocardiography—LV function, valve disease
  - CT—plain/pulmonary angiogram/high resolution
  - CT coronary angiography in selected patients ➲ p.429

Chapter 5

Palpitation

Diagnosing palpitation

Definition

Palpitation is the symptom of an increased awareness of the heartbeat. The term, however, is interpreted by patients to mean different things and it is important to elicit exactly what the patient's symptoms are.

The history is vital. A good history can often provide the diagnosis and may avoid the need for further investigation, especially if a non-cardiac cause is suspected. ECG documentation of the cardiac rhythm during an episode is proof of the diagnosis—if this is normal, an arrhythmic cause for the symptoms can be excluded.

In general, if the symptoms are brief (< 10 sec), not associated with other severe symptoms, and/or occur only at times of stress/anxiety, it is unlikely there is a concerning cause for them.

1. Clarify the symptoms—ask the patient to 'tap out' the rhythm

- Pounding heart—may be physiological
- Sudden one-off 'jump'—unimportant, likely to be ectopic beat
- Irregular heart beat—likely to be multiple ectopic beats or AF
- Fast heart rhythm—consider tachyarrhythmia

2. What is the pattern? Likely cause(s) (Box 5.1)

- Abrupt onset/cessation SVT, VT, AF
- Slow increase/decrease Sinus tachycardia
- At times of stress/anxiety Anxiety/emotion
- Related to exertion Sinus, AF, SVT if abrupt onset
- Early beat, pause, then heavy beat Atrial/ventricular ectopic beats
- Irregular rhythm AF, multiple ectopic beats

3. How often does it occur?

- Useful for determining impact on patient
- Guides choice of investigation

4. Duration of symptoms Likely cause(s) (Box 5.1)

- Brief (few seconds) Atrial/ventricular ectopics
- Several minutes/few hours SVT/AF
- Continuous Sinus tachycardia/thyrotoxicosis

5. Associated symptoms (warrant further cardiac investigation)

- Angina
- Syncope or near syncope
- Significant breathlessness

6. Previous history

- Known poor LV function—VT more likely
- Previous SVT/AF/VT—recurrence?

Investigations

12-lead ECG

Ideally during symptoms.

Blood tests

- FBC—anaemia → sinus tachycardia?
- Thyroid function—thyrotoxicosis?
- U&E—low/high K^+? (encourages arrhythmias)

Assuming that by this stage, you think a true arrhythmia may be present, further investigations may be undertaken:

Echocardiogram

Identifies any structural heart disease.

Ambulatory ECG monitoring

ECG documentation of an arrhythmia prior to management is crucial, treatment is only appropriate when you know what you're dealing with. Assuming this has not been obtained previously, it is worth considering ambulatory monitoring to attempt to document the rhythm during a symptomatic episode. It is worth persevering until an ECG is recorded during symptoms.

24/48-hour ECG monitor

Good for frequent symptoms, may need several before rhythm identified.

Patient-activated event recorder

The ECG is stored during an episode and can be downloaded to the ECG department over the telephone. The device may be kept for several weeks ∴ good for less frequent episodes. Patient needs to be alert during episode and capable of operating device.

Implantable loop recorders

A small device implanted under the skin in pectoral or axillary region. It typically records 40 min of ECG, 'frozen' by a patient-activated key or stored automatically. Good for infrequent but severely symptomatic events.

Wearable devices

Some wearable devices now have single-lead ECG functions allowing patients to make recordings of their heart rhythm at the time they have symptoms. Some devices also have automated alert functions to warn patients when an arrhythmia is suspected ➲ p.437.

General management

- Establish rhythm and treat accordingly (see Box 5.1, ➲ p.36, for relevant sections)
- Most investigations are best performed on an outpatient basis
- Admit if significant associated symptoms for further investigation and ECG monitoring:
  - Severe chest pain
  - Severe SOB
  - Syncope/near syncope ➲ p.37

Box 5.1 Causes of palpitation

Cardiac

- Tachyarrhythmia:
  - AF ➲ p.151
  - Atrial flutter ➲ p.157
  - SVT ➲ p.161
  - VT ➲ p.169
- Ventricular or atrial ectopic beats

Non-cardiac

- Sinus tachycardia—pain, anxiety, fear, exertion, hypoxia, infection, hypovolaemia (e.g. dehydration), anaemia, thyrotoxicosis, ➲ p.143
- Thyrotoxicosis—appropriate referral to endocrine team. Consider β-blockade (propranolol 40 mg QDS PO) ± carbimazole (40 mg daily PO) if severe (HR >140 bpm)
- Gastro-oesophageal reflux
- Anxiety/emotion
- Rare:
  - Phaeochromocytoma
  - Carcinoid syndrome

Chapter 6

Syncope

Introduction

Syncope: a transient, sudden loss of consciousness, usually leading to falling.

Syncope can be caused by a wide spectrum of conditions, ranging from the benign faint to potentially fatal cardiac arrhythmias. The challenge is to identify those that require specialist management.

The underlying mechanism is hypotension due to a failure of cardiac output or a loss of peripheral vascular resistance. This results in reduced cerebral perfusion and lost consciousness A 6–8 sec interruption to cerebral blood flow may be all that is required for syncope to occur. Syncope can occur without warning but in some, there are prodromal symptoms such as nausea, sweating, loss of balance, or altered vision. Patients with true syncope do not usually remember hitting the ground.

One in 3 of the population will have at least 1 episode of syncope during their lifetime.

Diagnosing syncope

The history and examination are the most important steps in differentiating syncope from non-syncopal causes of loss of consciousness.

- Conditions that mimic syncope, with a loss of consciousness include:
  - Epilepsy
  - Hypoglycaemia
  - Intoxication
- Some conditions without loss of consciousness may mimic syncope—falls, cataplexy, psychogenic syncope, stroke
- Remember that many elderly patients with syncope describe the episodes as falls or trips, often failing to recognize loss of consciousness

Box 6.1 Causes of syncope

Neurally mediated syncope and orthostatic hypotension are the cause of > 50% of cases of syncope. Cardiac causes represent 15% of cases. Neurological and psychiatric causes are found in 10%.

Neurally mediated (reflex) syncope

- Vasovagal syncope:
  - Classical (simple faints)
  - Non-classical (unprovoked)
- Situational syncope:
  - Swallow, cough, micturition
- Carotid sinus hypersensitivity

Orthostatic hypotension

- Autonomic failure:
  - Primary (e.g. pure autonomic failure, multi-system atrophy, and Parkinson-plus syndromes)
  - Secondary (diabetes mellitus)
- Drug induced (vasodilator therapy)
- Volume depletion (diuretics, fluid loss, and Addison disease)

Cardiac arrhythmia

- Sinus node dysfunction ➲ p.134
- AV block ➲ p.139
- Paroxysmal arrhythmias ➲ p.143
- Inherited syndromes e.g. long QT, Brugada syndrome (➲ p.349, p.351)
- Drug-induced bradycardia or prolonged QT interval (➲ p.134, p.173)

Other cardiovascular

- Obstructive valvular disease, e.g. AS (➲ p.281)
- LV outflow obstruction, e.g. hypertrophic cardiomyopathy (➲ p.343)
- Aortic dissection (➲ p.179)
- Pericardial tamponade (➲ p.201)
- Pulmonary hypertension (➲ p.213)
- Pulmonary embolus (➲ p.208)
- Atrial myxoma (➲ p.100)

Questions to ask

- Enquire about the 3 Ps:
  - *Provocative* factors (fatigue, dehydration, warm atmospheres, emotional circumstances, fear, pain)
  - *Prodromes* (nausea, sweating, giddiness, abdominal discomfort)
  - *Postural* components (standing, sitting, or lying)
- Try to obtain a witness account of the episode. Ask about the appearances of the patient during the episode. Was there pallor? Was there seizure activity and if so for how long? Remember that short-lived seizures and myoclonic jerks often occur in simple vasovagal syncope
- How long did the episode last? Arrhythmic syncope can be very brief with almost immediate recovery such in intermittent AV block (Stokes–Adams attacks). Vasovagal episodes tend to be a little longer although these too can be quite short lived
- How long did the patient take to recover and how did they feel? Was there confusion? Following vasovagal episodes patients may report nausea/vomiting and prolonged light headedness with recurrent syncope or presyncope if they stand too quickly. They may also feel profound tiredness which can last for hours or more, and often patients report sleeping in the immediate aftermath of episodes

Investigations

- 12-lead ECG. Abnormalities suggesting a cardiac cause include:
  - Q waves (prior MI)
  - LBBB or RBBB and left anterior or posterior hemiblock
  - AV block (2° or higher) ➲ p.139
  - Sinus bradycardia (< 50 bpm) or sinus pauses > 3 sec
  - Pre-excitation (short PR interval and delta wave) ➲ p.165
  - Prolonged QT interval ➲ p.349, p.313
  - Widened QRS (> 0.12 sec)
  - RBBB with ST elevation in V1–V3 (Brugada syndrome) ➲ p.351
- CXR—cardiac enlargement or aortic dissection ➲ p.179
- Routine blood testing (except plasma glucose) has a low yield
- Carotid sinus massage (Box 6.2)
- Implantable loop recorder in patients with recurrent syncope ➲ p.44
- *In selected patients*: echo, ambulatory ECG monitoring

Box 6.2 Carotid sinus massage

- Used to diagnose carotid sinus hypersensitivity
- Perform with continuous ECG recording and (ideally) beat-to-beat BP monitoring since BP changes are rapid
- With the patient supine, pressure is applied to each carotid sinus in turn for 10–20 sec. If no abnormal response is elicited, the procedure can be repeated with the patient tilted upright
- Avoid in patients with a history of recent stroke (< 3 months), carotid bruits, or known carotid vascular disease

Carotid sinus hypersensitivity is defined as a ventricular pause of > 3 sec or a drop in systolic pressure of > 50 mmHg.

Carotid sinus syndrome is the combination of syncope and carotid sinus hypersensitivity, in a patient in whom clinical evaluation and investigation has identified no other cause of syncope.

Box 6.3 Tilt-table testing

- A provocation test for neurally mediated syncope
- There are a number of protocols in use in clinical practice varying in the angle of tilt (typically 60°–70° head-up), the duration of tilt (20–45 min), and the use of additional provocation (sublingual GTN)
- Both false positives and false negatives can occur, but the test compares favourably with other non-invasive cardiac investigations
- Tilt testing is very likely to be positive in those with obvious classical vasovagal episodes
- However, the diagnosis is rarely in doubt in such patients and tilt testing has a much more important role in investigating patients with recurrent unexplained syncopal episodes and in the investigation of patients with a broad range of disturbances of consciousness where the cause is unclear (e.g. is it really epilepsy?)

Who needs ambulatory ECG monitoring?

The diagnostic yield of prolonged ECG monitoring is low in unselected patients with syncope and will be most beneficial in those with frequent symptoms or in whom you have a high suspicion of a cardiac cause. Factors which suggest a cardiac cause include a history of cardiac disease, an abnormal ECG, or abnormal echocardiogram.

Who should be admitted?

Most patients who present following a single episode of syncope can be investigated as an outpatient. In-hospital monitoring and investigation is warranted if the initial clinical evaluation suggests significant structural heart disease or when syncope is recurrent or disabling. Patients without clinical evidence of structural heart disease and no family history of sudden death who present with an isolated episode of classical vasovagal or situational syncope can be discharged back to their GP without the need for any specific follow-up. All other patients should be referred on for further evaluation as an outpatient.

Neurally mediated (vasovagal) syncope

- Loss of consciousness in vasovagal syncope is typically for < 30 sec although patients and relatives usually report longer
- Likely in the absence of cardiac disease and if there are provoking factors, associated prodromal autonomic symptoms or syncope occurs with head rotation (carotid sinus pressure)
- Situational syncope occurs when directly linked with swallowing, micturition, or coughing

Investigations

- Carotid sinus massage (Box 6.2)
- Tilt-table testing (Box 6.3)

If tests are negative and symptoms recur, then consider prolonged ECG monitoring or an implantable loop recorder (see Fig. 6.1).

Management

Carotid sinus syndrome usually responds well to dual chamber permanent pacing.

For other neurally mediated syncope, treatment is less straightforward, and patients should be referred for specialist advice.

- Non-pharmacological measures are the first-line treatments for patients with vasovagal syncope. These include education, reassurance, tilt training (enforced upright posture), leg crossing, or hand grips during prodromes (to delay or avoid loss of consciousness)
- Pacing for vasovagal syncope can reduce symptoms in selected patients but patients must be informed that it does not prevent attacks
- Pharmacological agents have an unpredictable response and include β blockers, fludrocortisone, midodrine, and fluoxetine

Orthostatic hypotension

Commonly occurs shortly after standing up, or after prolonged standing typically in a hot crowded room. Can occur after exertion. A systolic blood pressure drop of > 20 mmHg after 3 min of standing or a drop to < 90 mmHg is defined as orthostatic hypotension, irrespective of whether symptoms occur.

The commonest cause is vasodilator drugs and diuretic therapy, especially in the elderly.

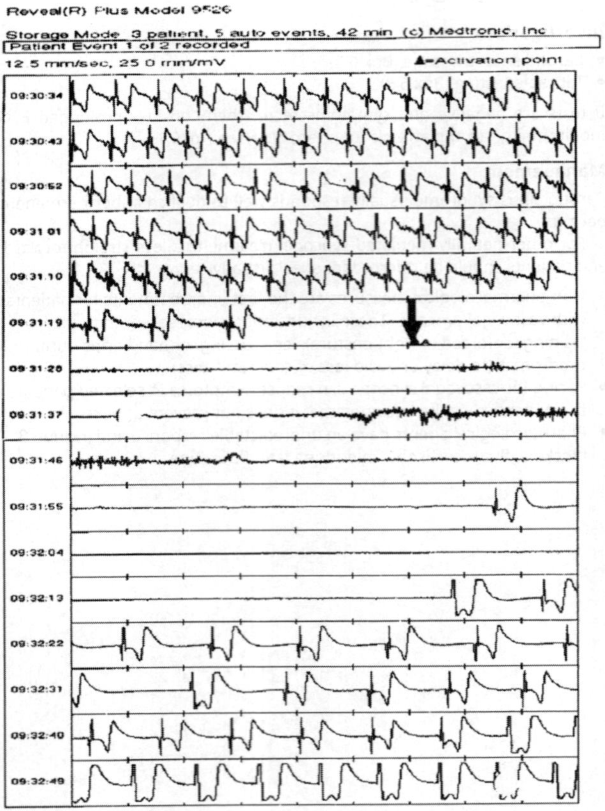

Fig. 6.1 ECG printout downloaded from an implantable loop recorder in a patient with neurocardiogenic syncope. The patient has activated the recorder (black arrow) soon after the onset of sinus arrest. After nearly 1 min of asystole, sinus rhythm returns. The early activation point suggests that the patient had a period of associated autonomic or hypotensive symptoms prior to bradycardia.

Cardiac syncope

- Likely if syncope occurs in the presence of severe structural heart disease, particularly severe LV impairment
- Syncope in patients with poor cardiac function confers a bad prognosis
- Symptoms can occur at any time
- May be provoked by exertion
- Can occur whilst sitting or supine
- Can be associated with palpitation or chest discomfort

Investigations

- Echocardiography
- Prolonged ECG monitoring
- *In selected patients*: electrophysiological studies
- Syncope occurring during effort should be investigated with echocardiography and exercise stress testing

Important causes of cardiac syncope

Urgent cardiology referral is required.

- *Severe LV impairment*: associated with monomorphic VT, atrial arrhythmias, postural or drug-induced hypotension
- *AS:* exertional syncope resulting from severe AS is associated with a high incidence of sudden death. ➲ p.96
- *Hypertrophic cardiomyopathy:* syncope occurs in up to 25% of patients and can be a risk marker for SCD. ➲ p.343
- *Long QT syndrome:* episodes of polymorphic VT can result in recurrent syncope. See ➲ p.349, p.173
- *Brugada syndrome:* a cause of SCD. ST elevation is seen in the right precordial leads (V1–V3) but changes can be dynamic. See ➲ p.351, 352

Driving and lifestyle restrictions

Documented advice on driving *must* be given to each patient presenting with syncope. Restrictions for driving should be reviewed according to national guidelines as updates are made frequently. In general, driving should cease for at least 4 weeks after an episode of unexplained syncope. If no cause has been identified then a period of at least 6 months without driving is usually recommended.

Weblink

In the UK, the Driver and Vehicle Licensing Agency issue guidelines for medical practitioners: ℘ https://www.gov.uk/guidance/assessing-fitness-to-drive-a-guide-for-medical-professionals

Other lifestyle restrictions

Patients should be advised to avoid situations where syncope would be hazardous, e.g. working up a ladder.

Reference

2018 European Society of Cardiology guidelines for the diagnosis and management of syncope https://doi.org/10.1093/eurheartj/ehy037

Part 2

Conditions

Chapter 7

Acute coronary syndromes

Introduction

Acute coronary syndromes (ACS) are a collection of clinical conditions involving acutely compromised myocardial perfusion (Table 7.1):

- ST segment elevation myocardial infarction (STEMI)
- Non-ST segment elevation ACS (NSTE-ACS) further subdivided into
  - Non-ST-segment elevation myocardial infarction (NSTEMI)
  - Unstable angina

Occurrence of myocardial injury determined by increased troponin levels differentiates NSTEMI from unstable angina.

Table 7.1 Classification of ACS

	Troponin	ECG
STEMI	↑ or ↑↑	ST elevation LBBB
Non-STEMI	↑ (occasionally ↑↑)	Normal Abnormal, but unchanged
Unstable angina	↔	ST segment depression T-wave inversion

Pathophysiology

Understanding the pathophysiology helps to explain the spectrum of presentation and underpins the rationale for treatment algorithms (see Box 7.1 for CCS risk factors).

Box 7.1 Risk factors for coronary atherothrombosis

- Tobacco smoking
- Family history
- Diabetes mellitus
- Hypertension
- High low-density lipoprotein (LDL)-cholesterol
- Low high-density lipoprotein (HDL)-cholesterol

Additional risk factors

- Inflammatory conditions, including rheumatological diseases
- Patients with elevated markers of systemic inflammation: high-sensitivity-CRP, interleukin-6, and tumour necrosis factor
- Central obesity
- Chronic kidney disease
- Sedentary lifestyle
- High apolipoprotein B (ApoB)
- Low apolipoprotein AI (ApoAI)
- High lipoprotein (a) [Lp(a)]
- High plasma homocysteine

Stable angina or chronic coronary syndromes (CCS) occur when fixed stenotic lesions in the epicardial coronary arteries, or in some cases the presence of coronary microvascular dysfunction, impede myocardial perfusion at times of increased oxygen demand (e.g. physical or emotional stress).

In contrast, ACS occur when erosion or rupture of the 'fibrous cap' overlying an atherosclerotic lesion exposes intensely thrombogenic material within the plaque milieu to platelets and coagulation factors in the bloodstream. The so-called culprit plaque is not necessarily stenotic prior to the acute presentation, which explains why many ACS events are unheralded. The nature of the occlusion (partial or total, transient, or fixed) and its location (proximally or distally within the coronary tree) largely determine the clinical presentation and course.

Non-atherosclerotic causes of acute MI

Myocardial infarction associated with an acute plaque event is also labelled as Type 1 myocardial infarction. In contrast to MI due to an acute coronary syndrome (Type 1 MI), Type 2 MI is defined as a mismatch in myocardial oxygen supply and demand that is not attributable to coronary atherosclerotic disease.

'Coronary artery-related', but non atherosclerosis-related causes accounting for Type 2 myocardial infarction are:

- Coronary Embolism (secondary to atrial fibrillation, paradoxical embolism through a patent foramen ovale or from vegetations in infective endocarditis)

- Spontaneous coronary dissection
- Coronary spasm (often encountered in cocaine abuse)
- Coronary arteritis, e.g. Kawasaki disease
- Thrombosis *in situ* in pro-coagulable states
- Trauma—avulsed coronary artery, *ab-extrinseco* (extrinsic) coronary compression in commotio cordis

'Non-coronary' causes of Type 2 myocardial infarction include:

- Tachyarrhythmias
- Severe bradycardia
- Severe arterial hypertension (hypertensive crisis)
- Severe anaemia
- Severe hypotension/shock
- Respiratory failure
- Heart failure

Type 1 and coronary artery-related Type 2 myocardial infarction can occur in the context of apparently healthy coronary arteries at invasive coronary angiogram. This entity goes under the name of 'myocardial infarction with non-obstructed coronary arteries' (MINOCA). It accounts for 6–8% of ACS presentation.

A special mention is required for Takotsubo syndrome, which presents similarly to ACS (e.g. chest pain, ECG changes, and troponin elevation) but with no objective evidence of myocardial infarction, as determined by magnetic resonance imaging. Adrenergic drive, possibly associated with microvascular dysfunction, can account for Takotsubo syndrome which typically features a reversible apical akinesia/diskinesia of the left ventricle causing the typical apical ballooning appearance. Rarer forms of basal or mid ventricle Takotsubo syndrome are also recognized.

Coronary artery anatomy

The origins of the coronary arteries can be seen in Fig. 7.1

The *left anterior descending* (LAD) coronary artery runs in the anterior interventricular groove supplying the anterior wall of the heart. It gives off *septal* branches that supply blood to the anterior 2/3 of the interventricular septum, including the left bundle branch; *diagonal* vessels to the lateral wall of the LV; and a terminal bifurcation that supplies the apex of the LV and sometimes wraps around to supply the inferior wall of the LV.

The *circumflex* (LCX) artery runs posteriorly in the left AV groove and gives *obtuse marginal* branches to the lateral wall of the LV, supplying the posterior wall of the LV.

The *right* coronary artery (RCA) runs in the right AV groove. It gives branches to the sinoatrial node, AV node, and RV. On reaching the posterior interventricular groove, it gives rise to the *posterior descending artery* that supplies the inferior wall of the LV, and the inferior 1/3 of the interventricular septum. This is the more common variant. In about 10% of patients, the circumflex gives rise to the posterior descending artery and is then termed 'dominant'.

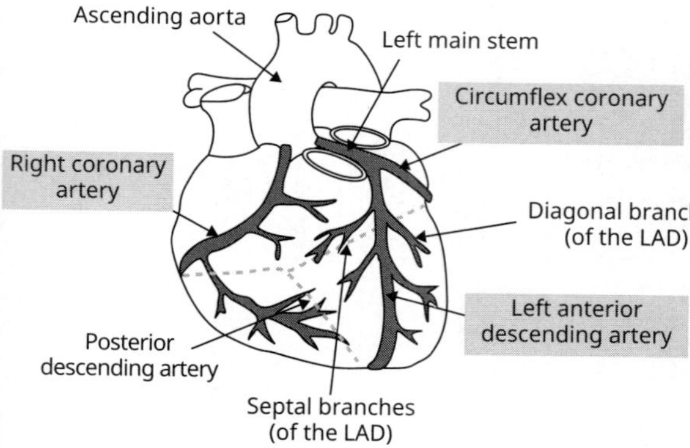

Fig. 7.1 Coronary artery anatomy. There are three principal coronary arteries. The left main stem arises from the left aortic sinus and soon gives rise to the (i) left anterior descending and (ii) circumflex coronary arteries. The (iii) right coronary artery normally has a separate origin in the right aortic sinus.

Table 7.2 Coronary artery territories

Site of arterial occlusion	Myocardial territory	ECG changes
LAD	Anterolateral	V4–V6, I, aVL
	Anteroseptal	V1–V4 LBBB
LCX	Posterior	Mirror image changes in V1–V2 or V3, i.e. ST segment depression ± inferior changes; tall R in V1 May be electrically silent on standard 12-lead ECG
RCA	Inferior wall of LV	II, III, aVF ST elevation in III > II
	RV	ST elevation V4R to V6R

Acute STEMI

This is a medical emergency usually caused by thrombotic occlusion of a major epicardial coronary artery. Irreversible ischaemic injury to the myocardium is threatened (or may have occurred at presentation). Prompt action conserves myocardium and prevents complications (mechanical, arrhythmic, heart failure) including death.

The optimal treatment of acute STEMI should be based on the implementation of an emergency system that is planned and agreed locally, taking into account local geography, ambulance provision, medical facilities, and expertise for the appropriate delivery of primary percutaneous coronary intervention (PPCI). Pre-hospital diagnosis is pivotal in most models of care.

Symptoms

- Severe 'crushing' central chest pain ± radiation to jaw, neck, or arms
- 'Autonomic' features: diaphoresis (sweating), nausea, and vomiting
- Breathlessness due to LV dysfunction
- Atypical presentations include pain in the back or abdomen, confusion
- MI may be silent (especially in the elderly and in patients with diabetes)

Determine

- Current haemodynamic status
- Timing of the onset of symptoms
- Can PPCI be provided within 2 hours from diagnosis?
- If not, are there contraindications to thrombolysis? (➲ Box 7.3, p.60)
- Has aspirin been given, e.g. in ambulance?
- Is there a history of coronary disease?

Signs

- Pain or distress
- Clammy (sweating and cutaneous vasoconstriction) and grey

Look for complications

- Hypotension
- Lung crepitations and other evidence of heart failure
- Rhythm disturbances—bradycardia, e.g. heart block; AF, sinus tachycardia (pain, anxiety, or compensatory
- Murmurs—MR due to papillary muscle ischaemia or chordal rupture; acquired VSD (➲ p.65)
- Fever < 38°C is common in the first 48 hours

Investigations

12-lead ECG (Fig. 7.2)

- If ST segment elevation is present, a rapid decision on revascularization is required. See ➲ Indications for revascularization, p.57
- In patients with inferior MI, right-sided ECG leads should be obtained, to identify possible RV infarction
- Where ECG diagnostic criteria are not met initially, but pain persists, obtain serial ECGs every 10 min and study for new or dynamic changes
- ECG monitoring should be initiated as soon as possible to facilitate immediate diagnosis and management of life-threatening arrhythmias

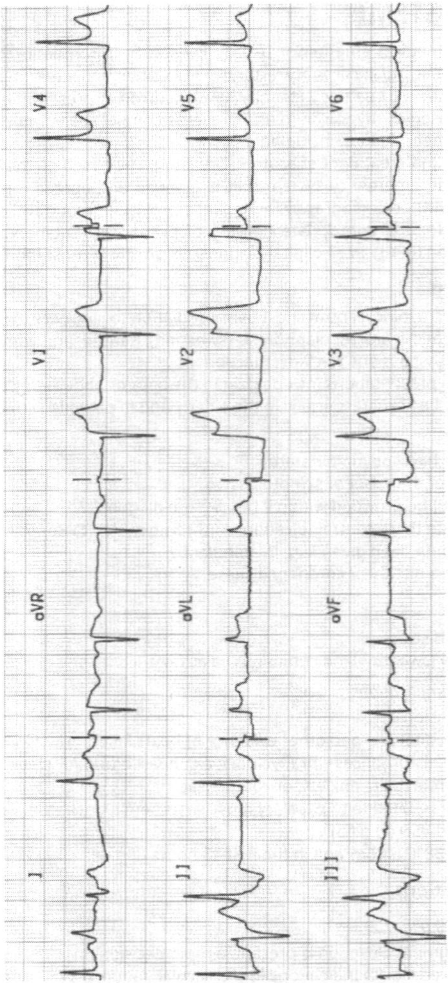

Fig. 7.2 ECG in acute anterolateral MI. There is marked ST segment elevation in leads V1–V4 and aVL. Reciprocal ST segment depression is present in leads II, III, and aVF.

Other investigations

- If diagnostic uncertainty persists, echocardiography can be helpful, since segmental hypokinesis occurs early in the course of acute ischaemia (though cannot be differentiated with certainty from chronic dysfunction). However, treatment should not be significantly delayed while waiting for an echocardiogram
- A portable chest radiograph may be helpful in selected patients such as for those with suspected pulmonary oedema or suspicion of other intrathoracic pathologies that could account for their presentation. It should not delay prompt revascularization where indicated
- Blood for troponin (Box 7.2), and repeated 12 hours after symptom onset. In acute MI, initial treatment decisions are *not* dependent only on blood test results, but are guided by clinical judgement
- FBC, U&E, serum cholesterol, and glucose. Remember that serum cholesterol may decrease after 24 hours and persist at lower level for several weeks following an acute MI

Immediate management

Your patient may be terrified. Provide reassurance where possible.

- Oxygen
- Aspirin 150–300 mg. Chewed for rapid buccal absorption
- Ticagrelor 180mg OR prasugrel 60 mg PO loading dose are preferred over clopidogrel
- IV access
- Diamorphine 2.5–5 mg IV or morphine 5–10 mg IV
- Metoclopramide 10 mg IV

► *Reperfusion therapy:* PPCI or thrombolysis (see ➲ p.57)

Important differential diagnoses

Aortic dissection (➲ p.179) can present with chest pain and ST segment elevation. The pain is usually distinguished by its abrupt onset, migration to the back, and tearing nature. Where ST segment elevation is recorded, it is usually in the inferior (i.e. right coronary) territory since dissection involving the left main stem is usually fatal.

Thrombolytic therapy in acute aortic dissection is potentially lethal. Where there is significant suspicion of dissection, further imaging (e.g. contrast CT aorta, TOE, or MRI) should be obtained.

Acute pericarditis (➲ p.198) may present with chest pain and ST segment elevation on the ECG. The pain is typically exacerbated by inspiration and relieved by sitting upright. The ECG changes are classically concave upwards (saddle shaped) and may be widespread, spanning the equivalent of multiple coronary territories.

Box 7.2 Interpreting the troponin measurement

Troponins are proteins involved in cardiomyocyte contraction. There are troponin isoforms specific to the myocardium, and elevated levels in the blood are indicative of myocardial injury. Levels rise within 12 hours of myocardial injury, peak at around 24 hours, and remain elevated for up to 14 days.

It is important to recognize that the diagnosis of ACS is, in the first instance, clinical—the initial management is *based on clinical diagnosis* and the ECG(s) and is not contingent on the troponin result.

The troponin may turn out to be elevated and in NSTEMI patients is one of the markers of risk (➲ Box 7.4, p.70) but, importantly, may be normal in patients with unstable angina who are at high risk of subsequent cardiac events, and the clinical diagnosis is crucial in these patients.

Furthermore, release of troponin T is not specific to coronary disease. Caution is necessary in interpreting an elevated serum troponin in the absence of a typical history and/or ECG changes, particularly where the rise is relatively modest. Other conditions that can lead to troponin elevation include:

- Myocarditis
- Pericarditis
- PE
- Sepsis
- Renal failure

Because of superior specificity, troponin measurement has largely superseded measurement of other biomarkers of myocardial damage—CK, AST, and LDH.

Reperfusion therapy for STEMI

Reperfusion therapy should be with PPCI in accordance with local policies unless unable to do so within the 2-hour window, in which case thrombolysis could be an alternative (see Fig. 7.3).

The goals are prompt restoration of coronary flow and myocardial perfusion. Rapid action is vital: the door-to-needle time (thrombolysis) should be < 10 min and the door-to-balloon time (for PPCI) should be < 60 min. Most hospitals have multidisciplinary teams to accelerate provision of reperfusion therapy. Delays increase myocardial necrosis, decrease the efficacy of eventual reperfusion therapy, and increase mortality.

Indications for reperfusion therapy

- Symptoms of myocardial ischaemia
- Onset within the prior 12 hours (or up to 24 hours if symptoms of ischaemia persist)
- ST segment elevation of > 0.1 mV (usually 1 mm) in at least two adjacent limb leads *or*
- ST segment elevation of > 0.2 mV (usually 2 mm) in at least two contiguous chest leads *or*
- New (or presumed new) LBBB *or*
- True posterior MI*

*Posterior MI is notorious for the absence of definitive ECG changes. ST segment depression in leads V2 and V3—particularly in the context of concomitant inferior and or lateral ST segment elevation—should suggest posterior MI, where the clinical syndrome fits. If the changes are inconclusive, an echocardiogram may help.

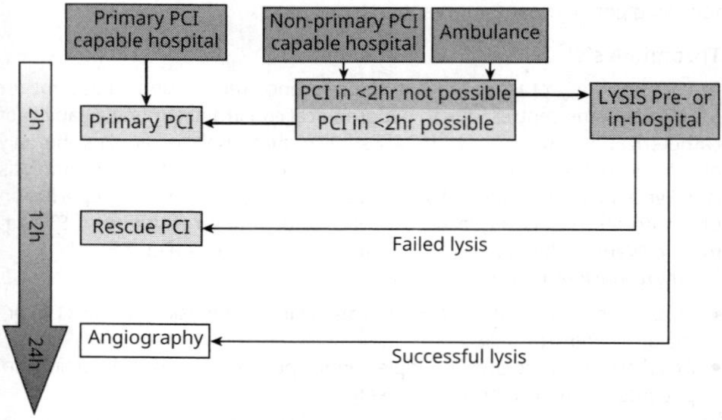

Fig. 7.3 Reperfusion strategy decision tree. PPCI should be delivered within 2 hours of diagnosis. Thrombolysis should only be given when this is not possible; following which urgent transfer to a PPCI centre should take place for subsequent invasive angiography.

Adapted with permission from Byrne RA, Rossello X, Coughlan J *et al.* 2023 ESC Guidelines for the management of acute coronary syndromes. *European Heart Journal* 2023; 44(38): 3720–826.

Primary PCI

PPCI refers to immediate PCI as the initial reperfusion strategy. It achieves high levels of vessel patency and, in experienced hands, may reduce mortality compared to thrombolysis. The risk of stroke is also lower compared to thrombolysis.

- Initiate immediate management measures (➲ p.55)
- Ticagrelor or prasugrel should be given to patients having PPCI. A loading dose should be given prior to PPCI
- Alert the cardiac catheterization laboratory/duty cardiologist at the earliest opportunity, ideally at 'first medical contact' and, if possible, before the patient has arrived in the hospital
- Ideally the patient is moved from the ambulance (or Emergency Department) directly to the cardiac catheterization laboratory
- Informed consent is usually obtained by the operator or a competent deputy

In the catheterization laboratory

- The purpose is restoration of myocardial perfusion as soon as possible, usually achieved by passing a coronary guide wire across the lesion, followed by balloon dilatation and stent deployment (Fig. 7.4)
- Other adjunctive intervention such as thrombus aspiration may also be performed

Although not given routinely, some patients may receive IV glycoprotein (GP) IIb/IIIa receptor inhibitors (e.g. tirofiban) by intravenous or intracoronary bolus injection with subsequent maintained intravenous infusion in the hours following PCI up to 18 hours, particularly in high-risk cases with large thrombus burden or when no or slow reflow occurs. (Slow or no reflow refers to poor or no visualization of contrast flow down the coronary artery following percutaneous intervention.)

Thrombolysis

In contemporary practice, PPCI is the reference reperfusion treatment for STEMIs. In some centres, due to geographical constraints or unavailability of catheterization laboratory with 24/7 service, thrombolysis remains the only alternative reperfusion treatment. In some areas, pre-hospital thrombolysis is delivered by community physicians or paramedics. Achieved reperfusion post thrombolysis is suggested by relief of pain and resolution of ST segment elevation. This is expected roughly in 50% of cases (Fig. 7.5).

When considering thrombolysis

- Exclude contraindications (Box 7.3) and warn of the risk of stroke (1%) or major bleeding (5–10%)
- Avoid arterial punctures, multiple venous punctures, and IM injections in patients where thrombolysis is likely

Following successful thrombolysis, patients should still be transferred to a centre for angiography ± PCI within 24 hours.

Choice of thrombolytic

Alteplase (rtPA) accelerated regimen (< 6 hours from symptom onset):

- If > 65 kg body weight (weight-adjust dose if < 65 kg)
- 15 mg by IV bolus followed by:

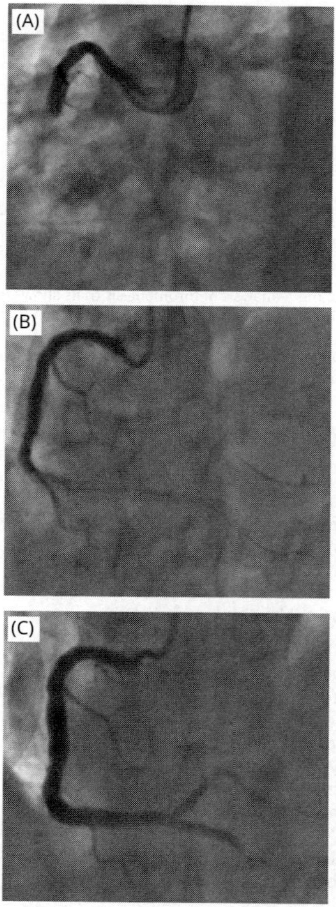

Fig. 7.4 (A) Inferior STEMI with occlusion of the RCA. (B) Coronary guide wires passed to the PDA and PLV branch of the RCA. Stent positioned at the distal RCA just before the bifurcation. (C) Restoration of flow following stent deployment.

- 0.75 mg/kg up to 50 mg over 30 min, then
- 0.5 mg/kg up to 35 mg over 60 min (i.e. total 100 mg over 90 min)

Alternatively:

- Streptokinase 1.5 million units IV over 60 min
- Tenecteplase (TNK) 500 mcg per kg (max 50 mg) IV over 10 sec
- Reteplase 10 units IV over not more than 2 min followed by 10 units 30 min later

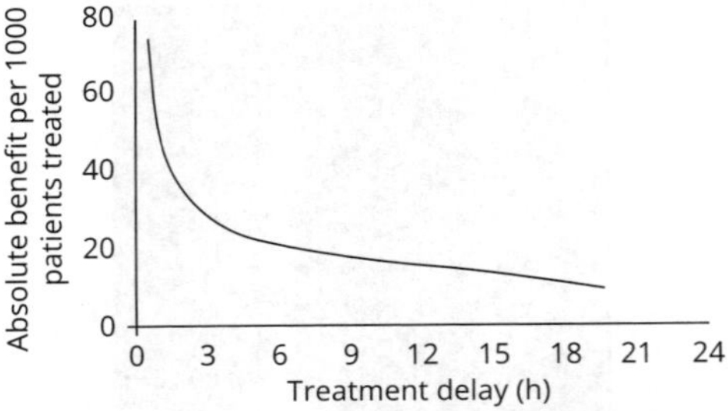

Fig. 7.5 Summary of meta-analysis of thrombolysis trials shows the marked time sensitivity of thrombolysis particularly within the first 'golden' 2 hours after the onset of pain.

Adapted with permission from Boersma E *et al.* Early thrombolytic treatment in acute myocardial infarction: reappraisal of the golden hour. *Lancet* 1996; **348**: 771–5.

Box 7.3 Contraindications to thrombolysis

Absolute

- Any prior intracranial haemorrhage
- Known intracranial structural vascular lesions (e.g. arteriovenous malformation)
- Known intracranial malignant neoplasm (1° or 2°)
- Ischaemic stroke within 3 months
- Active bleeding or bleeding diathesis
- Significant head trauma within 3 months

Relative

- Severe hypertension (systolic > 180 mmHg; diastolic > 110 mmHg) despite treatment
- Traumatic or prolonged CPR
- Major surgery within 3 weeks
- Non-compressible vascular punctures
- Recent (within 2–4 weeks) internal bleeding
- Pregnancy
- Active peptic ulcer
- Current anticoagulant use
- Pain for > 24 hours
- For streptokinase: prior exposure to streptokinase (persistent antibodies)

► N.B. Patients with contraindications to thrombolysis should be considered for PPCI

Modified from Antman EM *et al.* ACC/AHA guidelines for the management of patients with ST-elevation myocardial infarction. *Circulation* 2004; 110: 588–636.

Alteplase, tenecteplase, and reteplase have equivalent efficacy and are more efficacious thrombolytics, resulting in 10 fewer deaths per 1000 patients treated, but at the expense of 3 additional strokes compared to streptokinase.

Following thrombolysis, delayed (12–24 hours) administration of dual antiplatelet therapy, i.e. aspirin and ticagrelor (loading then maintenance) is recommended prior to PCI. For patients > 75 years or with higher bleeding risk, consider clopidogrel instead of ticagrelor.

Failure to reperfuse after thrombolysis

Ongoing ischaemic symptoms and/or persistent ST segment elevation (> 50% in the lead of greatest ST elevation, 60–90 min after thrombolysis) may result from a failure to achieve patency of the epicardial vessel or due to distal (microvascular) occlusion. In these circumstances, emergency (rescue) PCI should be undertaken (or, at least, considered), with transfer to the local PCI centre, if required (based on the findings of the REACT trial)

Additional treatments

The goals of treatment post MI are to:

1. Maintain stent patency and minimize risk of further thrombosis.

Dual antiplatelet therapy is recommended for 12 months followed by single antiplatelet lifelong. Ticagrelor or prasugrel is preferred over clopidogrel as the second antiplatelet therapy (in addition to aspirin). For patients at risk of GI bleeding, a proton pump inhibitor should be considered.

In some cases where the risk of further ischaemic events is high (e.g. patients with diffuse, multivessel disease, multiple treated lesions, long segments of stent), prolonged dual antiplatelet therapy (DAPT) beyond 12 months may be considered. Conversely, in patients with high bleeding risk or who may have unplanned or urgent surgery, the duration of DAPT may be shortened to 1 month. These decisions can be complex and require the weighing of thrombosis vs bleeding risks and are best guided by the interventional cardiologist.

2. Optimize myocardial remodelling and LV function

An ACE inhibitor (e.g. ramipril 2.5 mg BD) should be commenced within the first 24 hours following acute MI if the systolic BP is > 100 mmHg. There is particular benefit in the presence of LV dysfunction. The dose should be titrated upwards as BP permits.

In post-STEMI patients with LV ejection fraction < 40%, β-blockade and aldosterone blockade (unless significant renal dysfunction or hyperkalaemia) are recommended in addition to ACE inhibitors. For aldosterone blockade, the trial data were obtained using eplerenone

3. Retard atherosclerosis

High-intensity statin treatment should be instigated in almost all patients to achieve an LDL cholesterol < 1.4 mmol/L. Additional lipid-lowering therapies such as ezetimibe and PCSK9 inhibitors should be considered when statin alone is unable to adequately lower cholesterol levels, or where that patient is intolerant of statins.

In patients with diabetes, additional consideration should be given to achieve adequate glycaemic control according to local hospital guidelines. Glucose lowering therapies that confer cardiovascular benefit such as SGLT2 inhibitors and GLP1R analogues should be considered as a priority, with advice from the diabetes team, where needed.

Surgery

- CABG surgery is not usually undertaken in the acute setting

However, in a minority of patients, the extent and distribution of coronary artery disease, determined by angiography, might require CABG for optimal revascularization.

Where early CABG is planned or anticipated, it is usual to withhold the second anti-platelet agent to mitigate the risk of surgical bleeding, and continue aspirin 75 mg daily. In the absence of new stents, the short-term risk of monotherapy vs dual therapy outside of PCI is very small.

Risk stratification and prognosis

- An important predictor of 30-day mortality in acute MI is the presence (and degree) of heart failure, quantified by Killip[1] in 1967 and updated from GUSTO trial data for the thrombolytic era (see table 7.3)
- The extent of myocardial damage can be estimated from the magnitude of the rise in cardiac enzymes/troponin and from the appearances on echocardiography
- Cardiac magnetic resonance is highly accurate in assessing the extent of myocardial scar and ejection fraction, but can overestimate the extent of myocardial infarction in the first weeks after MI (Fig. 7.6)

Table 7.3 Acute MI, prognostic indicators

Group	Clinical feature	30-day mortality (%)
Killip class I	No S_3 and clear lungs	5.1
Killip class II	S_3 or crepitations in lungs	13.6
Killip class III	Crepitations > 50% of lung	32.2
Killip class IV	Shock	57.8
Anterior MI		9.9
Inferior MI		5.0
Age < 60 years		2.4
Age 60–75 years		7.9
Age > 75 years		20.5

Adapted with permission from Lee KL *et al*, Predictors of 30-day mortality in the era of reperfusion for acute myocardial infarction. Results from an international trial of 41,021 patients. GUSTO-I Investigators. *Circulation* 1996; 91: 1659–68.

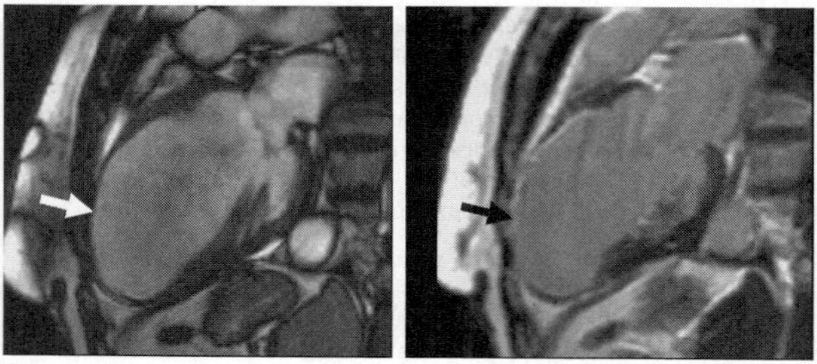

Fig. 7.6 Cardiac MRI following acute antero-apical MI. Note thinning of the LV anterior wall and apex (left, white arrow). Blood within the heart appears white on this still from a cine image. Right: delayed gadolinium enhancement imaging shows the full extent of the infarcted tissue—infarcted myocardium appears white (black arrow).

Reference

1. Killip T, Kimball JT. Treatment of myocardial infarction in a coronary care unit: a two-year experience with 250 patients. *American Journal of Cardiology* 1967; 20: 457–64.

Complications of acute MI

Immediate complications (within hours)

Ventricular arrhythmia

VT and VF are the principal causes of death early in acute MI. Patients in the immediate peri-infarct period should be managed on a specialized coronary care unit that is equipped to treat such arrhythmias.

Complete heart block

Usually occurring in the context of acute inferior MI, CHB is often transient, resolving with reperfusion. When haemodynamic compromise occurs, insertion of a temporary transvenous pacing wire may be indicated (➲ Box 11.1, p.133 and p.364). After an inferior STEMI, resolution of CHB may take several days, hence decision for a permanent pacemaker should not be rushed. CHB in the context of anterior MI, however, suggests extensive infarction, and adverse prognosis—temporary or permanent pacing should be considered.

Hypotension

Hypotension in the absence of signs of heart failure may respond to a fluid challenge, e.g. 250–500 mL normal saline given rapidly, particularly following an acute inferior MI which is can be accompanied by RV infarction (see below). Intravenous fluid in this case would maintain left-sided filling pressures.

Cardiogenic shock (➲ p.11)

Caution should be taken with fluid challenges in large myocardial infarction as hypotension may be indicative of incipient cardiogenic shock. Anticipation, or onset, of cardiogenic shock requires urgent expert attention (ITU/cardiology). Inotropic support ± vasopressors (➲ p.20) and/or mechanical ventricular support might be required. In addition to hypotension, signs of heart failure (such as pulmonary oedema, peripheral vasoconstriction, clamminess) and echo-evidence of severe LV impairment should alert to possible cardiogenic shock.

Pulmonary congestion and pulmonary oedema

Give oxygen, morphine, and IV loop diuretics, e.g. furosemide 40–100 mg IV. Infuse GTN 0.5–10 mg/hour IV if BP >90 mmHg systolic. Obtain a CXR. Insert a urinary catheter and monitor urine output hourly. Give oxygen and monitor HbO_2 saturation with pulse oximetry. In severe cases, CPAP or intubation and ventilation may be required. Anticipate these requirements and discuss early with the ITU physicians. Speak to the patient's relatives.

Right ventricular infarction

Occurs in 30% of inferior MI and carries an adverse prognosis. RV infarction is suggested by ST elevation > 1 mm in V4R. Often associated with hypotension, which may require robust fluid resuscitation to 'push' the RV and maintain left-sided filling pressures.

Early complications (within days)

New murmur

New murmur and abrupt haemodynamic deterioration suggest the possibility of papillary muscle rupture (or dysfunction) causing MR, or VSD, or free wall rupture. Obtain an echocardiogram urgently. In general, a structural problem needs a structural fix. Call the surgeons early.

Mitral regurgitation

Acute severe MR due to papillary muscle rupture is a cardiac surgical emergency. Stabilization can be attempted with IV diuretics, IV nitrates, ± mechanical ventricular support. These are all temporizing measures at best. Urgent surgical repair should be considered.

Ventricular septal rupture

Acquired VSD is life-threatening and requires urgent surgical repair. Stabilization can be attempted with IV diuretics, IV nitrates, and IABP insertion in cases of small VSD with limited interventricular shunts

Rupture of myocardial free wall

Abrupt deterioration within 3 days post MI may indicate myocardial rupture. If not fatal, urgent surgical repair should be considered.

Pericarditis

Common after MI. The associated pain is usually pleuritic, positional, and distinct from the ischaemia-related pain of the initial presentation. Pericarditis occurs > 12 hours after acute MI and is treated with high- (anti-inflammatory) dose aspirin, up to 650 mg 4–6-hourly in combination with colchicine if tolerated. There is some evidence that indometacin and ibuprofen may adversely affect myocardial remodelling early post MI, and are best avoided. Anticoagulation should be stopped if a pericardial effusion develops or enlarges.

Mural thrombus and systemic embolization

Oral anticoagulation (DOAC or warfarin) should be given to patients with known LV thrombus to reduce the risk of systemic embolization. The duration of therapy, initially 3–6 months, is guided by repeat imaging such as cardiac MR or echocardiography to assess resolution of thrombus and patient's clinical status such as bleeding risk

New (or coexisting) atrial fibrillation

Direct factor X inhibitors (apixaban, edoxaban, rivaroxaban) can be considered as an alternative to warfarin in patients with pre-existing atrial fibrillation or with post-MI established and not-spontaneously cardioverted atrial fibrillation. DOACs can be prescribed in combination with dual antiplatelet therapy. However, duration of triple therapy should be weighted according to the perceived individual patient bleeding and thrombotic risk profile and in conjunction with the interventional cardiology team. Current guidelines recommend 1 week to 1 month of triple therapy depending on ischaemic risk, followed by DOAC and single antiplatelet up to a year then DOAC monotherapy indefinitely

Late complications (several weeks)

Dressler syndrome

Autoimmune-mediated acute febrile illness that occurs 2 weeks to several months after acute MI. The incidence has fallen in the reperfusion era. Management is with aspirin or NSAIDs (non-steroid anti-inflammatory drugs). Large pericardial effusions may accumulate causing haemodynamic embarrassment or even tamponade. In Dressler syndrome management obtain an echocardiogram, stop anticoagulants to minimize risk of haemorrhagic transformation. Percutaneous drainage (➲ p.367) may be required if tamponade occurs (rare).

Ventricular tachycardia

Scar formation post MI predisposes to VT (➲ p.169). In selected patients' implantable cardioverter defibrillator (ICD) therapy is indicated. ICD is however considered if severe left ventricular impairment persists (EF < 35%) after 45 days from initial admission according to DINAMIT study results.

Left ventricular aneurysm

Infarcted tissue may become thinned and dyskinetic. Aneurysms are haemodynamically inefficient, predispose to thrombus formation, and may cause persistent ST elevation on the ECG.

Post-infarct management

- In the absence of complications or persistent ischaemia, patients should be mobile within 24 hours
- After successful PPCI with an uncomplicated course, patients may be discharged at ~48–72 hours
- After successful thrombolysis, current guidelines recommend inpatient diagnostic angiography (within 24 hours) as the best strategy

Inform the patient that there may be restrictions on driving depending on local authorities which is often guided by information such as success of revascularization and LV function.

Take the opportunity to implement education on 2° prevention, e.g. smoking cessation and diet (low saturated fat, low salt, promote Mediterranean-type diet). Introduction to a supervised, structured rehabilitation programme is generally beneficial.

Discharge medication

- Aspirin
- Ticagrelor or prasugrel
- β-blocker
- ACE inhibitor
- High-intensity statin
- Aldosterone antagonist (if ejection fraction < 40%; K^+ < 5 mmol/L)

Longer term

- For most patients, aspirin 75 mg daily will continue indefinitely
- The default recommendation is for dual antiplatelet therapy (aspirin and ticagrelor/prasugrel) for a year then aspirin lifelong. This duration may be extended or shortened determined by the balance between ischaemic and bleeding risk
- β-blockers are often given indefinitely in recovered STEMI patients, but evidence exists for the first year or two post-MI only
- Indefinite use of ACE inhibitors should be considered in patients with atherosclerotic disease (as 2° prevention). The benefit is greatest when there is LV dysfunction, and in these patients the dose should be titrated upwards as an outpatient
- LDL reduction with a statin shows marked benefit in 2° prevention. Targets for treatment for patients who present with ACS are for LDL-cholesterol < 1.4mmol/L
- Omega-3 fatty acids commenced within 3 months of acute MI have been associated with a mortality benefit
- Low-dose colchicine (0.5 mg OD) can be considered as a secondary prevention strategy in patients who are considered to have residual risk of developing further events

Further reading

Byrne, RA, Rossello X, Coughlan JJ *et al.* 2023 ESC Guidelines for the management of acute coronary syndromes. *European Heart Journal* 2023; 44(38): 3720–826.

Schüpke S, Neumann FJ, Menichelli M *et al.* Ticagrelor or prasugrel in patients with acute coronary syndromes. *New England Journal of Medicine* 2019 Oct 17; 381(16): 1524–34.

Tardif JC, Kouz S, Waters DD *et al.* Efficacy and safety of low-dose colchicine after myocardial infarction. *New England Journal of Medicine* 2019 Dec 26; 381(26) :2497–505.

Unstable angina and NSTEMI

In the absence of sustained ST segment elevation, ischaemic pain of abruptly worsening severity or occurring at rest is classed as 'unstable angina' or non-ST segment elevation MI (NSTEMI). The distinction depends on the eventual presence (NSTEMI) or absence (UA) of an elevated troponin measurement. The underlying pathology (ruptured or eroded coronary plaque with non-occlusive or intermittently occlusive thrombus) and initial management is the same. The immediate objectives are to relieve pain and to prevent progression to acute MI.

Symptoms

- Similar to STEMI
- Central chest pain/ache of variable severity and duration—may radiate to the jaw or (left) arm and typically not relieved by GTN
- There may be a history of prior chronic stable angina. Pain is sometimes accompanied by 'autonomic' features diaphoresis (sweating), nausea, and vomiting

Signs

- There may be no abnormal physical signs
- Pain or distress
- Clammy—a result of sweating and cutaneous vasoconstriction
- Occasionally accompanied by intermittent pulmonary oedema, depending on degree of ischaemia and underlying LV function

Investigations

At presentation, the diagnosis is clinical.

ECG

- The ECG may be normal
- ECG changes include ST segment depression and T-wave inversion, which may be 'dynamic'—coming and going with symptoms (Fig. 7.7)
- Exclude sustained ST-segment elevation (➲ p.54)
- If the ECG is normal but pain persists, obtain serial ECGs

Bloods

- Check FBC—to exclude anaemia
- Troponin at presentation and 12 hours after onset of pain

Immediate management

There are 4 principal categories of therapy:

- Agents to reduce ischaemia
- Antiplatelet agents
- Anticoagulants
- PCI

A general scheme is given here, but the precise management is determined in part by decisions on 'early conservative' management vs an 'early invasive' strategy (i.e. angiography ± PCI)

- Aspirin 150–300 mg. Chewed to achieve rapid buccal absorption

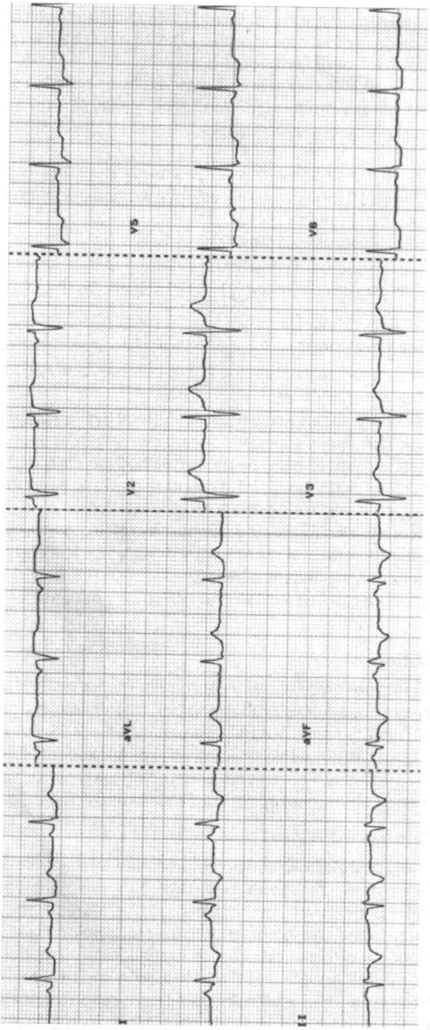

Fig. 7.7 ECG during chest pain. ST segment depression in leads I, V5, and V6 with T-wave inversion in leads II, III, and aVF is suggestive of ischaemia in the inferolateral territory.

- Ticagrelor 180 mg OR prasugrel 60 mg PO loading, followed by maintenance dose of 90 mg twice daily and 10 mg OR 5 mg (determined by weight and age of patient) respectively
- Anticoagulation: LMWH (enoxaparin 1 mg/kg twice daily SC) *or* factor Xa inhibition (with fondaparinux 2.5 mg daily SC—for early conservative group)
- SL or IV GTN
- Morphine 5–10 mg or diamorphine 2.5–5 mg IV analgesia as required
- Metoclopramide 10 mg IV as required (give with opiates if prescribed)
- ACE inhibitor, e.g. ramipril 2.5mg OD
- β-blocker, e.g. bisoprolol 2.5mg OD
- In-hospital PCI. Timing for invasive treatment depends on factors discussed below. TIMI risk score and GRACE score can be helpful (see Box 7.4)

Early invasive treatment

- With a view to revascularization (by PCI or coronary artery bypass as influenced by coronary anatomy)
- Clinical indications for an early invasive strategy include ongoing symptomatic ischaemia, especially dynamic ST segment depression on the ECG (i.e. changes with the pain), haemodynamic compromise, (recurrent) major arrhythmias, and recent (e.g. within 6 months) PCI
- Elevated troponin also suggests a high-risk category
- The TIMI score is a well-validated, simple risk calculator (see Box 7.4). As a guide, patients with TIMI score > 3 are at high risk and early invasive management may be beneficial
- The GRACE score can be calculated to risk stratify patients for urgent invasive angiography

Anticoagulation

- Anticoagulants are given to reduce thrombin-mediated thrombus formation and are administered in addition to antiplatelet agents
- Both unfractionated and LMWHs have been used in ACS. For patients undergoing an early invasive strategy, UFH or enoxaparin should be given immediately. For patients undergoing early conservative management, LMWH (enoxaparin) or fondaparinux may be given

P2Y12 inhibitors

Ticagrelor or prasugrel is currently recommended instead of clopidogrel as they have been shown to be more effective. However, clopidogrel can be used instead for patients with higher bleeding risk. More recently, emerging evidence suggest the use of prasugrel over ticagrelor in ACS, although widespread adoption to clinical practice is still lacking. The default recommendation is for dual antiplatelet therapy (aspirin and ticagrelor/prasugrel/clopidogrel) for a year then aspirin lifelong. The duration for dual antiplatelet therapy may be extended or shortened determined by the balance between ischaemic and bleeding risk.

Glycoprotein IIb/IIIa inhibition

Glycoprotein IIb/IIIa inhibitors are potent antiplatelet agents that block the common path of platelet aggregation. Routine administration prior to coronary intervention is no longer recommended but may be given in the cathlab in the event of no or slow coronary reflow.

Discharge medication and longer-term management

Similar to STEMI (p.67), typically:

- Aspirin
- Ticagrelor/prasugrel/clopidogrel
- β-blocker
- ACE inhibitor
- High-intensity statin

The score is determined by simply summing the number of risk factors as listed. For patients with TIMI score 0–1, the combined risk of death, (re)infarction, or recurrent severe ischaemia requiring revascularization is 75% while TIMI score 6–7 confers a risk of 41%. A score >3 is often used to indicate high risk worthy of an early invasive strategy.

Box 7.4 TIMI risk score for unstable angina/NSTEMI (1 point for each)

- Age ≥ 65 years
- ≥ 3 coronary risk factors
- Use of aspirin within 7 days
- Elevated cardiac markers
- ST segment deviation
- Prior angiographic evidence of coronary disease
- > 2 angina events within 24 hours.

Box 7.5 GRACE score for unstable angina/NSTEMI

The GRACE score was derived from a prospective multi-national observational study to predict risk of death and myocardial infarction at 6 months.

Factors affecting GRACE score calculation:

- Age
- Heart rate and systolic blood pressure
- Creatinine
- Cardiac arrest at admission
- ST segment deviation on ECG
- Abnormal cardiac enzymes
- Killip class (Signs/symptoms of cardiac failure)

Grace score of >140 in the context of unstable angina/NSTEMI suggest consideration of urgent invasive angiography within 24 hours.

Further reading

Byrne RA, Rossello X, Coughlan JJ *et al.* 2023 ESC Guidelines for the management of acute coronary syndromes. *European Heart Journal* 2023; 44(38): 3720–826.

Jobs A, Mehta SR, Montalescot G *et al.* Optimal timing of an invasive strategy in patients with non-ST-elevation acute coronary syndrome: a meta-analysis of randomised trials. *Lancet* 2017 Aug 19; 390(10096): 737–46.

Chapter 8

Acute heart failure

Introduction

Heart failure (HF) is a highly treatable condition in which prompt and effective treatment can make a huge difference to symptoms and prognosis. Establishing your patient onto the right medications as early as possible will avoid readmissions and will reduce mortality.

HF is defined as a clinical syndrome of signs and symptoms due to a structural or functional abnormality of the heart resulting in raised intracardiac pressures (congestion) and in cardiac output not meeting demand.

Acute heart failure can represent the first presentation of HF, or a decompensation of existing HF. In all cases, efforts should be made to identify any precipitants for the current presentation, and the underlying cause of HF ➲ p.89. HF is not a homogeneous condition and whilst some general principles apply, successful treatment depends upon accurate assessment of the aetiology and haemodynamic profile in each patient.

Aims of treatment of acute HF

- Immediate: Confirm diagnosis and make an initial assessment
- Initial stabilization
  - Restore oxygenation and treat congestion
  - Identify factors precipitating acute decompensation
  - Initiate treatment of congestion
- Intermediate
  - Continue or escalate diuresis
  - Assess underlying aetiology
  - Introduce disease-modifying prognostic therapies
  - Consider adjunctive therapies
- Pre-discharge
  - Ensure full congestion relief
  - Commence all disease-modifying prognostic therapies
  - Arrange appropriate follow-up

Clinical features of acute HF

These are of fluid overload and low cardiac output. Not all of the below features will be present in every patient. Older patients (> 60) are more likely to present with peripheral oedema, and younger patients can often present with ascites and pulmonary oedema.

Fluid overload/congestion	Low cardiac output
Orthopnoea	Tachycardia
Raised JVP	Low BP/narrow pulse pressure
Gallop rhythm/third heart sound	Cool extremities
Pulmonary inspiratory crackles	Poor capillary refill
Peripheral oedema*	Confusion/drowsiness
Ascites*	Oliguria/renal dysfunction
Hepatic distension/abnormal LFT*	Electrolyte disturbances
Breathlessness on bending over ('bendopnoea')	Poor tissue perfusion and elevated serum lactate
	Pulsus alternans (late stage)

Those marked with a * can be absent or hard to identify in acute HF.

The presence of cardiogenic shock (systolic BP < 90 mmHg with signs of reduced major organ perfusion) identifies a very high-risk situation. Urgent attention and treatment as described in Chapter 21 are needed.

Investigations

- Full clinical examination
- Pulse, blood pressure, oxygen saturations, respiratory rate
- Bloods:
  - FBC—anaemia, infection
  - U&E—renal failure as comorbidity or differential
  - Thyroid function—thyroid dysfunction can mimic cause of oedema or decompensate HF
  - Troponin—acute coronary syndrome, myocardial strain
  - NT-proBNP/BNP (brain natriuretic peptide)—see below
  - Lipid profile—assess coronary artery risk
  - HbA1c—exclude diabetes
  - Iron studies—exclude iron overload, identify iron deficiency
  - Consider D-dimer to exclude pulmonary embolism although likely to have very high false positive rate
- Arterial blood gas including lactate: low threshold to perform if concern about hypoxaemia or hypoperfusion
- ECG—ischaemia, MI, arrhythmia, suggestion of structural changes
- CXR—pulmonary oedema, tamponade, sepsis, dissection
- Echocardiography
- Focused/ point-of-care ultrasound if available—left-ventricular function, lung ultrasound to identify pulmonary oedema or effusions

BNP

- Can be useful as a rule out of heart failure, if under 400 pg/mL then heart failure is unlikely
- Limited positive predictive value as it is elevated by almost any other cause of acute illness causing strain on the heart, particularly including sepsis, infection, pulmonary embolism, acute coronary syndromes severe cardiac valvular disease, other cardiac structural abnormalities

Clinical presentation of heart failure

Four broad presentations of HF are seen and can be helpful in guiding treatment.

Acute decompensated heart failure: Most commonly caused by left ventricular dysfunction. Features of cardiac congestion with salt and water retention, generally onset over days, resulting in development of peripheral and pulmonary oedema. Treatment: diuretics, inotropes if concurrent shock.

Acute pulmonary oedema: Caused by most aetiologies of heart failure, more common in context of high afterload and left-ventricular diastolic dysfunction. Dominant feature is rapid onset of pulmonary oedema. Treatment: diuretics and consider vasodilators.

Cardiogenic shock: Caused by severe cardiac dysfunction with low cardiac output. Main feature is systemic hypoperfusion and shock. Treatment is predominantly inotropes and organ support.

Isolated right ventricular failure: Caused by right ventricular dysfunction (e.g. right ventricular infarction) or pulmonary venous obstruction (e.g. pulmonary embolism, adult respiratory distress syndome). High venous pressure with systemic hypoperfusion due to low right ventricular cardiac output. Treatment: treat cause, diuretics, cautious volume supplementation may be needed, inotropes.

There are major overlaps in these presentations, e.g. acute decompensated heart failure is often seen with concurrent pulmonary oedema.

Congestion and hypoperfusion

Congestion manifests as high intracardiac and venous pressures.

Hypoperfusion is seen as signs of shock and low cardiac output.

The presence or absence of these may be helpful in identifying groups of patients in HF and regarding treatment principles.

	No congestion	**Congested**
Normal perfusion	***Warm and dry*** Normal/adapted physiology; the target	***Warm and wet*** Most common Diuretics (including prognostic agents)
Hypo-perfusion	***Cold and dry*** Shocked and dehdrated Inotropes, consider cautious fluids	***Cold and wet*** Inotropes Diuretics

The NYHA classification (Table 8.1) can be unhelpful as the differences between class II and class III may be very subtle. Patients may not have symptoms because they do not exert enough to develop them.

Table 8.1 New York Heart Association (NYHA) classification of HF

Class	Features
I	Asymptomatic (though with abnormal heart). No limitation of physical activity.
II	Mildly symptomatic, with slight limitation of physical activity. Comfortable at rest but ordinary physical activity results in fatigue or dyspnoea.
III	Moderately symptomatic, with marked limitation of physical activity. Comfortable at rest but less than ordinary activity results in symptoms
IV	Severely symptomatic. Unable to carry out any physical activity without discomfort. Symptoms at rest.

Cause of presentation of heart failure

The below factors can cause decompensation of existing HF, or precipitate the acute presentation of HF which was already present or slowly developing.

C	Coronary syndrome: MI, ACS or complications of this
H	Hypertensive emergency
A	Arrhythmias: AF, VT, bradycardia/heart block
M	Mechanical cause (rupture, VSD, acute MR, acute valve degeneration, chest trauma, dissection, thrombosis)
P	Pulmonary embolism or other respiratory illness
I	Infection
T	Tamponade

Also consider:

- Non-adherence with medications or excess fluid intake
- Toxic substances (alcohol, recreational drugs)
- Drugs (e.g. cardiotoxic chemotherapeutics, corticosteroids, negative inotropic substances)
- High cardiac output states: e.g. severe anaemia, thyroid dysfunction, adrenal crisis
- Pregnancy and peripartum related problems (peripartum cardiomyopathy, pre-eclampsia)
- Cerebrovascular insult or head injury
- Acute native or prosthetic valve incompetence secondary to endocarditis, aortic dissection, or thrombosis

Differential diagnosis of heart failure

Is that of causes of breathlessness as per Chapter 4 ➲ p.29.

Causes of non-cardiogenic pulmonary oedema

- Acute respiratory distress syndrome (alveolar–capillary permeability):
  - Infection
  - Toxins
  - Aspiration of gastric contents
  - Disseminated intravascular coagulation (DIC)
  - Acute pancreatitis
- Drugs
- Other:
  - Lymphatic insufficiency
  - High altitude
  - Neurogenic
  - Post-anaesthesia

Acute management of HF

The aim of initial treatment is to stabilize the patient, and correct acute physiological derangements such as hypoxaemia or severe pulmonary oedema.

Treat hypoxaemia

- Sit patient up
- Oxygen to be given only if hypoxic (oxygen saturation less than 90%), no benefit and potential harm if given unnecessarily
- If respiratory distress (> 25 breaths/min, oxygen saturation less than 90%) then CPAP is indicated
- Consider NIV if type II respiratory failure, but involve anaesthetist/ITU if this is present as may progress rapidly to need for intubation
- Intubation likely to be needed if pO_2 < 8 kPa despite CPAP/NIV
- Opiates can result in dangerous sedation, use only if severe or intractable pain/anxiety

If hypotension and shock are present

(Also see Chapter 2 on cardiogenic shock ➲ p.11)

- Early specialist and intensive care assessment, consider inotropes
- Assess normal baseline blood pressure from shared care records or other resources as available: patients with chronic heart failure may have long-standing stable hypotension without adverse effects
- In dominant left ventricular failure, intravenous fluid is likely to worsen or cause pulmonary oedema and should be avoided
- In acute right ventricular failure, low ventricular preload may worsen cardiac output. If you are sure the presentation is acute right ventricular failure, consider very cautious use of intravenous fluid, almost always alongside inotropes

Treat congestion

- Loop diuretics (intravenous furosemide for most, consider oral furosemide/bumetanide if milder symptoms)
- Initial dose for acute heart failure should be at least 50 mg intravenous furosemide if diuretic naïve, or 2 times baseline diuretic dose
- 40 mg furosemide is equivalent to 1 mg bumetanide (or 20 mg torazemide); e.g. if on 1 mg twice daily bumetanide, starting dose of intravenous furosemide should be 80–100 mg twice daily
- Give IV diuretics every morning and early afternoon unless catheterized
- Consider assessing diuretic response with spot urinary sodium measurement (urine Na should be > 50–70 mEq/L at 2 h post diuretic; increase diuretic dose if not)
- Start SGLT2 inhibitor and aldosterone antagonist early (can be day 1) unless hypotensive or otherwise contraindicated, ➲ p.84

Consider vasodilators

- Only for significant hypertension: systolic BP >160 mmHg
- Nitrate e.g. glyceryl trinitrate 1–10 mg/hour titrated to maintain systolic blood pressure over 110 mmHg systolic
- Extreme caution if possibility of aortic stenosis or severe LV hypertrophy

Other adjunctive treatments

- Thromboembolism prophylaxis if not anticoagulated
- Involvement of specialist heart failure teams reduces adverse outcomes and benefit patients. Refer to your local heart failure team at admission/diagnosis of heart failure
- Consider plans for escalation and resuscitation status

Management of concurrent conditions

Arrhythmias

See Chapter 11 on arrhythmias ➲ p.131.

- Treat fast atrial arrhythmias: heart rate control generally the best strategy, digoxin is often preferred due to lack of hypotensive effect. Amiodarone may be considered
- Caution with β-blockers in acute HF, particularly if any signs of shock due to initial negative inotrope
- If shocked due to arrhythmia consider electrical cardioversion ➲ p.6

Acute coronary syndromes

- If ST elevation, for emergent revascularization with primary PCI ➲ p.53
- In non-ST elevation, consider urgent PCI if dynamic ECG changes and patient stable enough to lie flat
- Note that acute heart failure will often cause small troponin elevations in the absence of type I myocardial infarction

Acute ventricular septal defect/mitral valve or papillary muscle rupture

- Often responds poorly to conventional therapy
- Consider urgent surgery or percutaneous intervention

Recurrent admissions with 'flash' pulmonary oedema

- Consider renal artery stenosis, reversible ischaemia, intermittent arrhythmias

Severe aortic stenosis with heart failure

- Initial treatment is with diuretics plus SGLT2 inhibitors and aldosterone antagonists to treat initial pulmonary oedema. Vasodilators are contraindicated
- Assess for urgent percutaneous intervention or surgery

Severe mitral regurgitation with heart failure

- Treat as for heart failure with reduced ejection fraction. In this context mitral regurgitation is often functional and may resolve with treatment of heart failure
- In patients with persistent severe mitral regurgitation despite heart failure therapies, assess for percutaneous mitral valve intervention or surgery

Monitoring

Pulse, BP, ECG monitoring, pulse oximetry

- For all in first 24 hours
- Prolonged in the presence of arrhythmias, during inotrope therapy, or in the case of persistent haemodynamic instability

Arterial blood gases

- On admission in all cases with severe heart failure; if abnormal, repeat at appropriate intervals to monitor response to therapy and guide need for assisted ventilation
- Regularly in patients on CPAP (➲ p.80)
- Consider an arterial line if haemodynamically unstable or for frequent arterial blood gases

Electrolytes, creatinine, and renal function

- As required: alternate days is normally appropriate in patients on IV or combination diuretics
- Daily in patients who are haemodynamically unstable

Daily weights/fluid balance/urinary catheterization

- Fluid balance is impractical to achieve unless in ITU/HDU environment
- Daily weights are a practical if inaccurate way of assessing response to fluid offloading
- Consideration of urinary catheterization recommended in severe heart failure

CVP monitoring

- Not routinely required but useful in cardiogenic shock
- Caution in acute pulmonary oedema (lying patient flat may worsen respiratory failure)

Sub-acute management

Once the patient has been stabilized, the priorities are to establish the cause of HF if not known, continue to treat congestion, and to introduce medications with prognostic benefit.

Subtypes of HF

An echocardiogram is essential as soon as practical as an inpatient. This will differentiate between common subtypes of heart failure, in particular by measuring left-ventricular ejection fraction (EF) although other important findings may be identified.

- Heart failure with reduced EF:EF < 40%. Although further investigation as to the underlying cause of reduced ejection fraction is needed, this may well be appropriately considered as an outpatient
- Heart failure with moderately reduced ejection fraction (EF 40–60%)
- Heart failure with preserved ejection fraction (EF > 60%). Ejection fraction is within the normal range. To confirm the diagnosis, other cardiac abnormalities are required. Key echocardiographic abnormalities seen: dilated atria, high left ventricular filling pressures as demonstrated by E/E' ratio, left ventricular hypertrophy
- Valvular heart failure. Mitral or aortic valve disease are most common

Further treatment with diuretics

In the context of significant peripheral oedema, 1 kg weight loss per day is targeted. In the context of pulmonary oedema, resolution of oedema and pleural effusions should be the aim. Increase diuretic doses if targets are not being achieved within 1 to 2 days. Escalate treatment as below:

Initial treatment for all

- SGLT2 inhibitors ➲ p.83 and aldosterone antagonists have a prognostic benefit and a diuretic effect, and should be started alongside furosemide if any significant fluid overload

If not responding to loop diuretics

- Double dose of loop diuretic. Note furosemide must not be given at more than 4 mg/min, so iv bolus doses over 80 mg must be given as short infusions
- If not responding to bolus doses, consider switch to intravenous infusion, with total dose increased over previous e.g. 240 mg furosemide over 24 hours = 10 mg/h. Give a bolus immediately before starting e.g. 100 mg
- If not responding to furosemide plus SGLT2 inhibitor and aldosterone antagonist, consider adding adjunctive diuretics. Bendroflumethiazide, metolazone, and acetazolamide can be used; seek further specialist advice

Empirical treatment before an echocardiogram is available

Whilst an echocardiogram is vital whenever possible, practical constraints may mean that this cannot be arranged for some days. Empirical treatment is reasonable pending the result:

- Start SGLT2 inhibitor as indicated at any ejection fraction

- Start aldosterone antagonist if any significant congestion or oedema
- Treat iron deficiency as above

Acute use of SGTL2 inhibitors in heart failure

These are effective agents and are useful in acute HF as they have minimal blood pressure effect and act quickly. As above they can be started empirically and are indicated at any ejection fraction.

Whilst they are considered to be safe in acute HF, there are specific considerations to be aware of for SGLT2 inibitors:

- They are contraindicated in type 1 diabetes or those without intrinsic insulin production e.g. pancreatitis, pancreatectomy, genetic conditions. Caution in people with prior ketoacidosis
- In people with type 2 diabetes on insulin, gliclazide, or similar agents, the dose of these should be reduced by a clinician with specialist knowledge of diabetes.

People taking SGLT2 inhibitors can suffer euglycaemic ketoacidosis, in which glucose levels are not raised but there is a ketoacidotic state. Check ketone levels as well as glucose in unwell people on these agents. Avoid use in patients who are not eating and drinking.

Disease-modifying prognostic heart failure therapies

These should be started as soon as possible. The sequencing of agents should be personalized to the patient. Wherever possible all indicated agents should be started on the index admission.

Heart failure with reduced ejection fraction (EF < 40%)

Class	Effects	Notes
Aldosterone antagonists: *Eplerenone 25-50 mg od* *Spironolactone 25–50 mg od*	Mortality and symptom relief benefit Diuretic Increase potassium Minimal BP effect	Avoid in severe renal failure e.g. eGFR < 20–30 Caution if K+ > 5
SGLT2 inhibitor *Dapagliflozin 10 mg od* *Empagliflozin 10 mg od*	Mortality and symptom relief benefit Diuretic Slightly reduce potassium Minimal BP effect	See cautions above Avoid in type 1 diabetes or mimics*, caution in type 2 diabetes on insulin
ACE inhibitor (ACEi)/ angiotensin receptor blocker (ARB) *Ramipril, candesartan*	Mortality and symptom relief benefit Increase potassium Reduces BP	Avoid if hypotensive Caution in acute renal failure, e.g. eGFR < 20 Caution if K+ > 5
Angiotensin receptor antagonist with neprolysin inhibitor (ARNI) *Sacubitril/valsartan*	Replaces and superior to ACEi/ARB Consider first line use Mortality and symptom relief benefit Increase potassium Reduces BP	Must have 48-hour washout of ACEi Avoid if hypotensive Caution in acute renal failure, e.g. eGFR < 20 Caution if K+ > 5

Class	Effects	Notes
β-blocker *Bisoprolol, carvedilol, nebivolol*	Mortality and symptom relief benefit Reduces BP Significant negative inotrope Reduce heart rate	Avoid if shock or borderline Continue if already on a β-blocker. Caution in asthma Consider outpatient initation

*For example pancreatitis, pancreatectomy, genetic conditions. Caution in people with prior ketoacidosis.

Other drug therapies may be considered with expert input: ivabradine to slow heart rate, low-dose digoxin.

Heart failure with moderately reduced ejection fraction (EF 40–60%)

- As for HF with reduced ejection fraction
- Weaker evidence and less mortality benefit for all agents apart from SGLT2 inhibitors
- Very weak evidence for ARNI, not licensed for this in many countries

Heart failure with preserved ejection fraction (EF > 60%)

Class	Features	Class
SGLT2 inhibitors *Dapagliflozin 10 mg od* *Empagliflozin 10 mg od*	Mortality and symptom relief benefit Diuretic. Slightly reduce potassium. Minimal BP effect	As above
Aldosterone antagonists *Eplerenone 25–50 mg od* *Spironolactone 25–50 mg od*	No mortality benefit. Diuretic. Increase potassium Minimal BP effect	As above
ACEi/ARB/ARNI	No benefit of ACEi/ARB but may be considered to treat hypertension.	
β-blocker e.g. *bisoprolol, carvedilol*	No benefit, may worsen symptoms by reducing chronotropic competence. Cessation or reduction of β-blockers can be considered to improve symptoms.	

Other acute therapies for heart failure

- Iron deficiency is commonly seen in heart failure, and intravenous replacement of iron reduces readmissions with heart failure and improve symptoms. Intravenous iron is suggested in patients with acute heart failure and in this context:
  - Transferrin saturation less than 15%.
  - Transferrin saturation less than 15–20% in the context of anaemia.
  - Ferritin is an acute phase reactant and is unhelpful in acute illness.
  - Different (more lax) criteria apply in stable outpatients, see ESC guidelines.
- In the context of heart failure and anaemia with haemoglobin less than 90 g/L consider blood transfusion (higher threshold for transfusion in patients who may be a transplant candidate to avoid HLA sensitization)

- In select patients with reduced ejection fraction, acute use of cardiac resynchronization therapy devices may sometimes occasionally be appropriate – seek specialist cardiology advice if left bundle branch block is present
- Acute placement of an implantable cardioverter defibrillator (ICD) is not normally appropriate unless the patient has presented with ventricular arrhythmia
- In the presence of severe mitral regurgitation, consider urgent percutaneous mitral valve intervention

Reference

2021 ESC Guidelines for the diagnosis and treatment of acute and chronic heart failure. https://doi.org/10.1093/eurheartj/ehab368

Adverse signs and problems

Suggest deterioration/failure to respond to therapy.

Hypotension (systolic BP < 90 mmHg)

- Confirm what the patient's normal blood pressure is from shared care records, the patient, or family members
- Stop any unnecessary exacerbating drugs (e.g. nitrates, calcium-channel blockers)
- If any evidence of organ hypoperfusion (e.g. oliguria, prolonged capillary refill time, impaired consciousness), treat as cardiogenic shock—see Chapter 2

Impaired renal function

- Cardiorenal syndrome is commonly seen in acute heart failure. Careful clinical assessment is essential
- If the patient is congested and overloaded, renal dysfunction is probably due to high renal venous pressures and will respond to increased diuretic dosing
- If any signs of shock, may be due to low renal perfusion and impaired cardiac output, may need inotropic support
- Monitor urine output (aim > 20 mL/hour)

Confusion/drowsiness

- Often due to hypotension and inadequate cerebral perfusion: Treatment of the shock/hypotension is required
- Rule out hypoxia and hypercapnia: check SpO_2 and/or arterial blood gases and treat findings accordingly

Lack of response to therapies

- Requires thought and assessment as to future plans for the patient
- Are they a candidate for escalation of therapy with intravenous infusions and intensive care? If so, escalate to treatment of cardiogenic shock (➲ p.11) and with advanced heart failure therapies (➲ p.21)
- If not, consider whether symptom support and palliative care may be appropriate (➲ p.441)

Discharge and follow-up

The rate of readmission after heart failure is high. This is reduced significantly if patients are fully decongested before discharge, or cessation of intravenous diuretics, and if all indicated disease-modifying prognostic heart failure therapies have been started before discharge. Aim for patients with heart failure with reduced ejection fraction to be on all four indicated agents before discharge.

Ensure there is no residual pulmonary oedema or significant pleural effusions. Only minor peripheral oedema should remain—this can be slow to completely resolve.

If local arrangements allow, selected patients may be safely managed on an ambulatory basis with intravenous diuretics given at home or in a day unit.

Ensure the patient has been seen by a member of the heart failure specialist team before discharge, and appropriate follow-up with the specialist team has been arranged, ideally within 2 weeks.

Causes of heart failure

In general further investigation should be performed to try and establish the underlying cause of heart failure. In the elderly and frail empirical treatment alone may be appropriate.

Further investigations to consider, many of these may be appropriate as an outpatient:

- Additional blood tests to look for specific causes; should be personalized to the patient:
  - Plasma and urine electrophoresis and immunoglobulins with light chain levels—exclude AL amyloidosis.
  - Hepatitis B, hepatitis C, HIV—assess for chronic viral myocarditis.
  - Calcium level—exclude calcium disorders (can cause LV dysfunction.)
  - ANA, ANCA—assess for causative autoimmune conditions.
  - Serum ACE level—can be used to assess risk of sarcoidosis.
- Cardiac MRI: To assess myocardial function, presence of scar/fibrosis
- Coronary CT angiogram: To assess coronary arteries—not needed in many patients as below. Discuss with cardiologist before ordering

Ischaemic heart disease

Remains the most common cause of left ventricular dysfunction. In the absence of acute coronary syndrome, the benefit of revascularization in patients with left ventricular dysfunction is uncertain and should be carefully considered. Secondary prevention treatment is still indicated.

Non-ischaemic cardiomyopathy

Covers several underlying causes; no cause may be found. The degree of left ventricular dysfunction is variable.

Causes include:

- Idiopathic (may be familial)
- Long-standing or acute severe hypertension
- Chronic tachyarrhythmia or atrial fibrillation
- Alcoholic cardiomyopathy, other illegal drugs
- Previous use of cardiotoxic chemotherapies
- Cardiac amyloidosis
- Cardiac sarcoidosis
- Current or prior myocarditis
- Peripartum cardiomyopathy
- Autoimmune disease
- HIV cardiomyopathy
- Arrhythmogenic cardiomyopathy
- Haemochromatosis/iron overload

Valvular or structural heart disease

- Aortic stenosis or regurgitation
- Mitral regurgitation or stenosis
- Tricuspid regurgitation (tricuspid stenosis and pulmonary valve disease are rare)
- Combination of multiple valve lesions is commonly seen
- Septal wall defects
- Other congenital heart disease

Heart failure with preserved ejection fraction

Most commonly related to the effects of long-standing cardiometabolic disease and age. Closely related to:

- Hypertension
- Diabetes
- Atrial fibrillation
- Obesity
- Obstructive sleep apnoea
- Other chronic respiratory disease

Can also be caused by AL or TTR cardiac amyloidosis, hypertrophic cardiomyopathy.

A similar phenotype can be seen with pericardial constriction or myocardial restriction. These are challenging to diagnose: requires careful and expert cardiac imaging and invasive assessment.

Myocarditis

Mild myocarditis is common, severe myocarditis causing heart failure is rare but important to identify as specific treatment can be life saving.

- Viral—many causes have been identified
- Other infective—Borellia, Coxiella
- Giant cell myocarditis, eosinophilic myocarditis
- Other autoimmune disease
- Toxins/drugs: alcohol, cocaine, immune checkpoint inhibitors, anthracyclines, clozapine, 5- fluorouracil
- Idiopathic

Can present with signs of infection alongside cardiac dysfunction. Elevated troponin identifies a group with more risk. Observe in hospital and consider cardiac MRI. Rare fulminant form can be seen with rapid onset severe symptoms. Involve specialist support and consider myocardial biopsy.

Hypertrophic cardiomyopathy

See also (➲ p.343). Can present acutely with syncope, arrhythmias, or chest pain. Presentation with heart failure is less common and is often secondary to atrial arrhythmia or at a late phase of the disease 'burning out'. ECG abnormalities with signs of severe left-ventricular hypertrophy may suggest likelihood. Echocardiogram is the key initial investigation. Avoid vasodilators in acute heart failure. Involve a specialist team, longer-term management involves a risk assessment for sudden death, genetic counselling, and family screening.

Chapter 9

Valve disease

Acute valve disease

Acute valve problems require urgent diagnosis and treatment, as decompensated heart failure can occur rapidly.

Clinical presentation

Acute

- Rapid deterioration of valve function with a previously normal valve
- The patient is usually extremely unwell as the LV has not had time to compensate
- Nearly always regurgitation rather than stenosis

Causes

- Infective endocarditis—leaflet disintegration, perforation, vegetation (causing regurgitation or stenosis), dehiscence of prosthetic valve
- Ischaemia—usually MR caused by papillary muscle infarction, rupture, or tethering to infarcted myocardial wall
- Ruptured chordae tendinae, causing MR or, rarely, TR
- Aortic dissection—due to leaflet distortion or prolapse
- Trauma

Acute-on-chronic

- Worsening of pre-existing valve lesion, or acute decompensation

Causes—as for acute, plus

- Progressive deterioration of valve function, i.e. natural history
- Acute changes in haemodynamics—e.g. hyper/hypotension
- Arrhythmias—particularly tachyarrhythmias
- Other diseases affecting the myocardium—ischaemic heart disease, hypertensive heart disease, infiltrative diseases, etc

Clinical features

Symptoms

- Shortness of breath (most commonly)
  - Acute valve disease—onset over minutes/hours
  - Acute-on-chronic—onset over days/weeks (generally)
  - Cardiac decompensation—onset over hours–months
- Angina (AS, acute coronary ischaemia)
- Presyncope or syncope (in AS or PS)
- Explosive, tearing back pain (aortic dissection)
- Fever (in infective endocarditis; IE)

Clinical signs

- Cardiac murmur (see Boxes 9.1, 9.2, 9.3)
- Signs of cardiac failure
- Peripheral stigmata of IE
- Absent pulses or radio-radial delay in aortic dissection

Investigations

Echocardiography

Transthoracic echocardiography (TTE) is the investigation of choice where acute valve dysfunction is suspected. This includes unexplained SOB or

Box 9.1 Brief guide to the commonest murmurs

Aortic stenosis (see p.96)

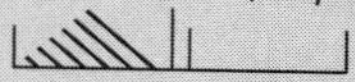

- Harsh, rasping, sometimes musical, ejection murmur
- Aortic region, radiating to carotids
- Slow rising pulse, soft/absent A_2, LVH

Aortic regurgitation (see p.97)

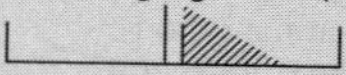

- Early diastolic, decrescendo murmur (± systolic flow murmur)
- Lower left sternal edge
- Collapsing pulse, displaced, hyperdynamic apex

Mitral regurgitation (see p.102)

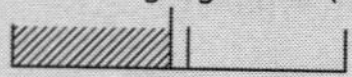

- Soft, blowing, monotonous, pansystolic murmur
- Apex, radiating to axilla
- Displaced, hyperdynamic apex

Mitral stenosis (see p.100)

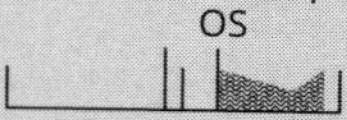

- Low-pitched, quiet, mid-diastolic rumble
- Apex, no radiation
- Opening snap, 'tapping' apex, AF, loud P_2 (pulmonary hypertension)

Box 9.2 Grading of systolic murmurs

Grade

1 Barely audible
2 Soft but readily detected
3 Prominent
4 Loud, usually with thrill
5 Very loud with thrill
6 So loud, can be heard with the stethoscope just off the chest

Box 9.3 How to recognize an innocent ('flow') murmur

- Soft ejection systolic murmur
- Grade ≤ 2
- Usually heard along left sternal edge/pulmonary region; occasionally at the apex
- Normal heart sounds
- No associated thrills or added sounds
- No signs of LV dilatation
- Normal ECG and no cardiac abnormalities on CXR

Innocent murmurs do not need echocardiography

Diastolic, pansystolic, or loud (grade 3+) murmurs are not 'innocent' syncope with signs of valve disease, or known valve disease with worsening clinical status. Severely unwell patients with suspected acute valve dysfunction need echocardiography urgently/emergently.

CXR

- To assess for pulmonary oedema/seek other causes of SOB

ECG

- Signs of chronic valve disease, e.g. LVH (AS); broad P wave (MS); AF (MS/MR)
- Fast AF/other arrhythmia—as a cause of acute decompensation
- Long PR interval—consider aortic root abscess in the context of IE
- Acute MI/ischaemia

Blood tests

- FBC—high WCC indicating infection (IE, chest, other)
- U&E—acute kidney injury, IE, high/low K^+ causing arrhythmia
- CRP/ESR—infection
- Blood cultures—if IE suspected, 3/6 sets over 24–48 hours

General management of acute valve presentations

- Identify and treat cause
- Take multiple sets of blood cultures prior to antibiotics
- Treat pulmonary oedema if present
- Diuretics (e.g. furosemide 80 mg IV or more)
- Consider intubation/ventilation if required for stabilization
- Consider inotropic support if signs of cardiogenic shock
- Vasodilators for *regurgitant* lesions (ACE inhibitors, or if severe, IV nitrates/sodium nitroprusside)
- Avoid β-blockers in AR—these lengthen diastole, worsening the AR, and also prevent a compensatory tachycardia
- Acute valve regurgitation may require urgent transfer to a tertiary centre with cardiothoracic surgical facilities: patients may be very unwell requiring ITU care ± emergency valve intervention
- For acute-on-chronic lesions with progression of symptoms or decompensation, most patients need inpatient referral to a cardiologist for consideration of transcatheter intervention or cardiac surgery

Chronic valve disease

Patients with chronic valvular heart disease are managed by active surveillance in the outpatient setting. In patients with severe valve lesions, the development of new or progressive symptoms (most commonly breathlessness or exercise limitation) is a trigger for considering valve intervention—either cardiac surgery or transcatheter valve intervention. In patients who are asymptomatic, the development of left ventricular dilatation or dysfunction should also prompt consideration of treatment. The timing and optimal approach to valve intervention should be discussed within a Heart Valve Team.

Further reading

2025 ESC/EACTS Guidelines for the management of valvular heart disease. *European Heart Journal* 2025; 46(44): 4635–4736

Aortic stenosis

The commonest valve lesion; prevalence 2% at > 65 years of age.

Causes

- Degenerative (most common)
- Bicuspid aortic valve (associated with coarctation and aortic dilatation ± dissection)
- Rheumatic heart disease
- Prior chest radiotherapy

Clinical features

Symptoms

- Exertional breathlessness, presyncope/syncope, angina, heart failure
- First presentation may be with acute decompensated heart failure

Signs

- Ejection systolic murmur, radiating to carotids
- If severe: slow-rising pulse, heaving non-displaced apex, absent S_2
- May be signs of pulmonary oedema/decompensated heart failure

Investigations

Echocardiography

- Aortic stenosis severity (peak velocity, gradient, valve area)
- Left ventricular function
- Concurrent valve disease

Cardiac CT

- Cardiac CT (gated) with peripheral vasculature is the key investigation for planning TAVI
- Provides assessment of valve morphology, annulus, coronary disease, peripheral vascular disease (for transfemoral vascular access)

Treatment

Medical therapy

- Diuretics for pulmonary/peripheral oedema
- In stable patients with left ventricular failure, consider guideline-directed medical therapy for heart failure
- Vasodilator drugs should be used cautiously (risk of hypotension)

Balloon aortic valvuloplasty

- Rarely used in contemporary practice but remains a salvage option for patients as a bridge to TAVI or surgical aortic valve replacement

Transcatheter aortic valve implantation (TAVI)

- Treatment of choice for older patients or those at increased surgical risk

Surgical aortic valve replacement

Treatment of choice for younger patients, those with complex bicuspid anatomy, multivalve disease, or concurrent coronary disease

Aortic regurgitation

Causes

- *Acute:* type A aortic dissection, infective endocarditis (IE), trauma
- *Chronic:* previous IE, aortic root dilatation (including Marfan syndrome), degenerative valve (native or bioprosthetic replacement), previous rheumatic fever, inflammatory disease (aortitis, SLE)

Clinical features

Symptoms

- Acute AR causes sudden severe SOB and pulmonary oedema
- In chronic AR, SOB may be the only symptom

Signs

- Early diastolic, decrescendo murmur heard at the lower left sternal edge, best in expiration
- ± ejection systolic flow murmur (forward flow across valve)
- In severe disease:
  - Collapsing pulse
  - Displaced, hyperdynamic apex (due to dilated LV)
  - Other eponymous signs, mostly due to widened pulse pressure (see Table 9.1).

Table 9.1 Eponymous signs in severe aortic regurgitation

Sign	Clinical features
Corrigan's	Visible carotid pulsation
de Musset's	Head bobbing with each pulse
Müller's	Visible uvula pulsation
Quincke's	Visible capillary pulsation in nail bed
Traube's	Systolic and diastolic femoral sounds ('pistol-shot' femorals)
Duroziez's	Compression of femoral artery proximally causes systolic bruit; distal compression causes proximal bruit

Management

Acute AR

- Patients are often in pulmonary oedema and extremely unwell
- Urgent cardiac surgery is required for valve replacement (± aortic root replacement if aortic dissection)
- Holding treatments include diuretics, vasodilators, inotropes, ventilation
- IABP is contraindicated—this worsens the AR
- Bioprosthetic aortic valve regurgitation can be treated by valve-in-valve TAVI (assuming no evidence of IE)

Chronic AR

- All patients with severe AR should be followed up at least yearly, and at 3–6 monthly intervals if the LV diameter or ejection fraction changes, or approaches the threshold for surgery (Fig. 9.1)

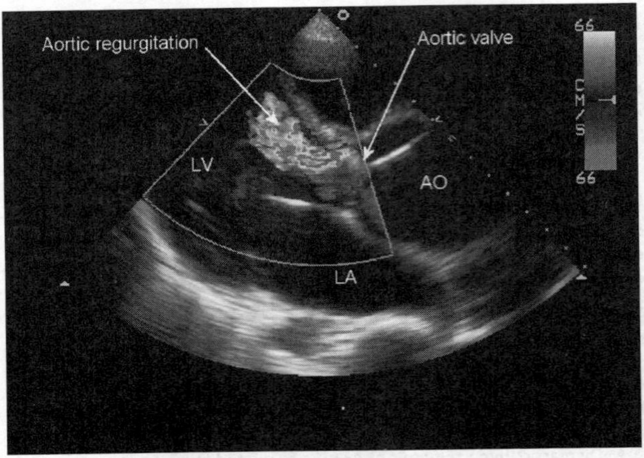

Fig. 9.1 Parasternal transthoracic echocardiogram demonstrating a broad jet of AR in a patient with a dilated aorta (AO).

- Patients who develop symptoms, or are asymptomatic but have evidence of reduced LV function (EF ≤ 50%) or LV dilatation (LVESD) > 50 mm) should be considered for surgical aortic valve replacement (AVR)
- Surgical AVR is the gold-standard treatment, but for patients at prohibitive surgical risk, there are now dedicated TAVI devices for AR (e.g. Jenavalve)

Mixed aortic valve disease

- True mixed aortic valve disease is distinct from (i) AR with increased systolic aortic flow velocity (due to increased stroke volume), and also (ii) AS with a mild regurgitation (not uncommon)
- The relative severity of each component (AS/AR) is variable, though predominant AS is more common
- The combination of a narrowed outlet and need for increased stroke volume places substantial demands on the myocardium, and the LV is often very hypertrophied and responds poorly to rapid changes
- Acute problems can therefore occur more readily, e.g. deterioration with the onset of AF

Causes

- Bicuspid valve, rheumatic heart disease, endocarditis on AS, previous (partially successful) valvuloplasty for stenosis

Mitral stenosis

Causes

- Rheumatic heart disease—now uncommon in developed world but remains prevalent in many low- and middle-income countries
- Degenerative (calcific) disease, with mitral annular calcification
- Rare causes: atrial myxoma, carcinoid, congenital, mitral valve thrombus/ vegetation, radiotherapy, metabolic disease

Clinical features

Symptoms

- Exertional SOB, fatigue, reduced exercise tolerance, haemoptysis
- Acute decompensation (pulmonary oedema, orthopnoea, PND) may be precipitated by new-onset AF, infection, pregnancy, anaesthesia
- First presentation may be with stroke

Signs

- Irregularly irregular pulse, prominent 'a' wave in JVP
- Auscultation: prominent S_1, opening snap, low-pitched mid-diastolic rumbling murmur
- If pulmonary hypertension (PH)—left parasternal heave due to RVH, loud P_2, malar flush (uncommon)

Investigations

ECG

- AF, P mitrale, signs of PH (right-axis, P pulmonale, RVH)

CXR

- Left atrial enlargement, signs of pulmonary congestion

Echocardiography

- Demonstrates typical doming of valve leaflets in rheumatic MS
- MS severity assessed by planimetry of valve, pressure half time, transmitral gradient, and pulmonary artery pressure

Management

Medical therapy

- Acute decompensation
  - Seek expert help urgently
  - Diuretics for acute pulmonary oedema
  - May need intubation/ventilation if respiratory failure
  - Rate control: digoxin for AF, β-blockers/verapamil/diltiazem in sinus rhythm (caution if decompensation)
  - Consider cardioversion for acute AF if no LA thrombus
- Chronic management
  - Anticoagulation (with warfarin, not DOAC) if AF, or sinus rhythm with prior thromboembolism, thrombus visualized in LA, spontaneous echo contrast, or marked left atrial enlargement
  - Rate control for AF
  - Surveillance echocardiography

Balloon mitral valvuloplasty

- Can be highly effective in rheumatic MS
- Durability of result is variable but can be many years
- Effective for patients presenting acutely in pregnancy
- Indications
  - Symptomatic moderate or severe MS
  - Asymptomatic moderate or severe MS with PA pressure > 50 mmHg at rest, or > 60 mmHg on exercise
- Contraindications
  - Moderate or greater mitral regurgitation
  - Left atrial thrombus
  - Severe or bi-commissural calcification
  - Absence of commissural fusion
- May be considered in suboptimal anatomy as a palliative approach

Cardiac surgery

- Mitral valve replacement (MVR) is the definitive treatment for symptomatic severe MS
- Consider MVR first line for symptomatic patients with unsuitable anatomy for BMV

Mitral regurgitation

The mitral valve is a complex structure, relying on the leaflets, papillary muscles, chordae tendinae, and myocardial function for effective coaptation

Aetiology

- Primary ('degenerative'): due to an intrinsic abnormality of the mitral valve apparatus, most commonly the leaflets (e.g. prolapse) (Fig. 9.2)
- Secondary ('functional'): due to changes in atrial or ventricular geometry or function, leading to mitral valve dysfunction

Mitral regurgitation (MR) can also be classified by onset

- Acute: infective endocarditis, MI (papillary muscle infarction, rupture, or tethering to infarcted LV wall), ruptured chordae, trauma
- *Chronic:* degenerative disease, mitral prolapse, dilated LV, myocardial dysfunction 2° to ischaemia, rheumatic heart disease

Pathophysiology

- MR leads to volume loading of the LV—if chronic this is initially well tolerated and is often asymptomatic
- Chronic MR leads to LV remodelling and an initial increase in ejection fraction (although a proportion of this is regurgitant)
- There is also volume loading of the LA, resulting in LA enlargement and fibrosis (which in turn predisposes to AF). If long-standing, elevated LA pressure leads to pulmonary arterial hypertension
- LV volume loading leads to LV dilatation, annular dilatation and further MR. Eventually there is impairment of LV function but this occurs late
- In contrast, acute severe MR leads to a sudden deterioration in cardiac output and raised LA pressure and is commonly associated with pulmonary oedema and cardiogenic shock

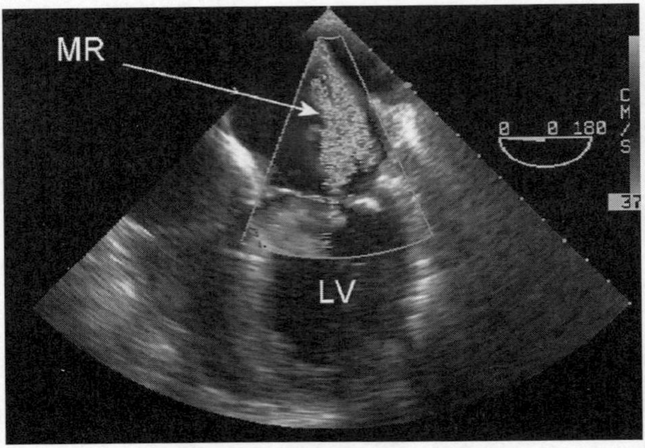

Fig. 9.2 Transoesophageal echocardiogram demonstrating MR.

Clinical features

Symptoms

- Acute MR causes sudden, severe SOB and pulmonary oedema
- Chronic MR may be asymptomatic for many years, but ultimately leads to exertional breathlessness, fatigue, orthopnoea, PND

Signs

- Pan-systolic murmur (soft, blowing) at apex, radiating to axilla
- If severe there may be a S_3, wide splitting of S_2 (early aortic valve closure), or a displaced, hyperdynamic apex

Acute presentation

Acute (new) regurgitation

- Commonest causes are post-MI, infective endocarditis and chordal rupture (leading to flail leaflet)
- Emergency valve repair/replacement is necessary
- Holding treatments include diuretics, inotropes, vasodilators, ventilation, IABP

Acute presentation of chronic disease

- Once symptoms develop in chronic disease, valve repair or replacement should be considered
- In secondary MR, optimization of HF medical therapy and consideration of coronary revascularization and/or cardiac resynchronization therapy should be undertaken prior to mitral valve intervention

Chronic presentation

Indications for valve repair/replacement are different in primary and secondary MR

Primary MR

— Symptoms
— Asymptomatic, with any of
  - LVEF ≤ 60%
  - **LV dilatation: LV end-systolic dimension ≥ 40 mm**
  - **New-onset AF**
  - **Pulmonary hypertension (PA systolic pressure > 50 mmHg)**
  - **Surgical repair may be considered in low-risk patients with LA dilatation if high likelihood of durable repair**

Secondary MR

— Mitral valve intervention should be considered in patients who remain symptomatic despite medical therapy
— If CABG is indicated, concurrent mitral repair (annuloplasty) should be performed to address secondary MR
— In patients at high risk of surgery, with anatomical criteria suggesting increased chance of response, transcatheter edge-to-edge repair (TEER) is indicated (see Box 9.4)

Box 9.4 Repair of mitral regurgitation

Cardiac surgery

- Surgical valve repair is the definitive treatment for primary MR
- The aim of surgical repair is to restore normal valve function by resection of abnormal/prolapsing leaflet segments and to stabilize the annulus, using a prosthetic annuloplasty ring
- Additional surgical techniques include implantation of neo-chords, chordal transfer/transposition, and palpillary muscle repositioning
- Repair is associated with better survival than mitral valve replacement. The most durable surgical repairs are in patients with isolated posterior leaflet prolapse
- Complex disease with leaflet or annular calcification, rheumatic valve disease, or prior radiotherapy is challenging and unpredictable for repair. In such cases replacement is usually the strategy of choice

Transcatheter edge-to-edge repair (TEER)

- The risks of cardiac surgery in elderly, comorbid patients have driven development of less invasive, transcatheter approaches
- TEER is a percutaneous (transfemoral) transeptal approach to mitral valve repair
- Under general anaesthesia with TOE guidance, the anterior and posterior leaflets are grasped and clipped together to create a double-orifice valve
- This approach is highly effective in selected anatomies, especially those with central mitral pathology (e.g. P2 prolapse)
- The two currently approved TEER devices are Mitraclip (Abbott) and Pascal (Edwards Lifesciences)
- In functional MR there remains ongoing debate about which patients derive benefit from TEER: in current guidelines, patients with severe MR on optimal medical therapy with an EF of 20–50%, LV ESD < 70 mm and the absence of severe pulmonary hypertension are deemed most likely to benefit

Transcatheter mitral valve replacement (TMVR)

- Development of TMVR devices remains an ongoing focus of clinical research and development
- The variability of disease affecting the mitral valve, challenges with sealing and anchoring and the proximity of surrounding structures (especially the LV outflow tract) have made device development and clinical trial recruitment difficult
- The transapical Tendyne TMVR device (Abbott) is commercially available, and several devices are in ongoing clinical trials

Pulmonary stenosis

Causes

- Congenital (may occur with other defects, e.g. Fallot's tetralogy)
- Rheumatic fever
- Carcinoid

Clinical features

- *Symptoms:* SOB if severe
- *Signs:* RV heave, prominent 'a' wave in JVP ± TR, quiet P_2, soft ejection systolic murmur at upper left sternal edge
- *ECG:* RVH, P pulmonale

Treatment

- Balloon valvuloplasty
  - Especially in children with congenital PS
  - Usual first-line treatment
  - Effective and may be repeated in future
  - PR is the main side effect and is well tolerated
- Surgical valvotomy
- Percutaneous valve implantation
- Surgical pulmonary valve replacement

Pulmonary regurgitation

Causes

- Congenital
- Infective endocarditis
- Pulmonary hypertension
- Previous balloon valvuloplasty or surgical valvotomy

Clinical features

- *Symptoms:* SOB if severe, or RV failure occurs
- *Signs:* RV heave, loud ± delayed P_2, ± soft pulmonary ejection murmur, diastolic decrescendo murmur, RV failure
- *ECG:* RVH

Treatment

- Usually none required—PR is tolerated very well
- Treat RV failure
- Treat cause of pulmonary hypertension, if driving PR
- If severe symptoms and/or RV failure, consider percutaneous/surgical pulmonary valve replacement

Tricuspid stenosis

Causes (rare)

- Mostly rheumatic heart disease (usually in association with MS)
- Carcinoid
- Rarely due to a pacemaker lead

Clinical features

- *Symptoms:* SOB, fatigue
- *Signs:* raised JVP with prominent 'a' wave, mid-diastolic murmur at left sternal edge—similar to MS but higher pitch, hepatomegaly and peripheral oedema if severe

Treatment

- Diuretics
- Balloon valvuloplasty
- Surgical valvotomy
- Surgical valve replacement

Tricuspid regurgitation

Causes

- Functional (arising secondary to RV dilatation)
- Pulmonary hypertension
- Congenital (including Ebstein's anomaly)
- Infective endocarditis
- Carcinoid

Clinical features

- *Symptoms:* SOB, exercise intolerance, fatigue, bloating
- *Signs*: Large 'v' waves in JVP, pulsatile hepatomegaly (peripheral oedema, ascites ± jaundice if significant RV failure), soft pan-systolic murmur at left sternal edge

Treatment

- Diuretics—furosemide, bumetanide, spironolactone
- If persistent symptoms on diuretics, consider
  - TEER
  - Transcatheter valve replacement (e.g. Evoque device)
  - Surgical tricuspid valve repair/replacement

Prosthetic valves

Surgical prosthetic valves

Bioprosthetic

- Most commonly leaflets made from bovine or porcine pericardium
  - Stented frame (e.g. Perimount, Magna Ease)
  - Stentless (e.g. 3F, Freestyle, BioValsalva)
- Sutureless—self-anchoring (e.g. Perceval, Intuity)
- Homograft—human tissue graft

Metallic

There are 3 designs of metallic valve

- Ball and cage (e.g. Starr–Edwards)
  - First artificial heart valve design
  - Metal cage with silicone elastomer ball
  - High risk of thrombus formation; no longer used
- Single tilting disc (e.g. Björk–Shiley, Medtronic Hall)
  - Multiple iterations, some early models prone to fracture of the outlet strut leading to embolization of the disc
- Bileaflet tilting disc (e.g. St Jude, ATS)
  - Now most common
  - Good track record
  - Low resistance to flow, and low thrombogenicity
  - Durable (can last > 20 years)

Transcatheter valves

There are 2 main designs of transcatheter (aortic) valve

- Balloon-expandable
  - a balloon-mounted, crimped valve deployed by balloon-expansion within the aortic annulus (e.g. SAPIEN 3)
  - leaflets are intra-annular, bovine pericardium
- Self-expanding
  - a nitinol frame valve which is released within the aortic annulus and returns passively to a fully expanded shape (e.g. Evolut, Navitor)
  - leaflets may be supra-annular or intra-annular

Prosthetic valve choice

- Bioprosthetic valves
  - — Do not require long-term anticoagulation
  - — Generally last 10–15 years
  - — Preferred in older patients (age > 70), those in whom anticoagulation is contraindicated, younger women considering pregnancy
- Metallic valves
  - — Preferred for younger patients (age < 60 years) who can tolerate lifelong anticoagulation (Box 9.5)

Clinical features

- Bioprosthetic valves often have a flow murmur but are otherwise like native valves

Box 9.5 Anticoagulation for metallic valves: acute issues

General approach to over-anticoagulation

- Identify the precipitating cause, e.g. drugs, liver failure
- Determine the degree of reversal required
- Decide how quickly reversal is necessary
- N.B.—the risk of bleeding on warfarin increases significantly with an INR of 5 and above
- In a non-bleeding patient, omitting warfarin is usually sufficient. If the INR is > 8, consider 3 mg of oral vitamin K

Major bleeding requiring immediate complete reversal

- This includes bleeding into a critical organ or space (e.g. intracranial, intraspinal, intraocular bleeding), or major haemorrhage with/without shock
- Seek expert haematology input
- Stop warfarin and reverse anticoagulation with prothrombin complex concentrate (PCC) and vitamin K (usually 5 mg IV)
- In general, the risk to the patient of an acute haemorrhage far outweighs the risk of thrombosis on a metallic valve, and warfarin should be reversed until the haemorrhagic risk has subsided
- Even the highest estimates of the risk of prosthetic valve thrombosis without any anticoagulation are around 30–50% *per year* (~0.5–1% per week)

Emergency surgery

- INR can be normalized with PCC to facilitate emergency surgery
- Once stable post-surgery, anticoagulation can be restarted, initially with LMWH

Elective procedures requiring cessation of anticoagulation

- Some procedures (e.g. dental extraction) can be done with a lowering of the INR to ~2.5 rather than cessation of warfarin
- For surgery or other procedures where anticoagulation needs to stop, bridging with low molecular weight heparin is performed
- A typical schedule for this is:
- Day – 6 evening: last dose of warfarin
- Day – 3 morning: commence LMWH
- Day – 1 morning: final dose of LMWH (at half dose if surgery is high bleeding risk)
- Therapeutic LMWH can be restarted when safe to do so after surgery; if stable restart warfarin
- Complex patients at high risk of thrombosis and bleeding may need to be managed in hospital with unfractionated heparin bridging

- Metallic valves have a distinctive 'click' as the valve either opens or closes. This should be a crisp sound—a dull or indistinct sound may suggest thrombus or vegetation on the valve
- Annual follow-up with echocardiography is routine for patients with prosthetic valves

- All patients with a prosthetic valve (bioprosthetic or metallic) are a high-risk group infective endocarditis
- Antibiotic prophylaxis should be considered prior to dental procedures (see p.130)
- Unexplained fever in a patient with a prosthetic valve should be taken extremely seriously, and multiple sets of blood cultures taken before use of empirical antibiotics

Echocardiography

- Systolic flow velocities are in general increased with a normally functioning prosthetic valve. Metallic valves can have high velocities (> 3 m/s) and the normal range for that size/design of valve needs to be taken into account
- Metallic valves cause echo 'shadows' which limit the available information. TOE may therefore be required on occasions to assess valve function in detail. With tilting-disc valves, it is normal to see tiny regurgitant 'washing jets'

Complications of prosthetic valves

Valve degeneration

- Structural valve degeneration (SVD) refers to the process of intrinsic valve degeneration (e.g. pannus growth, leaflet fibrosis, calcification, tears) affecting bioprosthetic valves, leading to valve stenosis or regurgitation
- The rate of SVD is highly variable: for surgical aortic bioprosthesis, SVD requiring re-intervention occurs in 10–50% of patients by 12 to 20 years after implant
- Predictors of SVD include patient factors (younger age, diabetes, end-stage kidney disease, hyperparathyroidism) and prosthesis-mediated factors (mitral position, small valve size resulting in patient–prosthesis mismatch)
- Options for treatment of SVD are a transcatheter valve-in-valve procedure (aortic or mitral) or redo surgery

Leaflet thrombosis

- Leaflet thrombosis affects bioprosthetic and metallic valves
- May be subclinical (e.g. high attenuation leaflet thickening or reduced leaflet motion on CT), or clinical
- Clinical valve thrombosis leads to symptoms associated with valve dysfunction (typically stenosis), and patients may present with heart failure or shock
- In a stable patient, anticoagulation with warfarin is recommended (at higher INR range if already anticoagulated)
- In a decompensated patient, commence treatment dose heparin anticoagulation. Thrombolysis can be considered
- If there is a failure to respond to anticoagulation, valve explant and surgical valve replacement is the definitive treatment

Haemolysis

- Small amounts of haemolysis are common with metallic valves Significant haemolysis is usually 2° to valve dysfunction—paravalvular leak, valve dehiscence, or infective endocarditis

- Bloods: anaemia, raised reticulocyte count, raised LDH, low haptoglobin
- Iron/blood transfusion may be required for symptomatic anaemia
- Paravalvular leak is often treatable with percutaneous plug closure or a transcatheter valve-in-valve procedure (i.e. TAVI)

Infective endocarditis

- See p.115

Acute rheumatic fever

- Immunologically mediated systemic inflammatory illness occurring several weeks after group A streptococcal (throat) infection
- Incidence now rare in developed world, but remains common in Indian subcontinent, the Middle East, and Oceania
- ARF commonly affects children aged 5–15 years, but chronic damage to cardiac valves leads to rheumatic heart disease in adulthood

Clinical features

Arthritis

- Most common feature. Rapid onset, over hours/days
- Large-joint, migratory polyarthritis—knees, ankles, wrists, elbows
- Can be exquisitely painful—one joint tends to predominate

Carditis

- Around 50% of cases have cardiac involvement
- Pancarditis—pericarditis, myocarditis, and endocarditis/valvulitis
- Valvulitis is most important—may cause acute heart failure, and long-term effects resulting in rheumatic heart disease (Box 9.6)
- Pericarditis ± effusion is common but usually benign
- AV block (usually 1°)
- Pansystolic murmur of MR is the commonest cardiac sign

Box 9.6 Rheumatic heart disease

- RHD is chronic valvular damage resulting from a single severe episode of ARF, or more commonly, recurrent episodes
- It typically manifests between the 2nd and 4th decade of life
- Mitral valve most commonly involved: typical pathology is leaflet thickening, chordal thickening, fusion, and retraction, fusion of the valve commissures, restricted leaflet motion
- Clinically, RHD manifests as heart failure, atrial fibrillation, embolic stroke, infective endocarditis
- Balloon mitral valvuloplasty is a safe and effective treatment for severe isolated mitral stenosis with favourable leaflet morphology (pliable, non-calcified valve with predominant commissural fusion). Symptom relief can last many years
- Mitral regurgitation or mixed mitral valve disease requires cardiac surgery, usually mitral valve replacement

Other

- Fever (common)
- Abdominal pain (rare)
- Sydenham's chorea ('St Vitus' dance')—rhythmic, involuntary upper limb movements. Usually after prolonged latent period (6 months) and resolves after 6 weeks; usually affects females
- Subcutaneous nodules—firm, painless, especially extensor tendons
- Erythema marginatum—transient, non-painful macular lesions with central clearing, serpiginous margins

Treatment

- Antibiotics (eliminate residual infection)
  - Benzylpenicillin (penicillin G) 1.2 g single dose IM *or* phenoxymethylpenicillin (penicillin V) 250 mg PO (adults 500 mg) QDS for 10 days; erythromycin if penicillin-allergic (adults 250–500 mg QDS)
- Anti-inflammatories
  - Naproxen/ibuprofen/aspirin (high-dose)
  - Corticosteroids are often still used, but evidence for benefit is low; prednisolone 40–60 mg/day, tapering after 2–3 weeks
- Treat heart failure
- Consider surgical valve repair/replacement if severe dysfunction

Secondary prevention

- Prevention of recurrent ARF is key to preventing RHD
- After ARF: benzylpenicillin 1.2 g IM every 3–4 weeks (preferred) *or* phenoxymethylpenicillin 250 mg BD twice daily
- Duration depends on age and severity of cardiac involvement
- Minimum duration: 5 years or until age 21 (whichever is later); if severe valve destruction, continue to age 40 or more

Revised Jones Criteria for the diagnosis of ARF (2015)

Evidence of preceding group A streptococcal infection		
Positive throat culture or rapid streptococcal antigen test; elevated or rising streptococcal antibody titre). ARF can be considered in cases of chorea and chronic carditis in the absence of evidence of group A streptococcal infection		
ARF	2 major manifestations *or* 1 major plus 2 minor manifestations (*or* 3 minor manifestations for recurrent ARF)	
	Moderate- or high-risk population	**Low-risk population (incidence ≤ 2/100 000 school-aged children)**
Major criteria	Carditis (clinical/ subclinical) Arthritis (monoarthritis or polyarthritis, or polyarthralgia) Chorea Erythema marginatum Subcutaneous nodules	Carditis (clinical/subclinical) Arthritis (polyarthritis) Chorea Erythema marginatum Subcutaneous nodules
Minor criteria	Fever (≥ 38.5° C) Monoarthralgia ESR ≥ 30 mm/h and/or CRP ≥ 3.0 mg/dl Prolonged PR interval (unless carditis is a major criterion)	Fever (≥ 38.5° C) Polyarthralgia ESR ≥ 60 mm/h and/or CRP ≥ 3.0 mg/dl Prolonged PR interval (unless carditis is a major criterion)

Chapter 10

Infective endocarditis

Introduction

Infective endocarditis remains a potentially lethal condition despite current intravenous antibiotics and cardiac surgery, with an in-hospital mortality of 15–20%. Patients with suspected or confirmed infective endocarditis should be managed by a dedicated team to deliver timely diagnosis, optimal treatment, and early surgery when required.

While cases of classical subacute endocarditis do still present with chronic symptoms and signs, acute presentations with more destructive organisms such as *Staphylococcus aureus* are increasingly common.

Infective endocarditis of a normal native valve can occur but more typically there is an underlying valve abnormality increasing susceptibility to infection. Risk factors which increase the likelihood of infective endocarditis include the following.

Cardiac risk factors

- Prior infective endocarditis
- Prosthetic heart valves (including transcatheter and surgical valves)
- Congenital heart disease
- Valvular heart disease
- Cardiac implantable electronic device (pacemaker, ICD)

Non-cardiac risk factors

- Central venous catheter
- Immunosuppression
- Haemodialysis
- Intravenous drug use
- Recent hospitilization
- Recent invasive dental or surgical procedures

Clinical presentation

Infective endocarditis should be considered in all patients with sepsis or unexplained fever in the presence of risk factors.

Patients can present with variable clinical features and to any medical specialty. The onset of symptoms may be sub-acute (over months), acute (1–4 weeks), or occasionally hyper-acute (hours to days).

Clinical features

Symptoms are often non-specific and can mimic other systemic diseases. A high index of suspicion in patients with risk factors is essential. The following symptoms/signs may be present:

Infection

- Fever—most common clinical feature
- Night sweats
- General malaise
- Weight loss
- Anaemia
- Clubbing
- Splenomegaly

Cardiac involvement

- New or altered murmur
- Signs of severe valve regurgitation
- Heart failure
- Prolonged PR interval if aortic root abscess

Signs of embolism

- Occur in 25%—cerebral, retinal, coronary, splenic, mesenteric, renal
- Pulmonary in right-sided endocarditis
- May develop into abscesses, or a mycotic aneurysm

Immune phenomena

- Rarer in acute presentations and in right-sided infective endocarditis
- Petechiae
- Splinter haemorrhages in nail beds
- Osler's nodes (tender nodules on finger pulps/palms/soles)
- Janeway lesions (painless palm/sole erythematous macules)
- Microscopic haematuria, glomerulonephritis, systemic vasculitis
- Arthralgia
- Roth spots (boat-shaped retinal haemorrhages with pale centre)
- Potential routes of infection should also be sought (e.g. teeth, skin)

Diagnosis

The diagnosis of infective endocarditis is based on clinical suspicion, evaluation of risk factors, blood cultures, and the findings on cardiac imaging.

Positive blood cultures are critical to both confirming a diagnosis of infective endocarditis and guiding appropriate treatment. A minimum of three sets should be obtained from peripheral veins at 30-minute intervals with a strict aseptic technique prior to antibiotic administration. Bacteraemia is continuous so timing of blood culture sampling with patient temperature is not required.

Transthoracic echocardiography is the first-line diagnostic imaging often supplemented by additional assessment by transoesophageal echocardiography, CT, MRI, and nuclear imaging (FDG-PET).

Diagnostic criteria for the diagnosis of infective endocarditis are well established, with a diagnostic sensitivity of around 80%. A confirmed diagnosis of infective endocarditis is based on either clinical criteria (see Box 10.1) or pathology obtained at the time of cardiac surgery.

A definite diagnosis of infective endocarditis based on clinical criteria requires either:

- 2 major criteria

or

- 1 major and 3 minor criteria

or

- 5 minor criteria

Modified Duke criteria

Box 10.1 Major criteria

Blood culture positive for infective endocarditis

- Typical organism for infective endocarditis from two separate blood cultures: *Staphylococcus aureus*, oral Streptococci, *Streptococcus gallolyticus*, *Enterococcus faecalis*, HACEK group
- Persistently positive blood cultures for organism consistent with infective endocarditis (drawn > 12 hours apart, or 3 positive cultures with first and last drawn > 1 hour apart)
- Single positive culture for *Coxiella burnetii*

Imaging positive for infective endocarditis

Valvular or perivalvular lesions typical of infective endocarditis detected by:

- Echocardiography—transthoracic/transoesophageal
- Cardiac CT
- FDG-PET
- SPECT-CT

Minor criteria

Predisposing heart condition or IV drug use

Fever > 38.0°C

Embolic vascular phenomena

- Major systemic or pulmonary emboli or abscess formation
- Osteoarticular septic complications—discitis
- Mycotic aneurysms
- Intracranial haemorrhage or ischaemic lesions
- Janeway lesions

Immunological phenomena

- Glomerulonephritis
- Osler's nodes
- Roth spots
- Positive rheumatoid factor

Microbiological evidence:

- Positive blood culture not meeting major criterion
- Serological evidence of active infection with organism consistent with infective endocarditis

(HACEK group: Haemophilus, Aggregatibacter Cardiobacterium, Eikenella, and Kingella spp.)

Investigations

Echocardiography

- Echocardiography should be performed as soon as possible once the diagnosis of infective endocarditis is suspected
- Transthoracic echocardiography (TTE) has a high specificity for vegetations (98%), but low sensitivity (60%). Transoesophageal echocardiography (TOE) may be required if suspicion is high
- Combined TTE and TOE have a negative predictive value of ~ 95%

Native valves

TTE should be the initial investigation. TOE is required when the TTE images are of inferior quality, when high clinical suspicion remains despite a normal TTE, or when a prosthetic valve is involved.

Prosthetic valves

TOE is usually required for better visualization, but valuable information can still be obtained from TTE, so it is normal to perform both.

Indications for echo

- Fever with
  - risk factor(s) for endocarditis, e.g. prosthetic valve
  - first manifestation of heart failure
  - new conduction disturbance or ventricular arrhythmias
  - typical immunological manifestations of endocarditis
  - multifocal/rapidly changing pulmonary infiltrates
  - cardiac risk factor(s) with recent invasive procedure
- New valve lesion (usually regurgitant murmur)
- Embolic events of unknown origin
- *Staphylococcus aureus* bacteraemia
- Positive blood cultures for organisms typical for endocarditis
- Sepsis (i.e. bacteraemia plus systemic features) of unknown origin

Echo findings in infective endocarditis

- Leaflet thickening
- Vegetations—intracardiac mass on a valve or intracardiac material
- Leaflet perforation—flow detected with colour Doppler
- Abscesses—echolucent paravalvular thickening
- Pseudoaneurysm—pulsatile echo free space
- Fistula—flow detected with colour Doppler between two cavities
- New prosthetic valve dehiscence

CT imaging

- Cardiac CT is more accurate than TOE for the diagnosis of perivalvular complications such as abscess formation and pseudoaneurysm. It is less accurate at identifying small vegetations
- Evaluation of the coronary arteries by CT can also provide useful information prior to surgical intervention although urgent valve surgery should not be delayed by waiting for coronary assessment
- Extending a cardiac CT to include the brain and abdomen can help identify systemic emboli which may aid in the diagnosis and prognostication in infective endocarditis
- CT may also identify potential sources of infection such as bowel lesions

Nuclear imaging

- FDG-PET CT is particularly helpful in patients with suspected prosthetic valve endocarditis but inconclusive findings on echocardiography
- Focal FDG avidity around a prosthetic valve is highly suspicious for prosthetic valve endocarditis. Diffuse homogenous uptake may suggest an inflammatory state rather than infection

Blood tests

- No specific blood tests or biomarkers are diagnostic for infective endocarditis, but the following should be completed to supplement risk stratification and monitoring of treatment:
  - FBC—anaemia, neutrophilia
  - ESR, CRP—non-specific but raised in 90% of cases
  - U&Es—renal function needs regular assessment
  - Serum for immunology for atypical organisms
  - LFT—relevant for some antimicrobials e.g. rifampicin

Urinalysis

- Microscopic haematuria ± proteinuria
- Red cell casts and heavy proteinuria if glomerulonephritis

ECG

- Lengthening PR interval (? aortic root abscess)

Management

Seek expert cardiology and microbiological advice—infective endocarditis is a serious condition that requires specialist management by a dedicated multidisciplinary team to ensure early recognition and treatment of complications.

Successful treatment of infective endocarditis requires complete eradiation of the causative organism by appropriate antimicrobial therapy of sufficient duration, and surgical removal of infected material if indicated. Haemodynamic consequences of valvar or peri-valvular destruction need prompt recognition and early surgery in most cases.

General principles

- Treat heart failure and shock as appropriate
- Ensure blood cultures are taken prior to starting antibiotic therapy
- Commence empirical antibiotic therapy in suspected infective endocarditis in unwell patients (i.e. sepsis, embolism, shock)
- Give tailored, prolonged antimicrobial therapy in adequate doses
- Monitor response to therapy—both clinically and biochemically
- Discuss early transfer to a surgical centre in patients who are unwell
- Consider surgery if significant complications arise

Antimicrobial therapy

Choice of therapy

This can be difficult and requires local knowledge of sensitivities. In all cases, discuss with microbiology/infectious disease specialists first. Therapy is guided by the organism (hence the importance of identification) (Box 10.2 and 10.3), and a general guide is shown in Table 10.1.

Treatment duration

All patients require initial treatment with high-dose IV antibiotics while response to therapy is assessed and any indication for surgery considered. In uncomplicated cases with sensitive organisms and no severe valve lesions or heart failure it may be appropriate to continue treatment with IV antibiotic therapy at home or oral antibiotic therapy.

- Shorter treatment regimens may be possible in selected patients:
  - Infection with fully sensitive *Streptococcus* on native valve
  - Rapid response to treatment within first 7 days with early fall in inflammatory markers and control of fever
  - Vegetations on echocardiography < 10 mm
  - No cardiovascular complications
  - Appropriate social circumstances and support

Prosthetic valve endocarditis requires treatment for a minimum of 6 weeks with intravenous therapy.

Antimicrobial therapy in native valve infective endocarditis

Box 10.2 Penicillin-susceptible oral *Streptococci* and *Streptococcus gallolyticus*

Intravenous treatment with one of:
- Benzylpenicillin for 4 weeks

or
- Amoxicillin for 4 weeks

or
- Ceftriaxone for 4 weeks

Intravenous treatment with one of:
- Benzylpenicillin + gentamicin for 2 weeks

or
- Amoxicillin + gentamicin for 2 weeks

or
- Ceftriaxone + gentamicin for 2 weeks

- If allergic to beta-lactams intravenous treatment with vancomycin for 4 weeks

Staphylococcus aureus **(meticillin sensitive)**

Intravenous treatment with one of the following:
- Flucloxacillin for 4 weeks

or
- Cefazolin for 4 weeks

If allergic to β-lactams intravenous treatment with one of:
- Cefazolin for 4 weeks

or
- Daptomycin for 4 weeks

Staphylococcus aureus **(meticillin resistant)**

- Intravenous treatment with vancomycin for 4–6 weeks

Enterococcus

Intravenous treatment with one of:
- Amoxicillin and ceftriaxone for 6 weeks

or
- Amoxicillin and gentamicin for 2 weeks

Antimicrobial therapy in prosthetic valve infective endocarditis

Box 10.3 Penicillin-susceptible oral *Streptococci* and *Streptococcus gallolyticus*

Intravenous treatment with one of:

- Benzylpenicillin for 6 weeks

or

- Amoxicillin for 6 weeks

or

- Ceftriaxone for 6 weeks

- If allergic to β-lactams intravenous treatment with vancomycin for 6 weeks

***Staphylococcus aureus* (meticillin sensitive)**

- Intravenous treatment with flucloxacillin or cefazolin for 6 weeks and gentamicin for 2 weeks

And oral treatment with:

- Rifampicin for 6 weeks

- If allergic to β-lactams intravenous treatment with cefazolin for 6 weeks and gentamicin for 2 weeks

And oral treatment with:

- Rifampicin for 6 weeks

***Staphylococcus aureus* (meticillin resistant)**

- Intravenous treatment with vancomycin for 6 weeks and gentamicin for 2 weeks

And oral treatment with:

- Rifampicin for 6 weeks

Enterococcus

Intravenous treatment with one of:

- Amoxicillin and ceftriaxone for 6 weeks

or

- Amoxicillin for 6 weeks with gentamicin for 2 weeks

Native valve endocarditis or prosthetic valve endocarditis > 12 months post surgery

Intravenous treatment with one of:

- Ampicillin and ceftriaxone

or

- Ampicillin with flucloxacillin and gentamicin

- If allergic to β-lactams intravenous treatment with cefazolin and gentamicin

or

- Vancomycin and gentamicin

Early prosthetic valve endocarditis or healthcare associated infection

Intravenous treatment with one of:

- Vancomycin with gentamicin and oral rifampicin

or

- Daptomycin with gentamicin and oral rifampicin

Antibiotic doses in adults with infective endocarditis

Table 10.1 Antibiotic doses in adults with infective endocarditis

Benzylpenicillin	7.2–14.4 g IV daily in 4–6 divided doses
Ceftriaxone	2 g IV daily in 1 dose
Gentamicin	3 mg/kg IV daily (max 240 mg/day) divided into 3 doses or Single higher dose titrated to blood levels as per local guidance
Amoxicillin	12 g IV daily in 4–6 divided doses
Flucloxacillin	8–12 g IV daily in 4 divided doses
Vancomycin	30 mg/kg IV daily in 2 divided doses (infused over 2 hours), titrated to trough levels
Rifampicin	300 mg BD PO
Cefazolin	6g IV daily in 3 divided doses

Treating infective endocarditis caused by other organisms

Infective endocarditis due to vancomycin-resistant enterococcus or organisms with high-level aminoglycoside resistance need early liaison with microbiology specialists to determine and appropriate regime.

Empirical treatment for endocarditis

While it is preferable to delay treatment until the causative organism has been identified, unwell patients with sepsis or heart failure and suspected infective endocarditis need prompt empirical treatment after cultures have been taken. The preferred empirical regime is based on the clinical scenario and presence of prosthetic material.

Cardiac surgery

Indications

- Heart failure—usually due to severe valve regurgitation or fistula formation
- Uncontrolled infection—persistent fever or sepsis despite medical therapy and evidence of abscess formation or enlarging vegetations
- High embolic risk—large vegetation (> 10 mm) and embolic events on appropriate medical therapy

Timing

- Timing of surgery is dependent on the clinical status of the patient and response to medical therapy
- Emergency surgery for cardiogenic shock secondary to acute severe regurgitation can be required in some patients, particularly with *Staphylococcus aureus* infection
- Urgent surgery (defined as within 3–5 days of diagnosis) for progressive heart failure is more common and should not be delayed once an indication for surgery is clear

Surgery after cerebral complications

- Patients who have sustained a cerebral insult—typically embolic infarction—with an indication for cardiac surgery need careful assessment to judge the optimal timing of surgery
- Delaying surgery by 10–14 days is widespread practice although evidence suggests the risk of cardiopulmonary bypass-related haemorrhagic transformation is lower than the risk of further embolic events while waiting

Prosthetic valve endocarditis

- Prosthetic valve endocarditis is more challenging to diagnose, more difficult to treat, and carries a worse prognosis
- Prolonged antibiotic therapy is required (6 weeks)
- Surgical treatment is more challenging and requires radical debridement of all prosthetic material
- Infective endocarditis of bioprosthetic valves can sometimes be treated with antibiotics alone but the need for redo surgery is still higher than for native valves
- TOE is mandatory in all cases to visualize the valve properly due to reduced sensitivity and specificity of TTE
- In patients with mechanical valves anticoagulation with warfarin is often replaced with low molecular weight heparin, for better control of anticoagulation and to facilitate potential surgery

Culture-negative endocarditis

The inability to culture a causative organism with standard blood cultures is usually caused by antibiotic administration prior to blood sampling, emphasizing the need for serial cultures before treatment. Culture-negative endocarditis can also be caused by fastidious bacteria and fungi.

Causes

- HACEK organisms—*Haemophilus*, *Aggregatibacter*, *Cardiobacterium*, *Eikenella*, and *Kingella*
- *Brucella*
- *Coxiella* (Q fever)
- *Legionella*
- *Bartonella*
- *Mycoplasma*
- *Tropheryma whipplei*
- *Aspergillus*
- *Candida*

Management

- Consider other causes for fever (antibiotic fever, line infection, autoimmune disease)
- If high clinical suspicion for infective endocarditis remains, consult with microbiology regarding:
  - Prolonged or special cultures
  - Serological testing
  - Molecular testing
- If valve replacement surgery is required, the excised valve should be sent for culture and molecular testing

Cardiac device-related endocarditis

Infective endocarditis of an implanted cardiac device such as a pacemaker or implantable defibrillator is a serious complication with a high mortality. As rates of device implantation increase the rate of device related infection will also increase.

Cardiac device infection can occur by either local infection introduced at the time of implantation or seeding onto the device during bacteraemia.

Microbiology

- Then commonest organisms encountered are *Staphylococcus aureus* and coagulase-negative *Staphylococcus*. Enterococcus infections are also frequent, with streptococcal infections being less common. HACEK group or fungal infections are extremely rare

Clinical presentation

The clinical presentation of cardiac device related endocarditis is with fever and malaise. There may be concurrent pocket infection (erythema, cellulitis, wound discharge) but the absence of overt pocket infection does not exclude the diagnosis.

Diagnosis

- Blood cultures and imaging
- Both TTE and TOE are often needed. Fibrinous masses on leads are also common and can be indistinguishable from vegetations
- FDG-PET CT can be particularly helpful to diagnose potential cardiac device infection in cases with limited or non-diagnostic echocardiography. Devices implanted within 6 weeks may demonstrate FDG activity without infection, so results require integration with microbiology and clinical criteria

Treatment

- The mainstay of treatment is early and complete extraction of the entire system, when possible, followed by prolonged antimicrobial therapy
- Large vegetations can be removed percutaneously, or if exceptionally large extraction by cardiac surgery may be required

Re-implantation should be delayed until surveillance cultures are repeatedly negative. In patients who are pacing-dependent a temporary tunnelled pacing lead should be implanted as a bridge to definitive re-implantation once treatment is completed. Any new device should be implanted at a separate site from the prior infected device.

Complications

Especially common with *Staphylococcus aureus*

Cardiac

- Abscess—usually requires surgical valve replacement and debridement with patch closure of the abscess
- Valve rupture, perforation, and/or regurgitation
- Sinus of Valsalva rupture
- Ventricular septal defect
- Left ventricular failure and/or pulmonary oedema
- Shock—cardiogenic and/or septic
- Conduction disturbance—new AV block suggests aortic root abscess
- Relapse—repeat episode caused by the same micro-organism
- Re-infection—further episode caused by a different micro-organism
- Late valve dysfunction—chronic valve regurgitation may lead to a requirement for future surgical valve replacement (20–40% of cases)

Non-cardiac

Emboli

- Can lead to stroke, peripheral arterial occlusion, or organ infarcts
- May also cause abscesses due to infected nature of embolic material
- Abdominal abscesses should be operated on prior to cardiac surgery
- Splenic abscesses are particularly prone to rupture and splenectomy may be required

Mycotic aneurysm

- Often caused by embolized infected material
- Common sites: sinuses of Valsalva; intra-cranial, mesenteric, and renal arteries
- Intracranial aneurysms have a high mortality (60%), if rupture occurs (sub-arachnoid haemorrhage: 80% mortality)

Renal failure

- Sepsis
- Dehydration
- Glomerulonephritis
- Emboli
- Antibiotic toxicity

Risk factors for adverse outcome

- Cerebral complications
- Peri-annular complications—abscess, fistula
- Prosthetic valve infection
- Haemodialysis
- Heart failure
- Older age
- Sepsis
- *Staphylococcus aureus* infection
- Unsuitability for cardiac surgery

Prophylaxis

Simple measures are important in preventing bacteraemia for patients at risk. Advice should be given regarding:

- Meticulous dental hygiene and twice-yearly dental review
- Good skin hygiene
- Wound disinfection and care
- Avoid self-medication with antibiotics
- Prompt treatment of focal bacterial infections
- Avoid tattoos and piercings
- Care with intravenous cannula during procedures
- Awareness of importance of persistent fever

Antibiotic prophylaxis

Routine administration of antibiotic prophylaxis prior to invasive dental procedures is recommended (see Table 10.2) in higher-risk groups which include:

- Prior treated infective endocarditis
- Prosthetic heart valves of any form including TAVI and valve repair
- Uncorrected congenital heart disease

Invasive dental procedures include extractions, periodontal surgery, root canal surgery, and oral biopsies. Routine dental checks and superficial descaling do not require prophylaxis.

Table 10.2 Antibiotic prophylaxis for patients at elevated risk undergoing invasive dental procedures:

1 hour before procedure:	
Standard	Amoxicillin 2 g PO Ampicillin 2 g IM/IV if cannot take orally
Penicillin-allergic	Cefalexin 2 g PO or clarithromycin 500 mg PO Ceftriaxone 1 g IM/IV if cannot take orally

Chapter 11

Arrhythmias

Bradycardia: general

- Definition: a heart rate of < 60 bpm
- May occur as a normal physiological variant (particularly nocturnally or in athletic individuals), 2° to a disease process, or because of drug therapy
- Broadly divided into sinoatrial node dysfunction, or a block at the AV node or His–Purkinje system
- Can be intermittent or persistent

Types

See Table 11.1.

Table 11.1 Types of bradycardia

Sinus node dysfunction	AV block
Sinus bradycardia (➲ p.134)	AV block (➲ p.139)
Sinus arrest (➲ p.136)	AV block associated with atrial fibrillation/ flutter (➲ p.142)
Junctional bradycardia (➲ p.137)	

Presentation

- Coincidental finding in asymptomatic patient
- Breathlessness on exertion
- Fatigue or lethargy
- Presyncope
- Syncope

Immediate management

Depends on:

- Haemodynamic status—BP, level of consciousness, urine output, signs of heart failure
- Associated medical conditions—MI, drug overdose, hypothyroidism, hypothermia
- Type of bradycardia

General principles

- Treat the patient rather than the ECG
- Identify and treat potentially causative factors—correct electrolytes, thyroid status, hypothermia, stop rate-slowing medications
- Patients with haemodynamic compromise should be considered for urgent treatment to improve heart rate
- Stable patients may require further cardiac monitoring; the decision regarding subsequent definitive treatment will depend on symptoms, type of bradycardia, and prognostic implications

Treatment options

- Pharmacologic—atropine, isoprenaline infusion (Table 11.2)
- Temporary pacing—transcutaneous or transvenous (Box 11.1)
- Permanent pacing—the precise pacing prescription (single or dual chamber, cardiac resynchronization, physiological pacing, leadless pacing) will depend on type of bradycardia, cardiac function, and clinical characteristics

Table 11.2 Drugs used to treat bradycardia

Drug	Mechanism of action	Dose (IV)
Atropine	Anti-muscarinic	500 mcg to a maximum of 3 mg
Isoprenaline	β-agonist	5 mcg bolus; 1–20 mcg/min infusion

Box 11.1 Indications for temporary pacing

N.B. Temporary pacing is often a bridge to permanent pacing. Ideally, a temporary pacing wire is only required if the patient cannot wait for a permanent system.

Definite

- Recurrent, frequent asystolic pauses causing syncope
- Any bradycardia with significant haemodynamic compromise despite medical therapy
- Bradycardia-induced ventricular arrhythmia

Can be considered

- Recurrent symptomatic pauses (> 3 sec)
- Incessant VT (for overdrive pacing)

No clear indication

- Asymptomatic AV block or sinus node disease

Sinus bradycardia

Symptoms

- Often an asymptomatic coincidental finding, especially if nocturnal
- Fatigue
- Exertional dyspnoea
- Less commonly, presyncope or syncope

Causes

- Physiological (fit, young patients at rest) in which case it is almost always asymptomatic
- Drug treatment, e.g. β-blockers, rate-slowing calcium antagonist, amiodarone
- Systemic illness, e.g. hypothyroidism, hypothermia
- Sinus node disease

ECG diagnosis

- Heart rate < 60 bpm (R–R interval > 5 big squares) (Fig. 11.1)
- P:QRS = 1:1

Immediate management

- Assess haemodynamic status—BP, level of consciousness, urine output, signs of heart failure
- Identify causative factors—drug history, thyroid status, electrolytes
- If haemodynamically compromised: give atropine 0.5 mg IV bolus

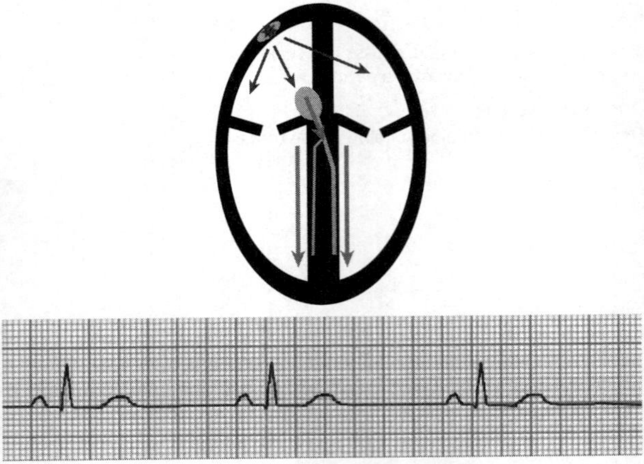

Fig. 11.1 Sinus bradycardia. The P wave and QRS have a constant relationship but the rate is slower than 60 bpm (R–R interval of > 5 large squares). Red arrows indicate a compulsory part of the rhythm/circuit; pink arrows indicate bystander (non-participating) pathways.

Prognosis and subsequent management

- Good prognosis
- Irreversible, symptomatic bradycardia may require permanent pacemaker insertion

Specific considerations

- It is very rare to require temporary transvenous pacing for sinus bradycardia, although it may be required for severe haemodynamic compromise in bradycardia that cannot be treated pharmacologically
- β-blocker and rate slowing calcium-channel blocker overdose (➲ p.292)

Sinus arrest

Presentation

- Sinus arrest is often intermittent with an adequate rhythm and haemodynamic status in between episodes
- Asymptomatic, coincidental finding, especially if nocturnal *(sinus arrest is only 'significant' if pauses are > 3 sec)*
- Presyncope or syncope—check sinus pauses occur simultaneously/just before the symptoms, to be certain that these are the cause

Causes

- Intrinsic sinus node disease
- Carotid sinus hypersensitivity or vasovagal reaction (➲ p.43)

ECG diagnosis

- A pause (significant if > 3 sec), not preceded by ectopic beat (Fig. 11.2)
- P:QRS = 1:1

Immediate management

- Dictated by frequency and severity of pauses
- Usually no immediate management is required, even though a permanent pacemaker may be indicated in due course
- Stop potentially exacerbating medications—β-blockers, calcium-channel blockers
- Very frequent pauses resulting in severe symptoms may require temporary transvenous pacing (see ➲ Box 11.1, p.133)

Prognosis and subsequent management

- Good prognosis
- Symptomatic sinus arrest may require permanent pacemaker insertion

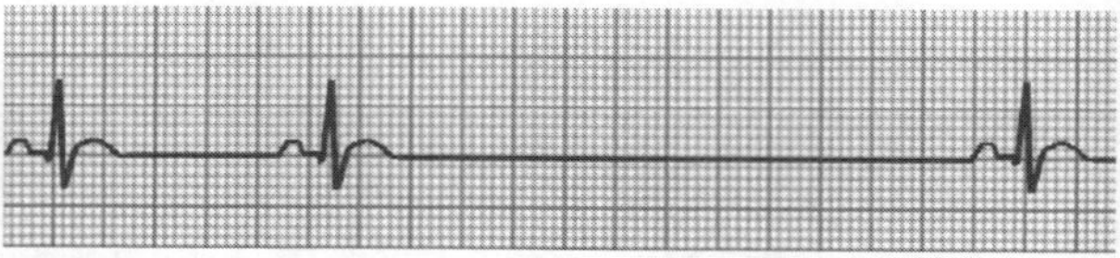

Fig. 11.2 Sinus arrest. The P waves slow or stop suddenly, resulting in a pause. Significant pauses are those > 3 sec, particularly when the patient is awake. Note that this pause is just under 3 sec, and is unlikely to result in symptoms, but longer pauses may occur at other times, especially if a precipitating factor (e.g. rate-slowing drug) is present.

Junctional bradycardia

Junctional bradycardia occurs when the sinus node fails and a low atrial or AV junction pacemaker takes over. Symptoms result from bradycardia and loss of the atrial contribution to ventricular filling, particularly if atrial and ventricular contractions are simultaneous.

Presentation

- Asymptomatic coincidental finding, especially if nocturnal
- Fatigue
- Exertional dyspnoea
- Less commonly, presyncope or syncope

Causes

- Drug treatment, e.g. β-blockers, calcium-channel blockers
- Systemic illness, e.g. hypothyroidism, hypothermia
- Hypokalaemia
- Sinus node disease with junctional escape

ECG diagnosis

- Retrograde P waves may be visible just before/after QRS complex
- (Fig. 11.3)
- No P waves may be visible (buried within the QRS complex)
- Regular QRS complexes (usually narrow) with rate < 60 bpm
- P:QRS = 1:1 if P waves visible

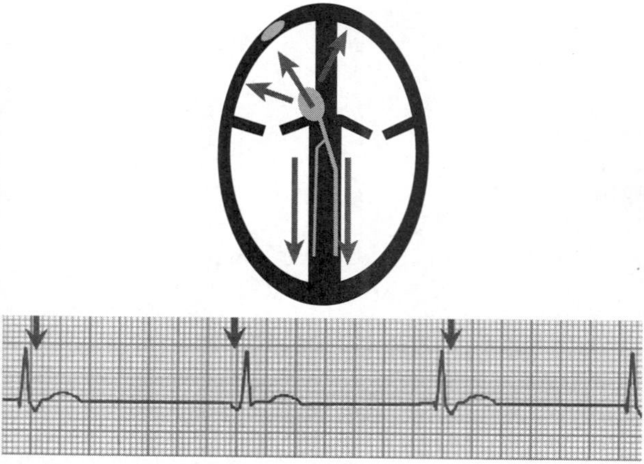

Fig. 11.3 Junctional bradycardia (see ➲ ECG, ➲ p.410). If the sinus node fails, the AV junction is the next in line in the pacemaker hierarchy. P waves originate from the AV node area and are therefore negative in leads II, III, and aVF. They occur just before, during, or after the QRS (arrows), depending upon which point in the AV junction they originate. There is a QRS complex, usually narrow, for every P wave.

Immediate management

- Assess haemodynamic status (blood pressure, level of consciousness, urine output, signs of heart failure)
- Identify causative factors (drug history, thyroid status, electrolytes)
- If haemodynamically compromised: give atropine 0.5 mg IV bolus

Prognosis and subsequent management

- Good prognosis
- Irreversible, symptomatic bradycardia may require permanent pacemaker insertion

Specific considerations

Temporary transvenous pacing for junctional bradycardia may be required for severe haemodynamic compromise. Single chamber ventricular pacing may not improve cardiac output and atrial or dual chamber AV sequential temporary pacing may be required.

Atrioventricular block

Conduction delay or block between the atria and the ventricles may be within the AV node (usually narrow QRS complex, benign, and responds to increase in sympathetic tone) or the His–Purkinje system (QRS may be wide, worse prognosis, and doesn't respond to autonomic changes).

Classification

By ECG criteria into:

1st-degree AV block

- Slight delay of AV conduction, but each atrial stimulus is still conducted to the ventricles

2nd-degree AV block (further divided into type I and type II)

- Increasing AV conduction block such that not all atrial stimuli are conducted to the ventricles

3rd-degree AV block (also called complete heart block)

- No atrial stimuli are conducted to the ventricles. Ventricular activity is driven by myocardial tissue below the region of block

Presentation

- Asymptomatic, coincidental finding
- Fatigue, exertional dyspnoea or low cardiac output state
- Presyncope or syncope

Causes

- High vagal tone—usually benign and asymptomatic, often has a narrow complex escape rhythm
- 1° conduction tissue disease
- Myocardial disease (ischaemia, infarction, fibrosis, infiltration)—usually affects His–Purkinje system and has a wide complex escape rhythm (Boxes 11.2 and 11.3, p.141)
- Congenital
- Drugs, e.g. β-blocker and calcium-channel blocker combination

ECG diagnosis

1st-degree AV block

- Prolonged PR interval (> 200 msec or 5 small squares; Fig. 11.4)
- 1:1 relationship between P and QRS
- QRS complex usually narrow

2nd-degree AV block (Mobitz type I/Wenckebach phenomenon)

- Progressive lengthening of PR interval until a P wave is not conducted. PR interval then returns to baseline (Fig. 11.5)

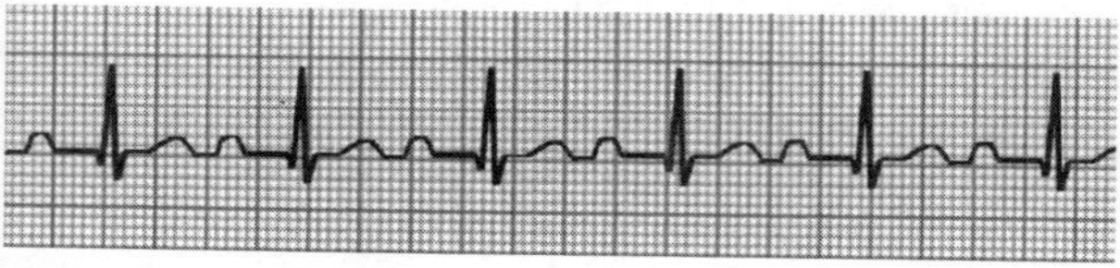

Fig. 11.4 1st-degree AV block.

- Narrow QRS (usually)
- P:QRS is > 1:1

2nd-degree AV block (Mobitz type II)

- No variation in PR interval but intermittent failure in conduction to ventricles, manifest as missing QRS complex(es) following P wave (Fig. 11.6)
- Narrow QRS (usually)
- Can be regular dropped QRS, e.g. 2 or 3 P waves for each QRS (termed 2:1 or 3:1 block, etc.)
- P:QRS >1:1, and can be 2:1 or 3:1

3rd-degree AV block (or complete heart block)

- Complete dissociation between P and QRS, i.e. no relationship (Fig. 11.7)
- P waves and QRS are usually regular but at different rates
- QRS complexes are often wide, but can be narrow if the AV block is high and the ventricular escape rhythm arises from the His–Purkinje system

Management

- Stop any rate-slowing medications
- Treat any precipitating causes—acute MI, drug overdose, abnormal electrolytes
- See Boxes 11.2 and 11.3 for management of AV block in the context of myocardial infarction and cardiac surgery respectively

1st-degree and Mobitz type I (Wenckebach) 2nd-degree block

- Do not normally require intervention

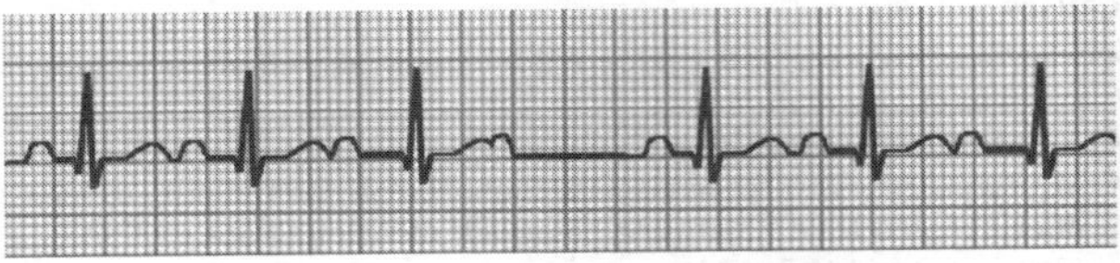

Fig. 11.5 2nd-degree AV block: Mobitz type I/Wenckebach phenomenon.

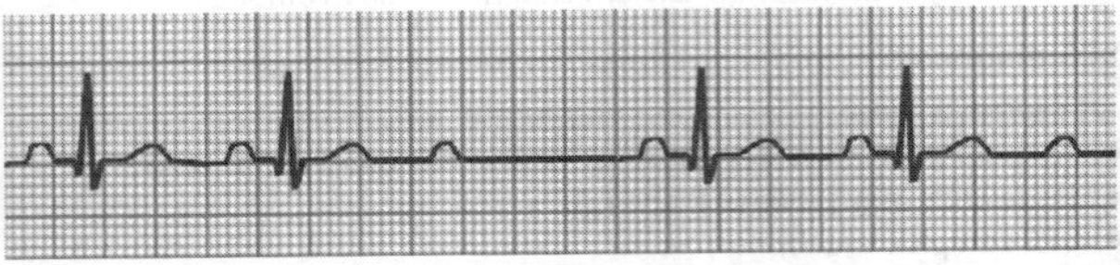

Fig. 11.6 2nd-degree AV block: Mobitz type II.

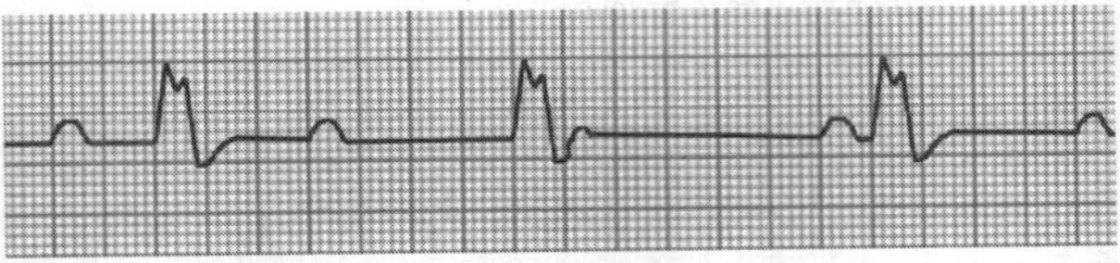

Fig. 11.7 3rd-degree AV block: complete heart block.

Mobitz type II 2nd-degree block and complete AV block

- Atropine (0.5–1.0 mg IV) will improve AV node conduction in the setting of high vagal tone but will have little effect on conduction disturbances due to His–Purkinje disease. Effects may last up to 3 hours
- Complete heart block with mild or infrequent symptoms may be observed until permanent pacing is performed, especially if the QRS complex is narrow
- In the presence of symptoms, IV isoprenaline or other sympathomimetic drugs can be trialled until permanent pacing is performed
- Temporary transvenous pacing may be needed if symptoms do no respond to medical therapy, and is required urgently if there is a low cardiac output state with reduced perfusion or recurrent syncope

Prognosis and subsequent management

- Good prognosis if due to AV nodal block (narrow QRS, escape rhythm > 45 bpm) and reversible cause
- Irreversible Mobitz type II 2nd-degree block or complete heart block due to His–Purkinje disease has a risk of asystole and usually requires permanent pacemaker insertion, whether symptomatic or not

Box 11.2 MI and AV block

Inferior MI

In the setting of acute inferior MI, 1° angioplasty (or thrombolysis) should not be delayed by the management of AV block. AV block is usually transient as the right coronary artery often supplies the AV node and reperfusion often results in restoration of normal conduction. If conduction returns to normal within 48 hours, permanent pacemaker insertion is not usually required. Temporary pacing is rarely required, and recovery of AV conduction can occasionally take > 1 week.

Anterior MI

2nd/3rd-degree AV block in the setting of acute anterior MI carries a poor prognosis as the extensive infarction involving the anteroseptal wall results in damage to the conduction system. Temporary transvenous pacing in the setting of acute MI carries a risk of myocardial perforation (of the pacing wire through the infarcted tissue). If pacing is indicated, then consideration should be given to placement of a permanent cardiac resynchronization device (potentially including a defibrillator component).

Box 11.3 AV block after cardiac surgery

Complete AV block is common after certain cardiac operations, e.g. aortic valve replacement. This may be due to damage to the AV conducting tissue during surgery or may be reversible due to oedema. Most patients would already have epicardial pacing leads *in situ* to facilitate temporary pacing if required, and transvenous pacing is needed only if the epicardial leads fail. Persistent high-grade AV block after 5–7 days usually indicates the need for permanent pacemaker implantation.

AV block and atrial fibrillation/flutter

High-grade AV block with atrial fibrillation/flutter may result in symptoms due to a slow ventricular response, either persistent bradycardia or symptomatic pauses. Pauses (R–R intervals) of < 5 sec are not usually significant (particularly at night or if asymptomatic).

Causes

- Intrinsic conduction tissue disease
- Coexisting cardiac disease—ischaemia, infarction, fibrosis, infiltration
- Drugs—particularly β-blocker and calcium-channel blocker combination (which should usually be avoided)

ECG diagnosis

AF and complete AV block

- No discrete P waves
- Often coarse, fibrillatory baseline—F waves
- Regular ventricular escape rhythm—QRS can be narrow or broad
- Differential diagnosis: junctional bradycardia

Atrial flutter with high grade AV block

- Saw-tooth baseline (flutter waves) especially in the inferior leads
- Flutter wave: QRS usually > 4:1
- Regular ventricular escape rhythm—QRS can be narrow or broad

Immediate management

- Treat any precipitating causes—acute MI, drug overdose, abnormal electrolytes
- Stop any rate-slowing medications
- Atropine (0.5–1 mg IV) will improve AV node conduction in the setting of high vagal tone but will have little effect on conduction disturbances due to His–Purkinje disease
- Temporary pacing is required only if there is a low cardiac output state with reduced perfusion or recurrent syncope
- Slow ventricular rates with mild or infrequent symptoms may be observed until permanent pacing is performed

Prognosis and subsequent management

- Discontinue exacerbating antiarrhythmic medications
- Irreversible high-grade AV block due to His–Purkinje disease has a risk of asystole and usually requires permanent pacemaker insertion, whether symptomatic or not

Tachycardia: general

- Definition: a heart rate of > 100 bpm
- Tachycardia may be broadly divided into appropriate (normal physiological response to certain conditions) or inappropriate (an arrhythmic process). The origin of the tachycardia may be from re-entrant circuits or foci in the atria (supraventricular) or ventricles. Symptoms are generally due to impaired cardiac perfusion and reduced cardiac output

To aid with diagnosis and management, a tachycardia is usually subdivided into (Table 11.3):

- Narrow complex—regular, QRS duration < 120 ms
- Broad complex—regular, QRS complex > 120 ms
- AF with rapid ventricular response—irregular rhythm, may be narrow or broad complex

Table 11.3 Types of tachycardia

	Narrow complex tachycardia	Broad complex tachycardia
Regular	Sinus tachycardia Atrial tachycardia AVNRT AVRT Atrial flutter (regular block)	VT Any regular narrow complex tachycardia with bundle branch block or antegrade conduction via an accessory pathway
Irregular	AF Atrial flutter (variable AV block)	Pre-excited AF Polymorphic VT Any irregular narrow complex tachycardia with bundle branch block

Presentation

- May be asymptomatic
- Breathlessness
- Chest pain
- Palpitation
- Presyncope
- Syncope

Immediate management

Depends on:

- Haemodynamic status—BP, level of consciousness, urine output, signs of heart failure
- Symptoms of cardiac ischaemia—chest pain, SOB
- Associated medical conditions—MI, drug overdose, hyperthyroidism, PE, heart failure
- Type of tachycardia

General principles

- Treat the patient rather than the ECG
- Treat potentially exacerbating factors—correct electrolytes, hypoxia, acid–base disturbances, dehydration, thyroid status
- Identify and treat underlying cause—MI, PE, heart failure
- Stable patients should have cardiac monitoring and treatment to control heart rate or restore sinus rhythm

Patients with haemodynamic compromise/significant symptoms due to the arrhythmia should be considered for urgent treatment to restore normal sinus rhythm.

Treatment options

- Vagal manoeuvres—carotid sinus massage, Valsalva
- Adenosine (➔ p.146)
- Antiarrhythmic drugs (➔ p.145)
- Synchronized DC cardioversion or defibrillation
- Overdrive pacing via implanted cardiac device or transvenous temporary wire (➔ p.175)

Pharmacological treatment of tachyarrhythmias

Drugs are used in the treatment of tachyarrhythmia for 3 main reasons:

- To aid diagnosis, e.g. adenosine
- To restore normal rhythm, i.e. antiarrhythmic drugs, adenosine (Box 11.4)
- To reduce heart rate, e.g. certain antiarrhythmic drugs acting on the AV node

Box 11.4 Administration of IV amiodarone

The IV bolus and infusion of amiodarone should be administered through a central venous catheter whenever possible. If it has to be given peripherally then ensure that amiodarone is given through a newly sited, large-bore cannula in a large peripheral vein (e.g. in the ante-cubital fossa) as extravasation of amiodarone may result in severe tissue damage. Thrombophlebitis is a recognized complication of peripheral amiodarone. Rapid loading with oral amiodarone (e.g. 400 mg three times a day for one week) is an alternative to consider.

Antiarrhythmic drugs

These drugs are classified according to their mechanism of action in the Vaughan–Williams classification (Table 11.4). They work by blocking certain ion channels or receptors in the heart to restore and/or maintain normal sinus rhythm.

General tips for choosing antiarrhythmic drugs

Ischaemia and heart failure

- Class I agents (flecainide and propafenone) are mostly contraindicated in patients with ischaemic or structural heart disease
- Caution with using calcium-channel blocker or β-blocker in acute decompensated heart failure
- Amiodarone and digoxin are generally safe in ischaemic or structural heart disease

Table 11.4 Vaughan–Williams classification of antiarrhythmic drugs

	Mechanism of action	Examples
Class I	Sodium-channel blocker	Lidocaine Flecainide Propafenone
Class II	β-blocker	Bisoprolol Atenolol Metoprolol
Class III	Potassium-channel blocker	Amiodarone Sotalol
Class IV	Calcium-channel blocker	Verapamil Diltiazem

Combinations

- The combination of β-blocker and calcium-channel blocker (especially when used intravenously) may result in bradycardia or even AV block and should be avoided
- Amiodarone potentiates the effects of digoxin and vice versa
- Digoxin has a slow onset of action and is less effective in hyper-adrenergic states, e.g. postoperation, sepsis, exertion, thyrotoxicosis

Remember—most antiarrhythmic drugs can have pro-arrhythmic effects. With the exception of digoxin, most antiarrhythmic drugs can lower BP. Commonly used antiarrhythmic drugs are listed in Table 11.5.

The role of adenosine

Adenosine is a very short-acting IV drug that specifically blocks the specialized conducting tissue of the AV node, with lesser effects on the sinus

Table 11.5 Commonly used antiarrhythmic drugs

Drug name	Dose
Amiodarone	Cardiac arrest dose 300 mg as IV bolus Slow IV bolus 150 mg over 10 min (in 100–250 mL 5% *dextrose*). IV infusion to total 1.2 g in 500 mL 5% *dextrose* over 24 hours through central line Oral loading: 400 mg TDS for 7 days *or* 200 mg TDS for 7 days followed by 200 mg BD for 7 days Oral maintenance: 200 mg OD
Digoxin	Oral loading 0.75–1.5 mg over 24 hours, split into 2–3 doses given 6- or 8-hourly Oral maintenance 62.5–250 mcg daily (depending on body weight and renal function) IV loading is rarely required but in cases of poor oral absorption can use 0.75–1 mg over 2 hours in 5% dextrose or 0.9% saline
Esmolol	Urgent IV bolus 1 mg/kg over 30 sec IV infusion 10 mg/mL in 5% dextrose or 0.9% saline. Load with 0.5 mg/kg/min for 1 min only. Maintenance with 0.05–0.3 mg/kg/min, starting at 0.05 mg/kg/min
Flecainide	IV 2 mg/kg to a maximum of 150 mg over 15 min Oral 50–150 mg twice daily
Lidocaine	IV bolus 50–100 mg over 1–2 min Infusion 4 mg/min for 30 min, 2 mg/min for 2 hours, then 1 mg/min
Magnesium sulfate	IV bolus 8 mmol (2g) over 10–15 min in 100 mL 5% dextrose Infusion 2–4 mmol (0.5–1 g)/hour. Concentration should not exceed 20%
Procainamide	IV loading 20 mg/min infusion up to a maximum total dose of 17 mg/kg. Maintenance infusion 20–80 mcg/kg/min
Verapamil	IV 5–10 mg over 2–3 min. Additional 5 mg after 5 min if necessary Oral 40–120 mg TDS

Table 11.6 Effects of adenosine on different arrhythmias

Arrhythmia	Effect of adenosine
Sinus tachycardia	Transient slowing of sinus rate. Transient AV block with ongoing P waves. As adenosine wears off sinus tachycardia rate may increase.
Atrial tachycardia	Up to 90% will show transient AV block with ongoing P waves. In some cases the atrial rate may also transiently slow. 10% of automatic atrial tachycardias are adenosine sensitive and will terminate.
Atrial fibrillation	Transient AV block. Fibrillatory baseline still visible up until AV conduction returns.
Atrial flutter	Transient AV block. Flutter waves become clearly visible up until AV conduction returns.
AVNRT	Tachycardia terminates and sinus rhythm returns
AVRT	Tachycardia terminates and sinus rhythm returns
AF and pre-excitation through accessory pathway	QRS complexes transiently widen and ventricular rate may increase further, possibly resulting in ventricular fibrillation
VT	Usually no effect, however some idiopathic VTs in normal hearts may terminate

node and atrial myocardium. It can be very useful in the treatment and diagnosis of tachyarrhythmia (see Table 11.6).

Termination of arrhythmias

- The principal effect is to cause transient AV nodal block. Any tachycardia dependent on AV node conduction will therefore terminate when AV node block occurs. (On rare occasions, the arrhythmia may reinitiate after a few beats of sinus rhythm, in which case a second dose of adenosine is often helpful.)
- Tachycardias that are not dependent on AV node conduction for their maintenance (AF, flutter) will continue, although the ECG appearance may transiently change, aiding diagnosis
- Rarer ectopic atrial tachycardias and idiopathic VTs may, however, be terminated with adenosine

Other effects

- High doses of adenosine may induce AF in 5–10% of patients
- Adenosine administration often results in ventricular ectopy but it is rare for it to provoke sustained VT
- To reverse the effects of adenosine, give IV aminophylline

Indications during tachycardia

Narrow complex regular tachycardia

- May terminate if AVNRT/AVRT. May reveal flutter waves if atrial flutter, or P waves if atrial tachycardia

Broad complex tachycardia

- When the patient is haemodynamically stable *and*
- No definite ECG/clinical characteristics to suggest VT *and*
- There is a likelihood of SVT with bundle branch block

Administration

Always record a continuous ECG (ideally a 12-lead rhythm strip) immediately before, during, and after adenosine administration.

- Administer as a rapid IV bolus through a large cannula placed as centrally as possible
- Follow immediately by a 20 mL flush of saline
- Ideally, connect the adenosine and flush syringes to the cannula through a 3-way tap to facilitate administration
- A 6 mg bolus is often insufficient and a 12 mg starting dose is recommended. In larger patients, 18 mg or higher may be needed. Wait a few minutes between doses
- Patients will experience transient chest tightness, sweating, and flushing during administration. Warn them!

Contraindications

- Severe asthma—adenosine is reported to be safe in mild asthmatics
- Dipyridamole use—inhibits adenosine uptake and potentiates its effect
- Pre-excited AF—adenosine can precipitate ventricular fibrillation
- Caution with severe sinus node disease and cardiac transplant recipients

Sinus tachycardia

- Sinus tachycardia is a physiological response, usually to physical, emotional, or physiological stress
- Heart rate is typically 100–160 bpm usually with subtle variation in rate
- There is almost always an identifiable underlying cause
- Inappropriate sinus tachycardia is a rare condition marked by dramatic increases in heart rate with minimal exertion and a mean resting rate >100 bpm
- Sinus node re-entrant tachycardia is also rare and may mimic sinus tachycardia but often has a sudden onset and termination and responds to IV adenosine

Common causes

- Exercise
- Pain
- Anxiety
- Dehydration
- Sepsis
- Shock
- Hypoxia
- PE
- Heart failure
- Anaemia
- Thyrotoxicosis
- Stimulants–caffeine, amphetamines, inotrope infusions

ECG diagnosis

- P waves are the same morphology as those in sinus rhythm—these may be hard to identify at a fast rate (Fig. 11.8)
- PR interval is usually normal
- P:QRS = 1:1

Treatment

Identify and treat the underlying cause—the tachycardia is 2° to this and is not itself a problem.

Atrial fibrillation

- The most common sustained clinical arrhythmia, affecting 1% of the general population, and up to 10% in those aged 80+
- Characterized by very rapid and disorganized atrial activity, usually resulting in a fast and irregularly irregular ventricular rate
- AF may be *paroxysmal* (will spontaneously revert to sinus rhythm); *persistent* (requires pharmacologic or electrical cardioversion to restore sinus rhythm); or *permanent* (no plan to restore sinus rhythm)

Main causes

Obesity, hypertension, valvular heart disease, cardiomyopathy (ischaemic, dilated or hypertrophic), acute infection, thyrotoxicosis, post-surgery, excess alcohol intake, genetic.

Presentation

- A wide spectrum. Patients may be asymptomatic, have palpitation, chest pain, dyspnoea, pre-syncope, syncope, or frank pulmonary oedema
- Symptoms result from a rapid, irregular ventricular rate and loss of atrial contribution to ventricular filling (and thus cardiac output)

ECG diagnosis

- Irregularly irregular ventricular rhythm (Fig. 11.9)
- No discrete atrial activity (although lead V1 often has a coarse, rapid fibrillatory baseline). See ➲ ECG, p.407

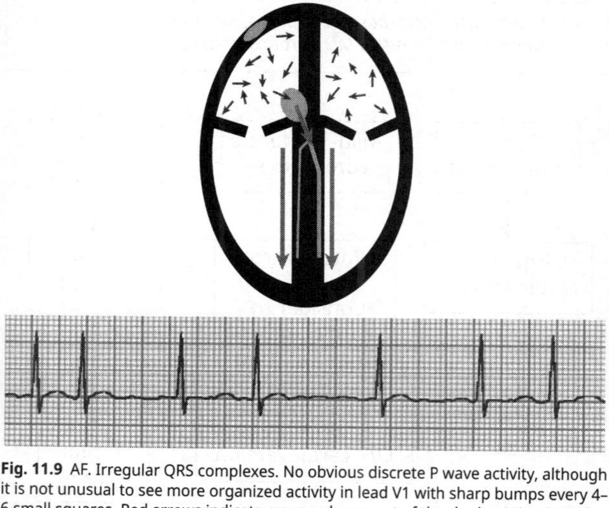

Fig. 11.9 AF. Irregular QRS complexes. No obvious discrete P wave activity, although it is not unusual to see more organized activity in lead V1 with sharp bumps every 4–6 small squares. Red arrows indicate a compulsory part of the rhythm/ circuit; pink arrows indicate bystander (non-participating) pathways.

Treatment: general principles

- Assess patient's haemodynamic status and symptoms
- Treat potentially exacerbating factors—correct electrolytes, hypoxia, acid–base disturbances, dehydration, thyroid status
- Identify and treat any underlying cause—acute MI, PE accessory pathway (Box 11.5, p.154)
- Post-surgical patients are often dehydrated, hypoxic, in pain, or any combination of these, and mostly respond to treatment of the underlying factors. They still require anticoagulation to reduce thrombus formation ± rate control if ventricular rate > 100 bpm, but rarely require cardioversion

The principal aspects of treatment are:

- Restoration of sinus rhythm vs ventricular rate control
- An assessment of thromboembolic risk

Specific treatment is highly dependent on the status of the patient (see ➲ Treatment: specific conditions, p.152).

Treatment

- Treatment is guided by symptoms and anticoagulation status (Fig. 11.10)

See Box 11.5 for specific management of pre-excited AF

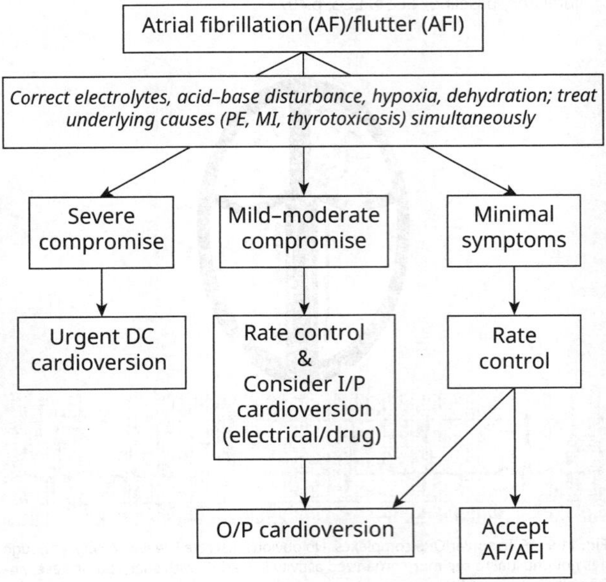

Fig. 11.10 Flowchart summarizing general treatment strategies for acute atrial fibrillation/flutter. DC—direct current; I/P—inpatient; O/P—outpatient.

AF with severe haemodynamic compromise

- Rare in individuals with a normal heart but can occur in the context of congenital heart disease or severe heart failure
- Hypotension and hypoperfusion, reduced conscious level, pulmonary oedema, or cardiac ischaemia due to AF mandate urgent treatment

Regardless of duration of onset

- Oxygen
- Therapeutic anticoagulation (if not already anticoagulated)—LMWH or a DOAC
- Synchronized DC shock under sedation/general anaesthesia using 200J biphasic energy

Symptomatic AF with mild–moderate compromise

(Breathlessness, palpitation and/or mild hypotension.)

Clear onset < 48 hours

- Easier to assess if high ventricular rate and symptoms are palpitation; caution needed if rates lower and dominant symptom is dyspnea or lethargy as AF may have been sub-clinical for some time
- Commence DOAC irrespective of CHA_2DS_2-VA if rhythm control being considered and continue for at least 4 weeks
- Consider pharmacological cardioversion with flecainide
  - Usually only if no known structural heart disease or significant coronary artery disease, and patient < 50 years
- Alternatively, synchronized DC cardioversion under sedation/GA
- Amiodarone is not preferred due to the side effect profile and because it takes longer to achieve rhythm control

Onset > 48 hours or unknown

- Commence DOAC irrespective of CHA_2DS_2-VA if rhythm control being considered and continue for at least 4 weeks
- Rate control:
  - β-blocker is the preferred option unless there is severe asthma or acute heart failure or pulmonary oedema
  - Rate-limiting calcium-channel blockers can be considered in severe asthma or other contraindication or previous side effects from β-blocker, but are contraindicated in heart failure
  - Digoxin is not a good first-line agent as it is slow to work, ineffective in high adrenergic states (e.g. postoperation, sepsis, thyrotoxicosis), and its effect may be lost once the patient becomes active and mobile; it is better used as an adjunct if the rate is not controlled on maximal tolerated dose of β-blocker or rate-limiting calcium-channel blocker
  - Amiodarone is not preferred for rate control
- If still highly symptomatic with uncontrolled ventricular rate, then TOE to exclude left atrial appendage thrombus followed by DC cardioversion can be considered
- If symptoms and ventricular rate are controlled, plan for discharge and consider outpatient DC cardioversion following a period of at least 4 weeks uninterrupted oral anticoagulation

Minimally symptomatic AF with no compromise

- Anticoagulation and rate control (if required) initially
- Consider elective DC cardioversion once anticoagulated
- In some cases, the decision may be made to accept AF as permanent

Box 11.5 Pre-excited atrial fibrillation

Pre-excited AF (➲ p.409) occurs in patients with an accessory pathway (➲ p.165) and can result in a very rapid, irregular, broad complex tachycardia producing severe symptoms. Sinus rhythm should be restored as soon as possible, usually with urgent DC cardioversion. Avoid drugs that block AV node conduction and increase accessory pathway conduction (e.g. bisoprolol, digoxin, verapamil, adenosine). Inpatient referral for ablation of the accessory pathway is usually recommended.

Box 11.6 Rapid control of ventricular rate in the Emergency Room or ICU

May be achieved with a continuous infusion of the IV β-blocker esmolol. This has the advantage of being short acting and can be titrated up and down depending upon heart rate and BP response.

Subsequent management

- Echocardiography to look for underlying heart disease
- If previous episodes of compromising AF, a future antiarrhythmic strategy may be appropriate (antiarrhythmic drugs or catheter ablation) to prevent recurrence
- Consider long-term anticoagulation based on CHA_2DS_2-VA score (Box 11.7, p.155)
- If AF is accepted as permanent, rate control to achieve a resting heart rate below ~90 bpm is recommended

Thromboembolic risk

The thromboembolic risk that results from the development of AF and following the restoration of sinus rhythm needs to be considered when assessing the various treatment strategies. Left atrial thrombus results from loss of atrial contractility, increased stasis, and pooling of blood in the left atrial appendage (Fig. 11.11). Restoration of sinus rhythm restores atrial contractile function over some weeks (there is a period of 'stunning') and this period is also associated with increased risk of embolism. This risk should be considered the same whether electrical or pharmacological cardioversion has occurred.

AF onset < 48 hours

- Safe to cardiovert patient without prior anticoagulation
- Usual to start anticoagulation and continue this for at least 4 weeks after cardioversion (if CHA_2DS_2-VA score < 2) or indefinitely (CHA_2DS_2-VA score ≥ 2)

AF onset > 48 hours or uncertain

- If there is a need to perform urgent cardioversion, it is safer after a TOE has excluded a left atrial appendage thrombus
- Otherwise, a 4-week period of therapeutic anticoagulation is necessary before scheduling outpatient cardioversion
- Usual to continue anticoagulation for at least 4 weeks after cardioversion (if CHA2DS2-VA score < 2) or indefinitely (CHA_2DS_2-VA score ≥ 2)

Long-term anticoagulation

- Oral anticoagulation can be used to reduce the risk of stroke or systemic embolism in AF, based on clinical risk assessment
- Embolic risk is easily assessed using the CHA_2DS_2-VA score—see Box 11.7 and Table 11.7
- In patients with AF and a high CHA_2DS_2-VA score, indefinite oral anticoagulation is recommended irrespective of current rhythm

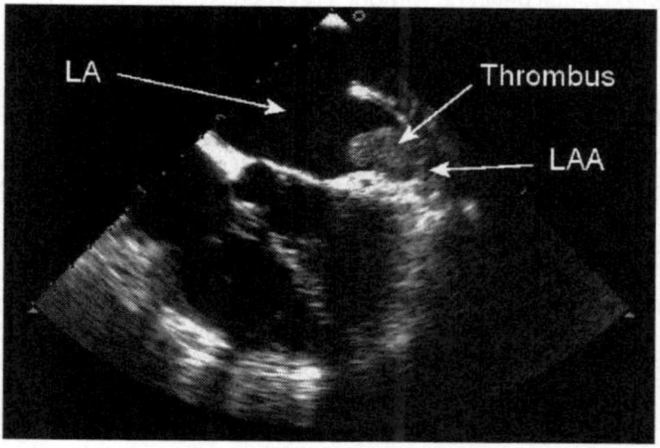

Fig. 11.11 TOE of the left atrium (LA) demonstrating a thrombus in the left atrial appendage (LAA). It is believed that > 90% of strokes in AF result from emboli originating in the LAA.

Box 11.7 Assessing thromboembolic risk: CHA_2DS_2-VA

The CHA_2DS_2-VA score is a quick and simple scoring system for assessing a patient's stroke risk. Points are scored according to risk profile to a maximum of 9:

- Congestive heart failure 1
- Hypertension 1
- Age > 75 years 2
- Diabetes mellitus 1
- Prior Stroke/TIA/embolism 2
- Vascular disease 1
- Age 65–74 years 1

The adjusted risk of stroke per year for each score is:

- 0: 0.0%
- 1: 1.3%
- 2: 2.2%
- 3: 3.2%
- 4: 4.0%
- 5: 6.7%
- 6: 9.8%
- 7: 9.6%
- 8: 6.7%
- 9: 15.2%

https://chadsva.org

- Direct oral anticoagulants (DOACs; apixaban, dabigatran, edoxaban, rivaroxaban) are generally preferred to warfarin as first-line therapy, except in patients with metallic heart valves or moderate/severe mitral stenosis or others with contraindications to DOACs (severe renal failure, interactions with some medications)
- There is no role for anti-platelet medications for embolic risk prophylaxis in AF
- In individuals with contraindications for long-term oral anticoagulation (e.g. intracranial bleeding without a reversible cause), left atrial appendage occlusion can be considered instead

Table 11.7 CHA_2DS_2-VA score, thromboembolic risk, and treatment

Score	Risk	Treatment
0 to 1	Low	No antithrombotic treatment
1 to 2	Intermediate	Oral anticoagulation should be considered (Class IIa)
≥ 2	High	Oral anticoagulation is recommended (Class I)

Atrial flutter

Atrial flutter is a re-entrant atrial tachycardia (in the right atrium) with an electrical wavefront that rotates around the tricuspid valve, although other less common circuits may present as atypical flutters.

- The atrial rate is usually a regular 280–320 bpm, with the ventricles activated in a 2:1 fashion due to filtering via the AV node
- Higher degrees of AV block may occur spontaneously or with the addition of drug therapy
- Rarely, 1:1 conduction may occur, leading to extremely rapid ventricular rates and severe symptoms
- Like AF, atrial flutter may be paroxysmal, persistent, or permanent
- As with AF, the thromboembolic risk needs to be considered when considering the various treatment strategies (see https://chadsva.org)
- AF and flutter often coexist and up to 50% of patients treated for typical atrial flutter will go on to develop AF in follow-up

Presentation

Patients may: be asymptomatic; have palpitations, chest pain, or dyspnoea; presyncope, syncope, or frank pulmonary oedema.

Principle causes

Obesity, hypertension, valvular heart disease, cardiomyopathy (ischaemic, dilated or hypertrophic), acute infection, postoperative, excess alcohol intake, lung disease, genetic

ECG diagnosis

- Typical atrial flutter has a 'saw-tooth' baseline with flutter waves at 300 bpm with mainly negative deflections in leads II, III, and aVF (Fig. 11.12)
- When there is 2:1 conduction to the ventricle, flutter waves may be hard to see as alternate flutter waves are hidden in the QRS complex
- Ventricular rate is usually regular at approximately 150 bpm (see ➲ ECG, p.410)

Treatment

- Essentially as for AF (but see Box 11.8)
- Two strategies are available—restoration of sinus rhythm, or ventricular rate control. Some pharmacological treatments may address both
- The treatment strategy should be based on duration of onset, haemodynamic compromise, and thromboembolic risk as for the management of AF (➲ p.154, 155)

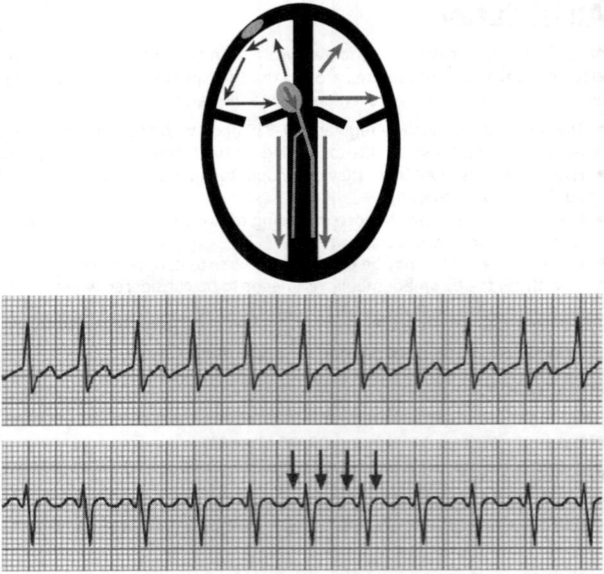

Fig. 11.12 Atrial flutter. Regular QRS complexes, typically at 150 bpm. Rapid, regular atrial activity usually between 280–320 bpm (1 flutter wave every large square). During 2:1 AV conduction alternate flutter waves may be hidden in QRS complexes. Lead V1 is often a good lead for spotting atrial activity (arrows). In typical flutter the flutter waves are negative in leads II, III, and aVF (saw-tooth pattern). Red arrows indicate a compulsory part of the rhythm/circuit; pink arrows indicate bystander (non-participating) pathways.

Box 11.8 Special considerations for atrial flutter

Flecainide and other Class I agents are contraindicated in isolation for the treatment of atrial flutter because they may slow the flutter rate within the atrium, allowing 1:1 conduction through the AV node and a paradoxical increase in ventricular rate with worsening of symptoms. These agents should also usually be combined with AV nodal blocking drugs (e.g. β-blockers) when used for patients in AF because of the risk of AF organizing into atrial flutter.

- Atrial flutter is easier than AF to cardiovert electrically but does not cardiovert easily with drugs
- Achieving adequate ventricular rate control in atrial flutter is often much more challenging compared to AF
- Atrial flutter can be readily treated with radiofrequency ablation of the cavotricuspid isthmus

Atrial tachycardia

- Sometimes called ectopic or focal atrial tachycardia and results from a discrete focus firing automatically at a rate greater than the sinus node
- Common sources of tachycardia are the pulmonary veins in the left atrium, the crista terminalis in the right atrium
- The ventricle is often activated in a 1:1 fashion unless the atrial rate is particularly fast (> 200 bpm) or AV nodal blocking drugs are being used
- Symptoms result from the rapid ventricular rate and usually manifest as palpitation, dyspnoea, presyncope, or chest pain

Principle causes

Often occurs in the setting of an acute illness or trauma (sepsis, surgery, injury). In children and young adults, the heart is often structurally normal. In older patients it is most likely to be associated with structural heart disease.

ECG diagnosis

- Discrete P waves, often a different shape to P waves in sinus rhythm (Fig. 11.13)
- Often has a normal PR interval (often categorized as a 'long RP tachycardia' when P to R wave shorter than R wave to next P wave)
- P:QRS is usually 1:1, but can be 2:1 or more (see ➲ ECG, p.411)

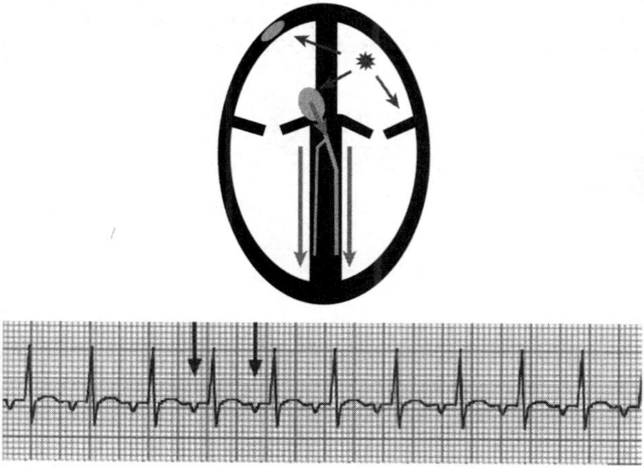

Fig. 11.13 Atrial tachycardia. A focal, automatic tachycardia producing a discrete P wave, although the shape is usually different from the P wave shape seen during sinus rhythm. Usually 1:1 AV conduction unless a very rapid atrial rate or drugs have been given. May have subtle variations in heart rate. Red arrows indicate a compulsory part of the rhythm/circuit; pink arrows indicate bystander (non-participating) pathways.

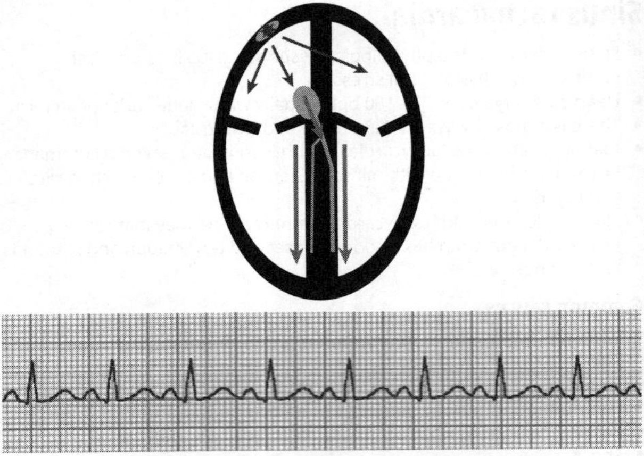

Fig. 11.8 Sinus tachycardia. The P wave is a normal shape and axis and precedes each QRS with a normal PR interval. There are often subtle variations in the heart rate. Red arrows indicate a compulsory part of the rhythm/circuit; pink arrows indicate bystander (non-participating) pathways.

Treatment

Treatment should address any underlying cause (e.g. infection, trauma) and optimizing electrolytes, fluid balance, hypoxia, acid–base balance

Severe haemodynamic compromise

- Rare in individuals with a normal heart but can occur in the context of congenital heart disease or severe heart failure
- Restore sinus rhythm with synchronized DC 200–360 J shock under sedation/GA
- However, if the underlying cause is still present, there is a high chance of recurrence. Hence, antiarrhythmic treatment is usually necessary:
  - Amiodarone—oral or IV
  - β-blockers, e.g. esmolol infusion (➲ p.146), especially in ITU

Mild to moderate haemodynamic compromise

- Attempt to cardiovert pharmacologically:
  - In general, amiodarone and β-blockers are safest
  - Flecainide may be considered if there is no known structural/ischaemic heart disease
- However, due to ongoing underlying cause (e.g. sepsis), acute cardioversion may not be successful and concurrent treatment to control rate is important:
  - β-blockers and calcium-channel blockers (if no hypotension or decompensated heart failure)
  - Digoxin is safe in LV dysfunction and can be added for better rate control
- If the atrial rate is > 200 bpm, atrial contraction can be impaired and thromboembolic risk is ↑ (i.e. like atrial flutter). Consider long-term anticoagulation with DOAC based on CHA2DS2-VA score

Atrioventricular nodal re-entrant tachycardia

- The commonest form of re-entrant tachycardia in adults
- The AV node is a critical component of the re-entrant circuit which comprises the 'fast' and 'slow' pathways within the AV node
- It may present at any age, with a bimodal distribution (young adults and middle-age); it is more common in females
- Heart rates are typically between 150–250 bpm
- In the typical form, the atria and ventricles are depolarized (and therefore contract) simultaneously
- Atrial contraction against closed AV valves can result in rapid, visible pulsation of the neck veins
- AVNRT is most often seen in a structurally normal heart

Presentation

Usual symptoms are rapid palpitations with sudden onset and termination, dyspnoea, chest tightness, and presyncope.

Principle causes

Attacks may be precipitated by exertion and physical or emotional stress, but are often spontaneous with no obvious cause.

ECG diagnosis

- Usually regular narrow complex tachycardia (may be broad complex if there is bundle branch block (RBBB/LBBB) or rate-related aberrancy
- P waves are usually hidden in the QRS and are not visible (Fig. 11.14)
- Sometimes, P wave may appear as a 'pseudo-R' wave at the end of each QRS complex (esp. lead V1). See ➲ ECG, p.412.

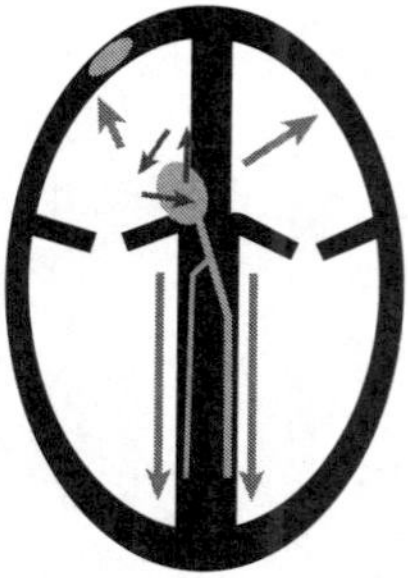

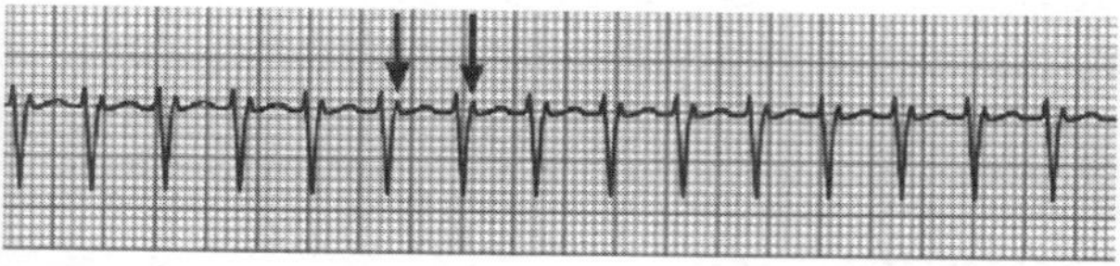

Fig. 11.14 AVNRT. A rapid, regular tachycardia. Usually narrow complex (unless bundle branch aberrancy occurs). Retrograde P wave occur during the QRS complex and are difficult to see, although typically appear as a 'pseudo-R wave' in lead V1 (arrows). Red arrows indicate a compulsory part of the rhythm/circuit; pink arrows indicate bystander (non-participating) pathways.

Treatment

- Tachycardia stops if the re-entrant circuit is interrupted, i.e. AV nodal block:
  - Vagal manoeuvres—carotid sinus massage, Valsalva manoeuvre, ocular pressure, ice application
  - Adenosine IV bolus (see ➲ p.156 for dose and administration)
- If 12 mg or 18 mg adenosine has no effect after being given appropriately, reconsider the diagnosis
- If tachycardia reinitiates immediately after terminating transiently with above treatment, consider IV verapamil/esmolol (caution in hypotension or LV dysfunction) followed by oral verapamil/B-blockers
- Other possible antiarrhythmic drugs:
  - Flecainide, sotalol (consult cardiologist)
- Rarely, DC cardioversion if pharmacological treatment fails or if there is severe haemodynamic compromise

Subsequent management

- First episodes do not usually require prophylactic drug therapy
- Referral for radiofrequency ablation if frequent symptomatic episodes as procedure is low risk and has high success rates (> 90%)

Atrioventricular re-entrant tachycardia

- AVRT is the result of an accessory pathway that connects the atria to the ventricles across the tricuspid or mitral valve annuli
- The AV node is also a critical component of the re-entrant circuit which comprises the AV node, the accessory pathway, and the adjoining atria and ventricular tissue
- Approximately 1/2 of accessory pathways conduct antegradely from the atrium to the ventricles during sinus rhythm, producing ventricular pre-excitation (see Wolff–Parkinson–White syndrome ➲ p.165)
- The remaining 1/2 only conduct retrogradely from ventricles to atria meaning there is no pre-excitation ('concealed' accessory pathways)
- The usual form of tachycardia is antegrade conduction from atria to ventricles through the AV node and bundle branches (with normal ventricular depolarization) and retrograde conduction from the ventricles to the atria through the accessory pathway (orthodromic reciprocating tachycardia, Fig. 11.15)
- Antidromic reciprocating tachycardia (Fig. 11.16) is much less common and results from antegrade conduction from the atria to the ventricles through the accessory pathway and retrograde conduction up through the AV node. Antidromic tachycardia can therefore only occur in those patients with ventricular pre-excitation
- Usually in structurally normal hearts, although there is an association with Ebstein's anomaly and hypertrophic cardiomyopathy

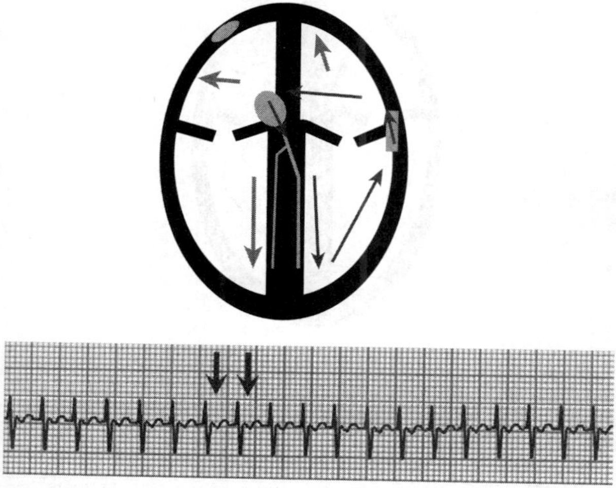

Fig. 11.15 Orthodromic tachycardia. A rapid, regular rhythm. The circuit goes from atrium to ventricle through the AV node and bundle braches so any delta wave disappears and the QRS is narrow (unless there is bundle branch block aberrancy); then from ventricle to atrium through the accessory pathway. The retrograde P wave occurs after the QRS (arrows). Red arrows indicate a compulsory part of the rhythm/circuit; pink arrows indicate bystander (non-participating) pathways.

Presentation

Usual symptoms are rapid palpitations with sudden onset and termination, dyspnoea, chest tightness, and presyncope or, rarely, syncope.

Principle causes and symptoms

Attacks may be precipitated by exertion and physical or emotional stress, but are often spontaneous with no obvious cause.

ECG diagnosis

- Usually regular narrow complex tachycardia
- May be broad complex if there is bundle branch block, rate-related aberrancy, or antidromic AVRT
- Retrograde P waves are often visible in the ST segment (sometimes categorized as a 'long RP tachycardia' when P to R wave shorter than R wave to next P wave). See Figs 11.15 and 11.16; also ➲ ECG, p.414.

Treatment

As for AVNRT (see ➲ p.161)

Subsequent management

- As for AVNRT (see ➲ p.161)
- In patients with ventricular pre-excitation see ➲ p.165

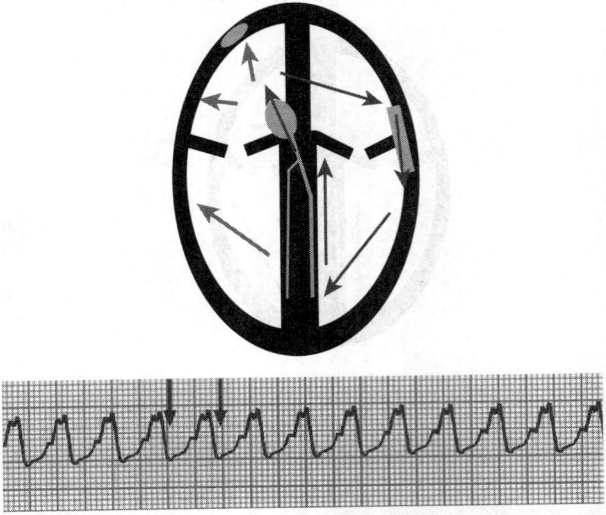

Fig. 11.16 Antidromic tachycardia. Much less common. A rapid, regular rhythm. The circuit goes from atrium to ventricle through the accessory pathway so the ventricle is totally pre-excited and the QRS is very wide; then from ventricle to atrium through the bundle branches and AV node. The retrograde P wave occurs at the end of the QRS (arrows). Red arrows indicate a compulsory part of the rhythm/circuit; pink arrows indicate bystander (non-participating) pathways.

Ventricular pre-excitation and Wolff–Parkinson–White syndrome

- Ventricular pre-excitation occurs when there is an accessory pathway capable of antegrade conduction. A portion of the ventricle becomes activated before AV conduction, which creates the delta wave. This fuses with the normal activation through the AV node, forming the resultant QRS complex (see Fig 11.17 and ➲ p.414)
- The accessory pathway may form part of a re-entrant circuit, resulting in AVRT (➲ p.163)
- WPW syndrome refers to patients with:
  - Ventricular pre-excitation due to an accessory pathway *and*
  - Palpitation 2° to SVT (AVRT)
- The accessory pathway capable of antegrade conduction may also result in atrial activity during atrial tachyarrhythmias being conducted rapidly to the ventricles (e.g. pre-excited AF, see ➲ p.154)

Presentation

- Asymptomatic ventricular pre-excitation
- Symptoms due to AVRT (➲ p.163)
- May be presyncope/syncope/sudden death with pre-excited AF (Fig. 11.18)

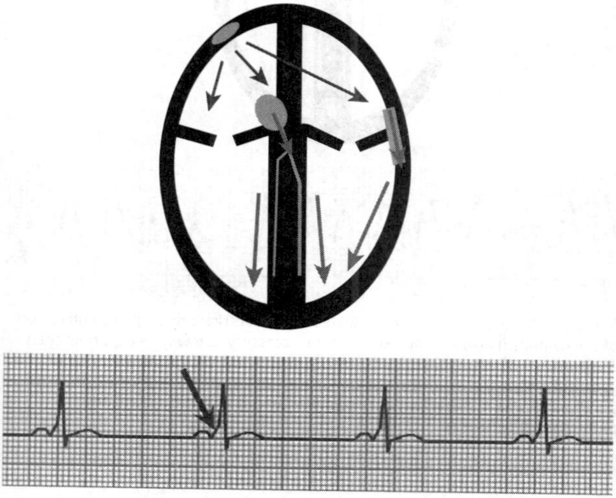

Fig. 11.17 Sinus rhythm and pre-excitation. There is a short PR interval and delta wave at the beginning of the QRS (arrow). Red arrows indicate a compulsory part of the rhythm/circuit; pink arrows indicate bystander (non-participating) pathways.

ECG diagnosis

Ventricular pre-excitation

- Short PR interval (< 5 small squares 0.2 sec)
- Delta wave (slurred onset of QRS) resulting in broader QRS complexes

Prognosis and subsequent management

- Patients with WPW syndrome have an *increased* risk of AF, which can lead to VF
- The risk of sudden death in patients with WPW is about 0.15%/year
- Asymptomatic ventricular pre-excitation has a much better prognosis
- Avoid AV blocking agents in maintenance treatment
- Patients with WPW syndrome should be referred for risk stratification and consideration of electrophysiological studies ± ablation of accessory pathway

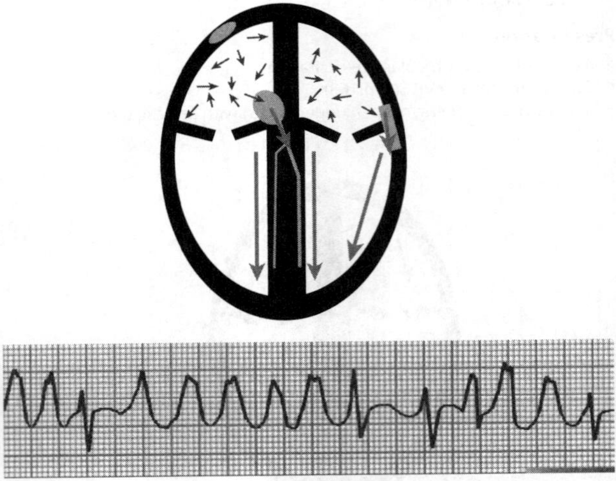

Fig. 11.18 Pre-excited AF. AF is conducted to the ventricles through a combination of the AV node (narrow complexes) and the accessory pathway (wide, pre-excited complexes). The accessory pathway tends to dominate producing a very rapid ventricular rate (➲ p.409). Also see ➲ Management, ➲ p.154. Red arrows indicate a compulsory part of the rhythm/circuit; pink arrows indicate bystander (non-participating) pathways.

Ventricular fibrillation

Presentation

Complete cardiovascular collapse/cardiac arrest.

Causes

- Often 2° to ischaemic heart disease (ACS, MI); structural heart disease (HCM, cardiomyopathies) and ion channelopathies (Brugada syndrome, ➲ p.351)
- Other cardiac precipitants include:
  - Pre-excited AF (➲ p.154, p.409)
  - VT (➲ p.169)
  - Bradycardia/long QT induced torsade de pointes (➲ p.173)
- Non cardiac causes include:
  - Metabolic—severe electrolytes/acid–base disturbance
  - Respiratory—PE, tension pneumothorax
  - Neurology—massive intracranial event

ECG diagnosis

Coarse irregular deflections—varying morphology, amplitude, and frequency (Fig. 11.19).

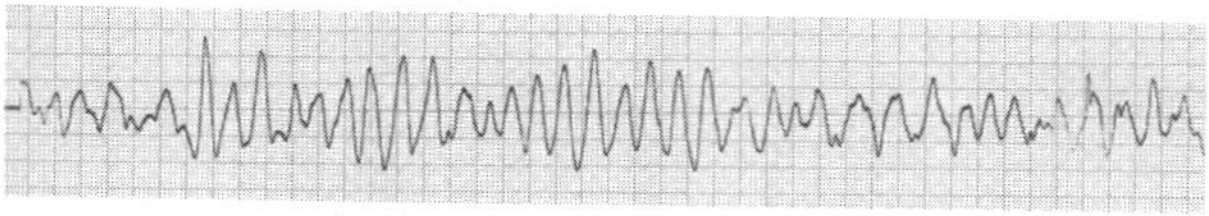

Fig. 11.19 Ventricular fibrillation. There is chaotic electrical activity with no discrete QRS complexes.

Immediate management

- Needs immediate defibrillation using standard ALS algorithms (➲ p.5)
- If VF is resistant to attempts at defibrillation then consider giving amiodarone 300 mg IV and using 2 defibrillators to give rapid sequential shocks
- Treat reversible causes—correct K^+, Mg^{2+}
- Repeated episodes of VF (electrical storms) require specialist input (see ➲ p.175)

Brugada syndrome

A collection of inherited defects in cardiac cell membrane ion channels which cause increased susceptibility to ventricular tachyarrhythmias (VT, VF), and can result in syncope or sudden death. The commonest affected gene is the SCN5A gene, encoding one of the sodium ion channels. The 12-lead ECG can show characteristic features of partial RBBB and right precordial (V1–V3) ST-segment elevation (see ➲ p.408), though there are several variants and some require provocation with sodium-channel blockers (e.g. ajmaline or flecainide) to reveal the changes (N.B. this is a specialized procedure for expert hands!). There is some evidence that environmental factors (e.g. exercise, dehydration) contribute to the arrhythmogenic potential. Implantable defibrillators may be required for selected patients.

Inherited long QT syndrome

A group of inherited defects in cardiomyocyte ion channels (predominantly the potassium channel) which lead to prolongation of the QT interval on the ECG, and a predisposition to ventricular arrhythmias, causing syncope or sudden death. It can be associated with Romano–Ward or Jervell–Lang–Nielsen syndromes. Several ECGs ± ambulatory ECG monitoring may be required for diagnosis. Exercise may be a precipitant for arrhythmias, and strenuous exertion should be avoided. Treatment is with β-blockers to reduce adrenergic drive and propensity to arrhythmias, pacemakers to prevent significant bradycardia, and/or implantable defibrillators. See also ➲ p.313 for drug-induced QT prolongation.

Ventricular tachycardia

VT is usually a re-entrant arrhythmia that results from diseased or scarred myocardium 2° to ischaemic heart disease or non-ischaemic cardiomyopathy. It may also occur in the setting of acute myocardial ischaemia or even a 'normal heart', where the mechanism may result from automaticity or triggered activity (abnormal 'firing' of a ventricular focus). Both ECG features and clinical characteristics can help to differentiate VT from SVT with bundle branch block (see Table 11.8).

- The ventricular rate may be anywhere between 100–300 bpm
- Tachycardia may be sustained (> 30 sec) or non-sustained
- The majority of episodes of VT are monomorphic, i.e. the circuit is consistent and stable and the QRS morphology does not change
- There is a subgroup of idiopathic monomorphic VT (including fascicular and RVOT tachycardia) that are believed to have a more benign prognosis (see Box 11.9)
- Polymorphic VT results in a beat-to-beat variation in QRS morphology and in the setting of a prolonged corrected QT interval (QTc) on the sinus rhythm ECG is called 'torsades de pointes'
- Polymorphic VT usually causes collapse and is more often non-sustained although it may sustain and degenerate into VF

Box 11.9 Other types of ventricular tachycardia

Fascicular VT

- Typically has a QRS of 0.12–0.14 msec
- RBBB and leftward axis
- Usually responds to IV verapamil

RVOT VT

- Typically has a QRS of 0.12–0.15 msec
- LBBB and inferior axis
- Usually respond to β-blocker therapy
- Can respond to IV adenosine

Table 11.8 VT vs SVT with bundle branch block

	Definitely VT	Probably VT	May be SVT with BBB
ECG criteria	AV dissociation Capture or fusion beats	Extreme axis deviation Concordance QRS duration > 160 ms QRS not typical of RBBB/LBBB	Typical RBBB/LBBB QRS morphology and axis identical to that in sinus rhythm
Clinical characteristics	Older patient Known ischaemic or structural heart disease Impaired LV function		Younger patient (< 35 years) Terminated with adenosine/vagal manoeuvres

BBB, bundle branch block

ECG diagnosis of broad complex tachycardia

Δ The differential diagnosis of a regular broad complex tachycardia is:

- VT
- SVT with bundle branch block (BBB), rate-related aberrancy, or antegrade conduction via an accessory pathway

A broad complex tachycardia should be assumed to be VT until proven otherwise. If in doubt, it is safer to mistreat an SVT as VT rather than treat a VT as an SVT.

►80% of broad complex tachycardia will turn out to be VT; this increases to 95% if there is a prior history of MI or IHD.

Always make the diagnosis on a 12-lead ECG, not a rhythm strip.

Clinically, the rate and the degree of haemodynamic compromise are not good discriminators.

- The following clinical characteristics support a diagnosis of VT:
  - Increased age
  - History of ischaemic or structural heart disease
  - Impaired LV function
- The following ECG features suggest VT (Table 11.8, p.169):
  - AV dissociation (P and QRS complexes at different rates)
  - Capture beats (when the sinus node transiently 'captures' the ventricles during AV dissocation, to produce a narrow QRS complex)
  - Fusion beats (when a sinus and ventricular beat coincide to produce a hybrid QRS complex of intermediate width)
  - 'North-west' axis (negative in leads I and II, positive in aVR)
  - Negative or positive concordance in the chest leads
- Typical RBBB/LBBB, especially if the QRS morphology and axis is identical to that in sinus rhythm, is more in keeping with SVT
- Adenosine is sometimes useful for diagnosis (see ➲ p.146)

Monomorphic ventricular tachycardia

Presentation

Symptoms range from none to palpitation, chest pain, and dyspnoea; presyncope to haemodynamic collapse and cardiac arrest.

Principle causes

- Ischaemic heart disease—acute or chronic
- Non-ischaemic cardiomyopathies—DCM, HCM, ARVC
- Idiopathic—fascicular, RVOT

ECG diagnosis

Regular broad complex tachycardia (Fig. 11.20). See ➲ p.169, Table 11.8 for ECG diagnosis of broad complex tachycardia).

Management

- Correct electrolytes (K^+, Mg^+) and treat underlying cause, e.g. MI
- VT that appears well tolerated has the potential to deteriorate rapidly, particularly in patients with known or suspected impairment of LV function

Severe haemodynamic compromise

(Reduced conscious level, pulmonary oedema, cardiac ischaemia, hypotension with poor perfusion.)

- Oxygen
- Immediate synchronized DC shock under sedation/GA
- If pulseless, follow ALS algorithm (➲ p.5)

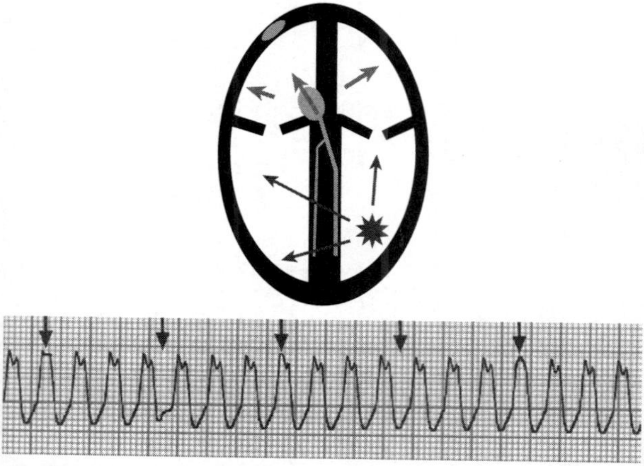

Fig. 11.20 Monomorphic VT. A regular, wide complex tachycardia. The QRS shape is constant although may be distorted by the independent P-wave activity if there is visible AV dissociation (arrows). Red arrows indicate a compulsory part of the rhythm/circuit; pink arrows indicate bystander (non-participating) pathways.

Mild–moderate haemodynamic compromise

(Adequate perfusion, mild chest tightness or SOB, alert and orientated.)

- Only consider adenosine if the arrhythmia is well tolerated and there is a high likelihood of SVT based on history or ECG
- Inform anaesthetist and prepare for back-up synchronized DC cardioversion
- In the meantime, attempt cardioversion with:
    - IV β-blockers or amiodarone
    - Consider lidocaine if BP stable

For recurrent episodes of VT, see ➲ Electrical storm ➲ p.175.

Subsequent management

- Cardiac investigations, e.g. echocardiography, coronary angiography, cardiac MRI
- Consider maintenance drug therapy with β-blockers and/or amiodarone
- In cases of RVOT or fascicular VT (➲ p.169, Box 11.9), consider verapamil
- ICD therapy may be indicated
- Catheter ablation for VT may be an option

Polymorphic ventricular tachycardia/ 'torsades de pointes'

Torsades de pointes is associated with long QTc, bradycardia, or pauses and is typically initiated following 'R on T' ectopic phenomenon.

Presentation

- Usually haemodynamic collapse/cardiac arrest if sustained
- May still be cardiovascularly stable if episodes are non-sustained

Causes

- Congenital—long QT syndrome (see ➲ p.349)
- Drugs—see Box 11.10 and ➲ p.313
- Electrolyte abnormalities—low K^+, low Mg^{2+}
- Bradycardia/pause-induced
- Myocardial ischaemia
- Others—significant metabolic derangement, subarachnoid haemorrhage

Box 11.10 Common QT prolonging drugs (see ➲ p.349)

- Antiarrhythmic drugs—class I agents, sotalol
- Antimicrobials—macrolides, moxifloxacin, ketoconazole
- Psychiatric drugs—phenothiazines, tricyclic antidepressants, lithium

ECG diagnosis

- Irregular broad complex tachycardia (Fig. 11.21)
- Regular variation of QRS morphology and axis ('twisting of the point' about the isoelectric baseline)

Immediate management (Fig. 11.22)

Haemodynamic collapse is usually present or imminent if the arrhythmia is sustained. Urgent DC cardioversion is indicated. If pulseless, follow ALS algorithm (➲ p.5).

Even if conscious and stable, or polymorphic VT is repetitive and non-sustained, prompt treatment is required as patients may deteriorate quickly:

- Check and correct electrolytes, especially Mg^+, K^+ (aim > 4.5 mmol/L)
- Treat possible underlying causes simultaneously, e.g. cardiac ischaemia

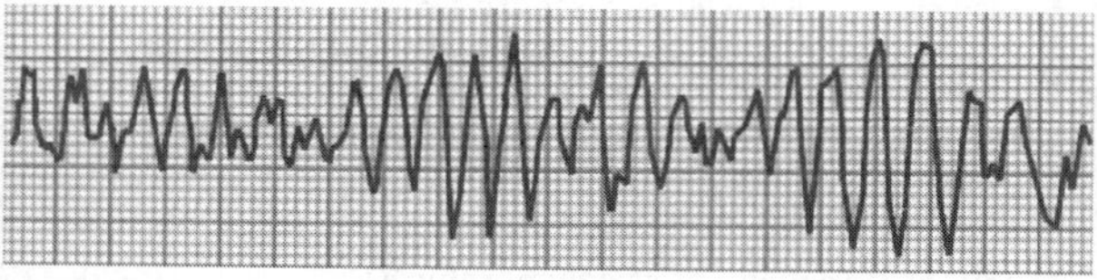

Fig. 11.21 Polymorphic VT. An irregular, broad complex tachycardia. With torsades des pointes QRS axis twists around the baseline.

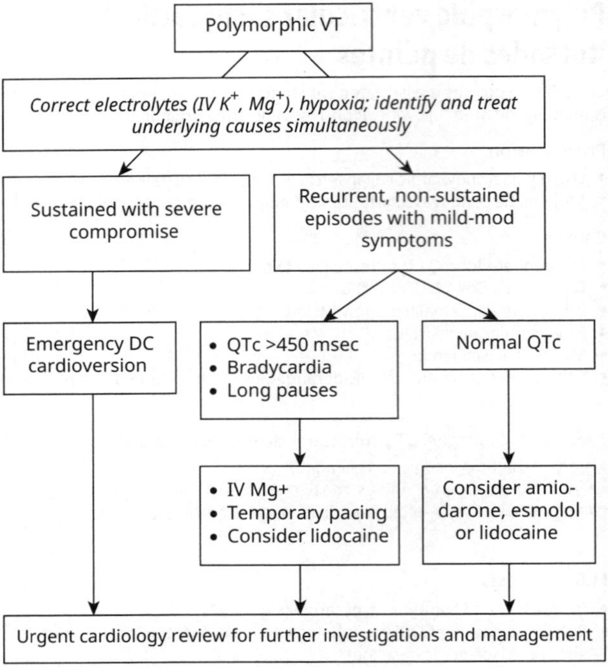

Fig. 11.22 Flowchart of management of polymorphic VT.

- If there is evidence of bradycardia/pause-initiated VT or if QTc in sinus rhythm > 0.45 msec, treatment is geared towards increasing heart rate and reducing QTc:
  - Stop any precipitating drugs
  - IV magnesium is useful even if there is no hypomagnesaemia—give 1–2 g (4–8 mmol) over 5–10 min in 100 mL 5% dextrose, then 0.5–1 g/hour infusion
  - Consider atropine/isoprenaline as a temporary measure
  - Temporary pacing at 90 bpm (see ➲ p.175)
- Amiodarone is contraindicated if sinus rhythm QTc is prolonged
- If the sinus rhythm QTc is normal and no bradycardia (in this case, usually due to myocardial ischaemia or obvious systemic cause):
  - Consider IV amiodarone or esmolol
  - Lidocaine can also be considered

Subsequent management of polymorphic VT

- Potassium should be kept > 4.5 mmol/L
- Avoid QT prolonging drugs
- Seek urgent cardiology review
- ICD therapy may be needed

Electrical storms

Seek early expert cardiology advice.

- VT or VF electrical storms are characterized by multiple, frequent, repetitive episodes of VT or VF, usually associated with significant haemodynamic compromise

Immediate management

- Correct the correctable—electrolytes, myocardial ischaemia, drug intoxication
- Sedation with anaesthetist cover, often requires intubation and ventilation to alleviate distress, increase oxygen delivery, and reduce the hyper-adrenergic state that may accompany repeated cardioversion
- Episodes may need to be terminated by repeated electrical cardioversions
- Antiarrhythmic drugs should be given, often > 1 is necessary:
  - IV amiodarone and β-blockade are the mainstays of treatment
  - Alternative antiarrhythmic therapies include lidocaine or procainamide as an IV infusion (see ➲ p.146)

► Amiodarone/sotalol/procainamide should be avoided in torsade des pointes 2° to prolonged QTc

- Temporary pacing for overdrive and antitachycardia pacing (see Box 11.11)

Box 11.11 Overdrive pacing

- Sustained monomorphic VT may be terminated painlessly by antitachycardia pacing in 80–90% of cases
- In patients with an implantable cardioverter defibrillator with VT below the treatment zone, manual anti-tachycardia pacing can be undertaken using the device programmer
- In other patients, placement of a temporary transvenous pacing wire in the right ventricle is necessary (➲ p.364)
- Pacing is performed at a rate 15–20 bpm faster than the VT
- On many temporary pacing boxes there is a '× 3' setting on the rate for this reason
- A high output (5–10 V) may be required
- Capture of the VT is indicated by a change in QRS morphology and an increase in heart rate on the monitor to the pacing rate
- Pacing is abruptly terminated after 5–10 sec of ventricular capture
- There is a risk that acceleration of the VT may occur with degeneration to pulseless VT or VF so operators must be prepared for immediate defibrillation
- Once sinus rhythm has been restored, constant background pacing at 90–110 bpm may be performed to prevent recurrent attacks. This is particularly useful with polymorphic VT and a prolonged QT interval, especially in the setting of pauses or bradycardia
- Constant ventricular pacing may result in low cardiac output due to the loss of AV synchrony, particularly in the setting of poor LV function. This may be overcome with dual chamber AV sequential pacing

Subsequent management

- Seek urgent cardiology advice
- If there is ongoing cardiac ischaemia, consider insertion of IABP ± coronary intervention
- Rarely, it is necessary to put patients on bypass/ECMO to allow electrical storm to settle

Implantable cardioverter defibrillators in the emergency room

ICDs are increasingly being implanted in certain patients (esp. ischaemic cardiomyopathy) to reduce the risk of sudden death due to ventricular tachyarrhythmia. They are programmed to recognize ventricular rates that exceed programmed parameters and are also able to deliver antitachycardia pacing (ATP), which is painless, or shocks (which can be painful) within seconds of the tachycardia commencing.

- It is common to programme ICDs to attempt ATP for VT that is more likely to be haemodynamically tolerated, e.g. rates between 150–190 bpm. Shocks will be delivered if ATP fails or the VT accelerates
- Fast VT (> 190 bpm) or VF is often treated by shock therapy
- ICDs can deliver up to 6 shocks during a single VT or VF episode; however, if sinus rhythm is transiently restored the counter returns to zero and recommences if VT or VF reinitiates
- Although ICDs try to distinguish between SVT and VT, if the device is uncertain, it will always assume the worst and treat as if it is VT. Patients may therefore receive inappropriate shocks for sinus or atrial tachycardias with rapid ventricular rates

Presentation

- Usually well between shocks
- In addition to experiencing shocks, patients may be unwell with chest pain, dyspnoea, syncope, fever, etc

Immediate management (Fig. 11.23)

- A magnet can be used to disable ICD shocks if necessary (see Box 11.12)
- Patients who are completely well after 1 isolated shock do not require hospital admission, particularly if this is not the first time. They can be seen in the ICD clinic within a few days
- It is important to exclude possible exacerbating causes especially for patients with multiple shocks or additional symptoms
    - Correct electrolytes, thyroid status
    - Treat myocardial ischaemia, sepsis, etc
- Interrogation of the ICD is then useful to determine if shocks are:
    - Appropriate (therapy for ventricular tachyarrhythmia) *or*
    - Inappropriate (device or lead failure, failure to recognize sinus/atrial tachyarrhythmia)

Box 11.12 Use of a magnet

ICD shocks may be disabled by placing a magnet over the generator and securing with tape. This may be useful with repetitive inappropriate shocks due to device or lead failure or rapidly conducted atrial arrhythmias. It may also be appropriate as a temporary measure during electrical storms when VT is haemodynamically tolerated but resulting in frequent painful therapies.

The patient must be monitored once a magnet is used as episodes of VF will not be treated by the ICD. The magnet does not disable the bradycardia functions of the ICD.

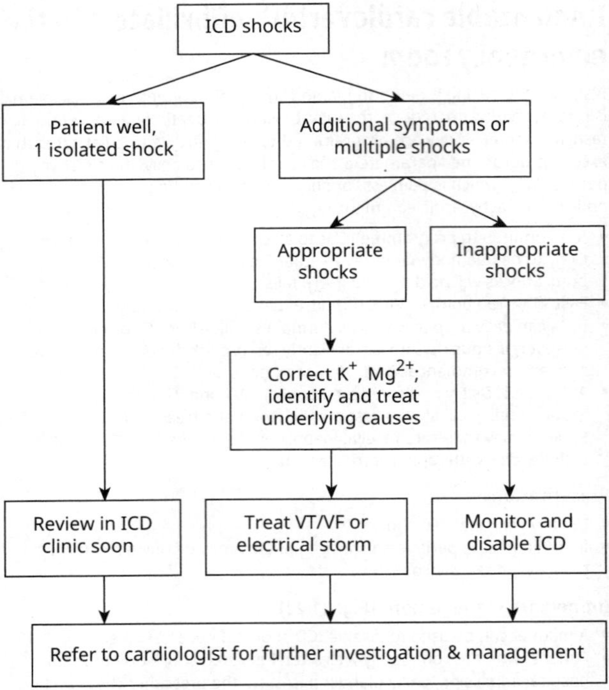

Fig. 11.23 Flowchart of the management of patients presenting with shocks from their ICD.

- Patients with inappropriate shocks should be monitored and the ICD may need to be temporarily disabled via the programmer whilst the underlying cause is addressed
- Patients with multiple appropriate shocks should be treated for electrical storm (Electrical storms, ➲ p.175). It is often useful to temporarily disable the ICD with a magnet (Box 11.12)

Subsequent management

- Refer to cardiologist—may need new leads, programming changes, etc
- Patients with appropriate shocks usually require drug changes

Chapter 12

Aortic dissection

Introduction

A tear in the aortic intima through which blood enters the aortic wall and strips the media from the adventitia.

- The dissection may result in fatal aortic rupture or propagate distally generating a blood-filled space between the dissected layers
- The blood supply to major branches (including the coronary arteries) may be compromised
- If the aortic root is involved, the aortic valve may become incompetent and retrograde propagation to the pericardium may result in cardiac tamponade
- The commonest site for aortic dissection is in the proximal ascending aorta within a few centimetres of the aortic valve or in the descending aorta just distal to the left subclavian artery. See Box 12.1 for causes
- Classification is usually made according to the Stanford classification (Fig. 12.1) that influences subsequent management:

Type A aortic dissection involves the ascending aorta and management is usually a surgical emergency. Don't dawdle! (Fig 12.2)

Type B aortic dissection spares the ascending aorta and management is initially medical (Fig 12.3)

Box 12.1 Causes and associations

- Hypertension (70%)
- Bicuspid aortic valve (7–14%)
- Marfan syndrome (5–9%) (➲ p.193), Box 12.5
- Aortic coarctation (➲ p.247)
- Trauma—particularly deceleration injury
- Iatrogenic—angiography

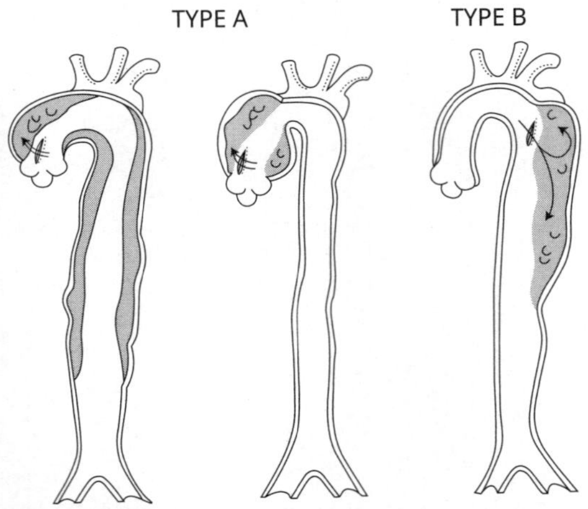

Fig. 12.1 Stanford classification of aortic dissection. Type A: all dissections involving the ascending aorta. Type B dissection does not involve the ascending aorta.

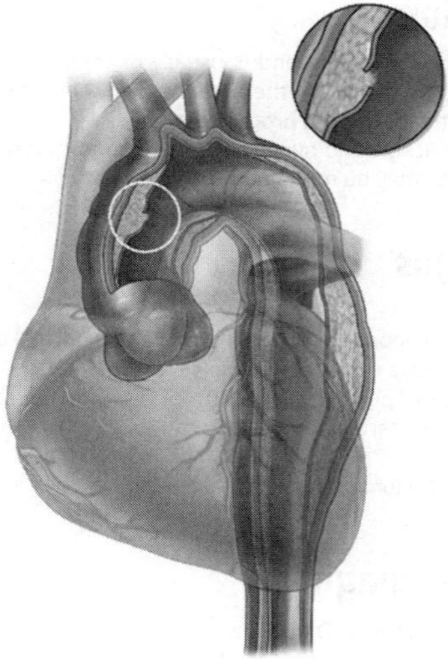

Fig. 12.2 Type A: the dissection involves the ascending aorta with or without involvement of the arch and the descending aorta.

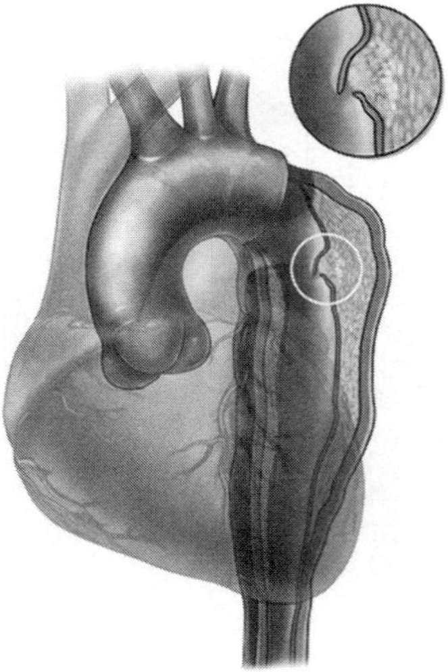

Fig. 12.3 Type B: the dissection involves the descending aorta (distal to the left subclavian artery).

Presentation

The cardinal symptom is *pain* and is usually instantaneous, of cataclysmic severity, pulsatile or tearing, in the anterior thorax or interscapular region, and migrates as the dissection propagates.

The history ± background hypertension are important for suspecting the diagnosis, as signs may be minimal.

Clinical signs

- There may be none
- The patient may appear shocked, but BP can be normal or elevated
- Pulmonary oedema can occur due to severe AR
- Absent or reduced pulses occur in 20% of patients (but can fluctuate)
- Signs of AR or pericardial tamponade can occur in type A aortic dissection
- A left pleural effusion is occasionally seen

Differential diagnosis

- Intramural haematoma (➲ p.195)
- Penetrating atherosclerotic ulcer (➲ p.196)
- Acute coronary syndromes (➲ p.47)

Risk scores

The Aortic Dissection Detection (ADD) risk score (Fig 12.4) stratifies patients according to risk markers relevant to:

- Pre-existing high risk conditions (such as aortopathies, family history of aortic disease)
- High-risk pain features (abrupt onset, severe, and ripping or tearing), and

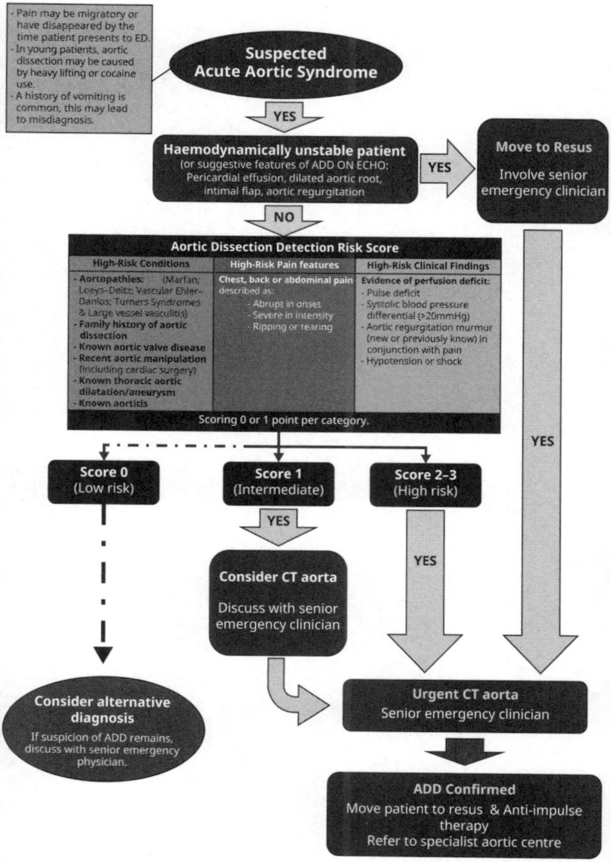

Fig. 12.4 Aortic Dissection Detection (ADD) risk score adapted with permission from NHS England Southwest Supra-regional SOP on the acute management of aortic dissection.

- High-risk exam features (perfusion / pulse deficits, differential blood pressure, neurological features, murmur, shock)

Intermediate and high-risk scores should guide urgent CT aortogram of high quality (i.e. ECG gated or using fast scan protocol, 2 mm slices, extent to include common carotid arteries proximally to common femoral arteries distally) to confirm or exclude an aortic dissection.

Investigations

CXR

- An abnormal aortic silhouette appears in up to 90% of cases (N.B. 10% of CXRs will appear normal)
- Separation of the intimal calcification that occurs in the aortic knob by > 1 cm (the 'calcium sign') is suggestive of aortic dissection
- Left-sided pleural effusions can occur and are more common with descending dissections

ECG

- Non-specific ST and T wave changes are common
- ECG changes of LV hypertrophy may occur in patients with long-standing hypertension
- Coronary artery involvement is uncommon but more commonly affects the right coronary artery (resulting in inferior ST elevation)

Blood tests

See Box 12.2.

Box 12.2 Blood tests

- May delay diagnosis so do not await results before arranging further imaging.
- Blood should be taken for FBC, D-dimer, creatinine, cardiac enzymes, and group and save
- A mildly raised white cell count is common
- Haemoglobin level may be reduced if there has been a significant bleed
- Lactate dehydrogenase can be elevated if there has been significant haemolysis
- D-dimers are usually elevated and can increase the pre-test probability of the aortic dissection detection score
- Cardiac troponin levels may be elevated and are associated with a worse in-hospital outcome
- Immunoassays of monoclonal antibodies to smooth muscle myosin heavy chains have a high sensitivity and specificity for the diagnosis of aortic dissection but are rarely available in the time required

Imaging

Imaging should be performed as quickly as possible using the most accessible and accurate modality that your hospital can provide. This is usually with CT and TTE. Aspects to look for are:

- The entry site of the dissection—ideally, but not always seen
- If the aortic valve is competent
- If there is a pericardial effusion or tamponade
- Any involvement of the coronary arteries

Computed tomography

With modern multi-slice scanners, CT has a sensitivity and specificity of 96–100% and is the standard investigation for suspected aortic dissection.

Magnetic resonance imaging

Sensitivity and specificity of nearly 100%. Non-invasive. Availability and reduced access to an unwell patient are the main limitations on its use. See Fig. 12.5.

Transoesophageal echocardiography

Useful for imaging the proximal ascending aorta, identifying involvement of coronary ostia, and examining the aortic valve (Fig. 12.6). Sensitivity of 98% and specificity of 95%. Patients usually require sedation. It is usually performed immediately prior to surgery after surgical consent has been obtained.

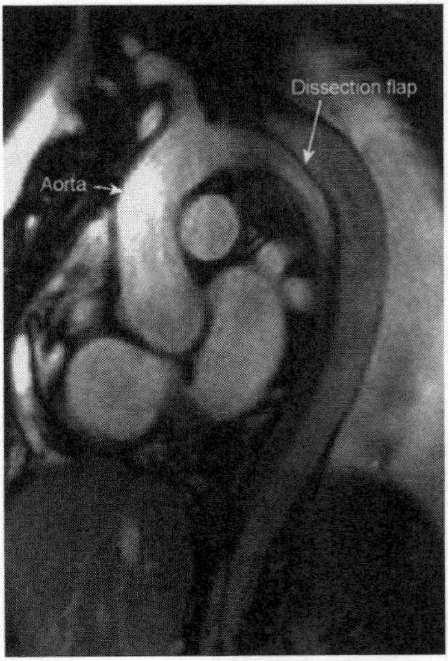

Fig. 12.5 MRI of a type B aortic dissection. There is a dissection flap in the descending aorta.

Transthoracic echocardiography

Can determine the involvement of the aortic valve, LV function, and identify pericardial effusions. Sensitivity of 59–85% and specificity of 63–96% for identifying dissection.

A normal transthoracic echocardiogram does not exclude aortic dissection.

Aortography

Invasive procedure with associated risks. Requires contrast material and takes time to perform. Sensitivity of 77–88% and specificity of 94%. It is now rarely performed as other imaging techniques are quicker and safer.

Coronary angiography

Not routinely performed in patients with aortic dissection. Chronic coronary disease is seen in a quarter of patients with aortic dissection, but this has not been shown to have a significant impact on outcome.

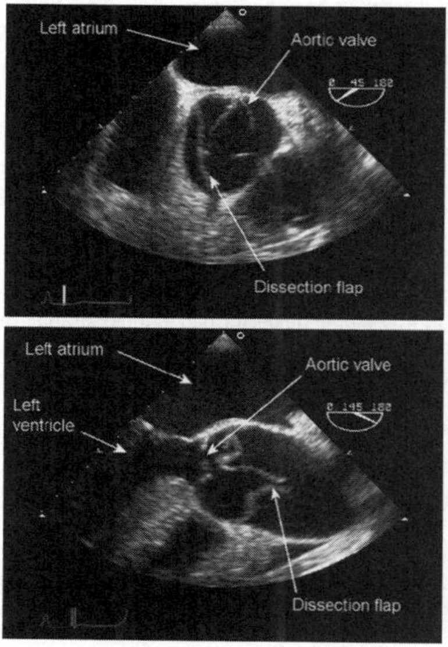

Fig. 12.6 TOE showing a type A aortic dissection. Just above the aortic valve in the proximal ascending aorta is a dissection flap. Top: transverse view. Bottom: longitudinal view.

Management

Immediate management

- Opiate analgesia should be given to eliminate pain
- Anti-impulse therapy to lower systolic BP to < 120 mmHg and heart rate < 80 bpm to prevent propagation of the dissection and rupture
- Intravenous β-blockers are the traditional first-line therapies (see Box 12.3)
- IV isosorbide dinitrate and oral nifedipine are alternatives in patients with contraindications to β-blockers but can increase heart rate

Box 12.3 IV antihypertensive therapy

- Labetalol is a β-blocker with α-blocking effects at high doses. It is given as an IV injection of 50 mg over 1 min followed by a continuous infusion of 1–2 mg/min.
- Esmolol is a short-acting β-blocker. It is administered as a bolus of 500 mcg/kg and as an infusion of 50–200 mcg/kg/min.
- Propranolol is given as an IV injection of 1 mg over 1 min and repeated every 5 min until an adequate response has been achieved or a total of 10 mg has been given. Additional propranolol should then be given every 4 hours.
- Sodium nitroprusside is given as an infusion of 0.5–1.5 mcg/kg/min increasing in steps of 0.5 mcg/kg/min every 5 min. Dose range 0.5–8 mcg/kg/min. It is usually given with a β-blocker to prevent reflex tachycardia.

- In hypotensive patients, it is important to exclude pericardial tamponade and check the BP in both arms before commencing fluid resuscitation
- Pericardiocentesis should be performed in the operating theatre if possible as it can precipitate irretrievable haemodynamic collapse
- Cross-match blood (at least 6 units)
- Urinary catheter and monitoring of urine output
- Transfer patient to ICU for close observation

Subsequent management of Type A aortic dissection

- *Type A* aortic dissections (involving the ascending aorta) should be considered for emergency surgery
- Discuss type A dissections with the cardiothoracic team
- Surgery usually involves excision of the intimal tear in the ascending aorta and interposition of a graft
- Where possible, preservation of the root with resuspension of the aortic valve is recommended (Fig 12.7)
- In those cases where a safe reconstruction of the proximal dissected segment cannot be achieved, aortic root replacement (modified Bentall procedure) is indicated (Fig 12.8)

Subsequent management of type B aortic dissection

- *Type B* aortic dissections are usually managed medically
- Surgery for type B dissections should be considered if there is evidence of proximal extension, progressive aortic enlargement, or ischaemic

complications from major branch artery involvement, though is rarely undertaken as an emergency
- Surgical risk is high, with paraplegia from spinal artery damage a particular concern

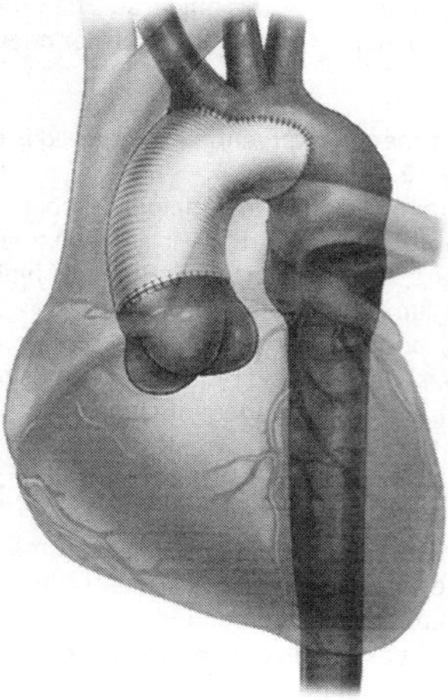

Fig. 12.7 Ascending aorta and hemiarch replacement.

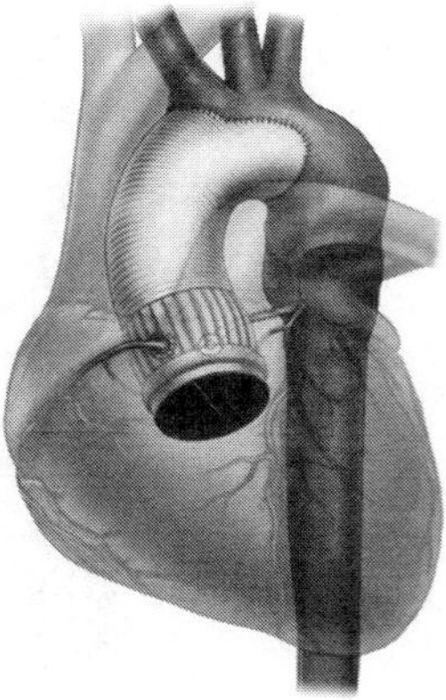

Fig. 12.8 Aortic root, ascending aorta, and hemiarch replacement.

Box 12.4 Endovascular aortic stenting

Endovascular stenting is a percutaneous procedure that may be considered for aortic dissection starting distal to the left subclavian artery or to treat the complications of penetrating aortic ulcers. A large covered stent can be delivered within the descending aorta to cover the intimal tear (Fig. 12.10). In suitable cases this obliterates flow into the false lumen, relieving branch ischaemia and preventing further aneurysmal dilatation.

- An alternative treatment if intervention is required is endovascular stenting—see Box 12.4 and Fig. 12.4
- Patients with contained rupture and malperfusion in type B dissections are defined as 'complicated' and thoracic endovascular repair (TEVAR) is the standard of care, especially in the presence of high-risk features such as increased false lumen and total aortic diameter (> 22 mm and > 40 mm, respectively), primary entry >10 mm
- Suitable anatomy is essential and retrograde extension of a type B dissection into the arch or an inadequate landing zone, may necessitate open surgical repair (± second-stage endovascular procedure) that could include the arch, if involved, such as the frozen elephant trunk technique (Fig. 12.9)
- For those patients with absence of high-risk features, optimal medical therapy, and close surveillance with CT for early detection of adverse morphological features is recommended
- Contact the local tertiary cardiac centre for advice about type B dissection management if necessary

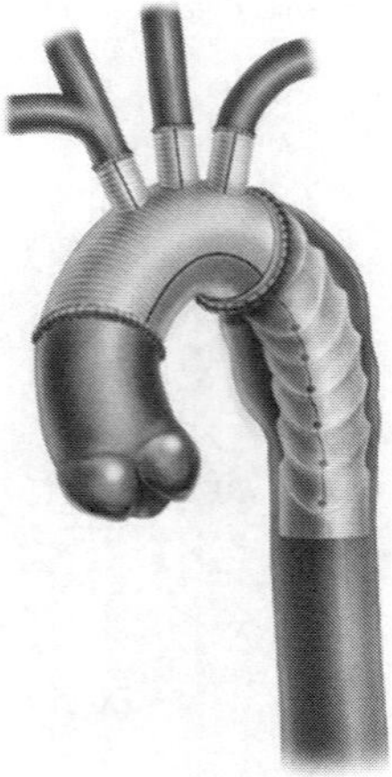

Fig. 12.9 Total aortic arch replacement with the frozen elephant trunk technique

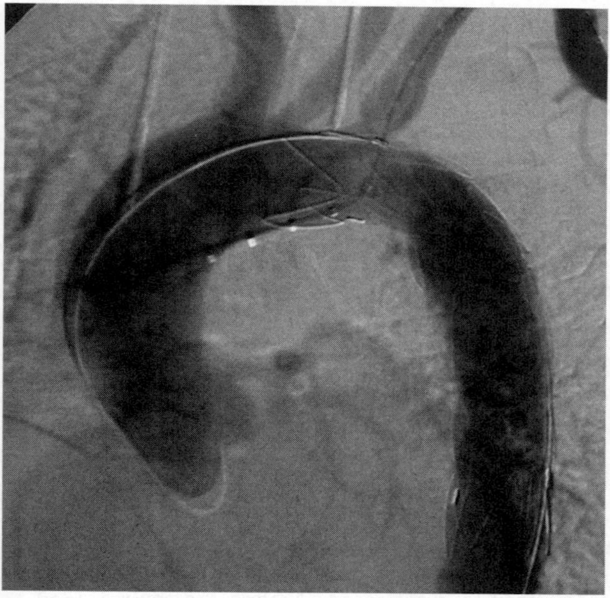

Fig. 12.10 Aortography during implantation of a covered stent in a patient with limited rupture of the descending aorta. The stent is carefully positioned just distal to the left subclavian artery.

Complications

Type A dissection

- Death from aortic rupture
- Myocardial ischaemia/infarction
- Pericardial tamponade
- Aortic valve incompetence
- Cerebrovascular event

Type B dissection

- Visceral ischaemia
- Limb ischaemia
- Renal failure

Prognosis

- The mortality from aortic dissection is initially as high as 1% per hour within the first 48 hours
- The in-hospital mortality for type B aortic dissection is correlated to the aortic diameter
- The surgical mortality is about 10–15% for type A dissection and slightly higher for type B
- The long-term survival for patients with either surgically treated type A or medically-treated type B dissections is about 75% at 5 years
- The false lumen commonly remains patent during long-term follow-up
- For patients who survive an aortic dissection, long-term medical therapy is essential to reduce the risk of aortic expansion and dissection recurrence
- The primary goal is to control blood pressure and reduce the mechanical stress on the aortic wall

Follow-up

- Long-term oral antihypertensive therapy should be initiated to maintain a systolic BP < 120/80 mmHg
- Drug therapies include β-blockers (reduces aortic wall stress by decreasing the force of contraction and heart rate), ACE inhibitors and angiotensin receptor blockers, as well as calcium antagonists
- Surveillance is recommended for all patients using the imaging modality with which there is the most local expertise, particularly in the first 2 years after presentation
- Surgery or endovascular stenting should be considered if there is evidence of progressive aortic enlargement

Box 12.5 Marfan syndrome

- Autosomal dominant connective tissue disease with a prevalence of at least 1 in 10,000
- Common cardiovascular features include:
  - Mitral valve prolapse (75%)
  - Dilatation of the aortic sinuses (90%)
- Aortic dilatation is usually limited to the proximal ascending aorta (Fig. 12.11) with loss of the sinotubular junction and a flask-shape appearance

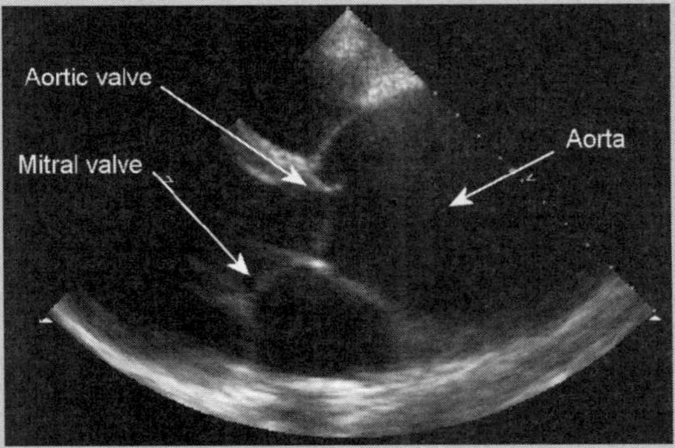

Fig. 12.11 TTE of an enlarged ascending aorta in a patient with Marfan syndrome

- AR is common when the aorta reaches 50 mm in diameter (normal diameter < 40 mm)
- The risk of dissection increases with the diameter of the aorta but occurs relatively infrequently below a diameter of 55 mm. Aortic dissection in Marfan syndrome is usually type A and begins just above

(Continued)

Box 12.5 (*Contd.*)

the coronary ostia. 10% of cases begin distal to the left subclavian artery (type B)

- Long-term β-blockade has been shown to reduce the rate of aortic dilatation and reduce the risk of aortic dissection
- Angiotensin receptor blockers such as losartan can reduce aortic dilatation
- Surgery is usually considered when the aorta reaches 50 mm

Weblink

The Marfan Foundation: www.marfan.org

Acute thoracic syndromes

See Fig. 12.12.

Intramural haematoma

- The result of haemorrhage within the media and adventitia of the aortic wall. The aortic intima remains intact
- Believed to be due to rupture of the aortic vasa vasorum
- Presentation can mimic aortic dissection
- Patients are typically elderly, with a history of hypertension and many have aortic atherosclerosis
- The diagnosis is made by excluding an intimal tear
- CT or MRI is the investigation of choice. A non-contrast-enhancing crescent along the aortic wall with no false lumen or associated atherosclerotic ulcer is usually demonstrated

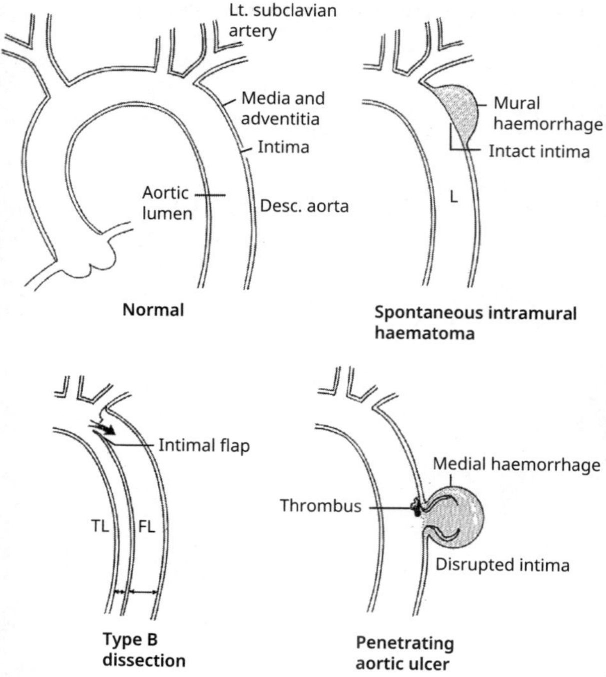

Fig. 12.12 Acute thoracic syndromes. An intramural haematoma is characterized by an intact intima. Type B aortic dissection usually starts distal to the left subclavian artery. A penetrating aortic ulcer involves a disrupted intima and haemorrhage into the media.

- There is evidence that an intramural haematoma may be a precursor of aortic dissection
- Treat as for aortic dissection with analgesia and IV antihypertensive agents
- Surgery is indicated when the ascending aorta is involved

Penetrating atherosclerotic ulcer

- Ulceration of an atherosclerotic lesion of the aorta that penetrates the elastic lamina of the aorta allowing haematoma formation within the media
- Usually in the descending aorta in elderly smokers
- Clinical presentation is similar to aortic dissection with chest or back pain
- In up to 25% of cases, penetration through to the adventitia results in false aneurysm formation and transmural aortic rupture occurs in up to 10% of cases
- CT or cardiac MR is used for diagnosis
- Standard treatment is surgery, but this is not often required and there has been increasing success with endovascular stenting

Chapter 13

Pericardial disease

Pericarditis

- Inflammation of the layers of the pericardium
- Characterized by typical chest pain often with particular ECG changes
- Sometimes associated with pericardial effusion (rarely tamponade) or inflammation of the adjacent myocardium (peri-myocarditis)
- Often idiopathic
- Usually self-limiting and benign, but can recur

Causes

Infections

- Viral, e.g. coxsackievirus, parvovirus B19, Epstein Barr virus, COVID-19—may be viral prodrome
- Bacterial, e.g. *Mycobacterium tuberculosis, Borrelia burgdorferi*

Non-infectious

- Uraemia
- Hypothyroidism
- Autoimmune—SLE, rheumatoid arthritis
- Post-cardiac injury—post MI (acute or Dressler syndrome if within 2–8 weeks), post-cardiac surgery or intervention, e.g. ablation
- Cancer-related—either metastasis (lung/breast cancer or lymphoma) or after radiotherapy or immune checkpoint inhibitor treatment
- Trauma

Presentation

- Chest pain—retrosternal, can be sharp or ache, often pleuritic or positional (worse lying flat), can radiate to shoulder/scapula/back
- Mild breathlessness
- History of recent febrile illness or associated autoimmune conditions or recent cardiac procedure

Clinical signs

- May be none
- Often uncomfortable with mild sinus tachycardia
- Pericardial rub—friction between 2 inflamed pericardial layers, 'footsteps in snow' crunching sound in time with cardiac cycle

Investigations

ECG (can be normal in 10%)

—2 main patterns due to inflammation of the epicardium/adjacent myocardium (Fig. 13.1):

1. 'Scooped' or 'saddle-shaped' ST elevation in several leads; may not correspond to coronary artery distribution
2. Non-specific T-wave inversion

Look for PR segment depression. It is highly specific for pericarditis and believed to be due to underlying atrial myocarditis.

Blood tests—FBC, CRP, ESR, U&E (? uraemia), thyroid function (? hypothyroid), troponin—may be raised in pericarditis; more common if ECG changes and represents peri-myocarditis

CXR—consider to assess cardiothoracic ratio, or signs of pleural as well as pericardial inflammation

Echo—should be considered in all patients with acute pericarditis, but in particular those who are unwell (? pericardial effusion or poor LV function) or who have significantly elevated cardiac troponins (? myocarditis) or if there is diagnostic uncertainty. Small-moderate pericardial effusions usually resolve with standard treatment.

Cardiac MRI—can show thickened and inflamed pericardium, pericardial effusion and myocardial inflammation, but is usually reserved for resistant or recurrent cases

Diagnostic clues

- Positional element to symptoms unusual in ACS
- Patients often younger with few coronary risk factors
- Widespread ECG changes without reciprocal changes
- Troponin is not specific to either peri-myocarditis or ACS—can be significantly elevated in inflammation

Management

- Acute uncomplicated pericarditis—first-line treatment is with anti-inflammatories (colchicine 500 mcg BD for 3 months plus ibuprofen 800 mg TDS for 1–2 weeks)
- If resistant to baseline treatment (no improvement after 4–6 weeks), or recurrent episodes (further episode after freedom for symptoms for > 4 weeks), consider prednisolone 0.2–0.5 mg/kg per day for 2–4 weeks added to colchicine for 6 months
- May be a role for an IL-1 receptor blocker, e.g. anakinra if difficult or recurrent episodes

When to ask for help

Specialist advice should be sought if there is evidence of cardiogenic shock, myocarditis, immunosuppression or use of immunotherapy, trauma or anticoagulation, or more than a small pericardial effusion

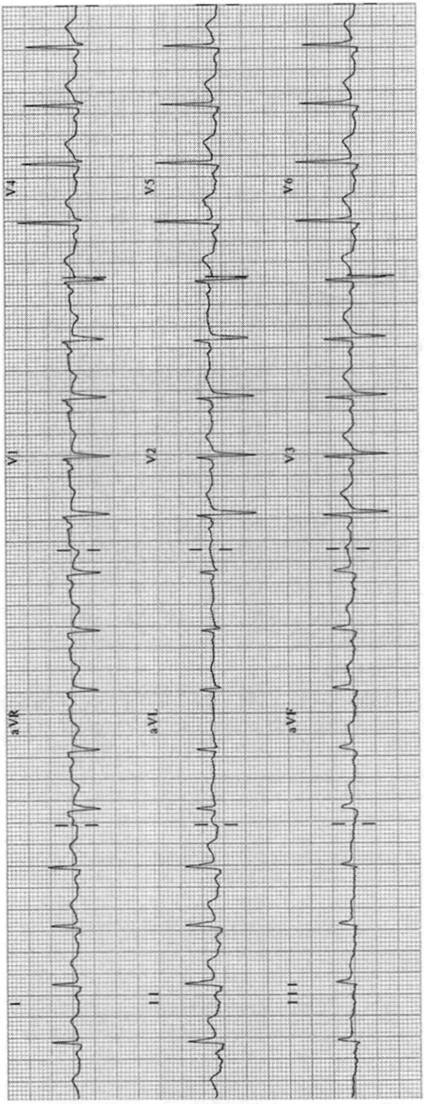

Fig. 13.1 Characteristic ECG changes of pericarditis.

Pericardial effusion and tamponade

Pericardial effusion: abnormal fluid accumulation in the pericardial sac

Cardiac tamponade: when a pericardial effusion causes haemodynamic compromise by restricting cardiac filling—usually occurs when fluid accumulates fairly fast, so even a very big pericardial effusion does not necessarily cause tamponade

Causes of pericardial effusion

- Inflammation (acute or chronic pericarditis as above)
- Trauma (injury to myocardium, aorta or coronary vessels)
- Post-MI: acute—free wall rupture; chronic—Dressler syndrome
- Type A aortic dissection
- Malignancy
- Post cardiac procedures, e.g. pacemaker, PCI or ablation
- Heart, liver, or renal failure

Presentation (depends on cause)

- Can be asymptomatic (identified on imaging for another indication)
- Chest pain
- Symptoms of heart failure (breathlessness, peripheral/abdominal swelling, fatigue)
- Light headedness
- History of recent procedure/trauma or relevant comorbidity

Clinical signs

- All signs below indicate some degree of haemodynamic compromise
- Tachycardia
- Hypotension with low-pulse pressure
- Jugular venous distension
- Muffled heart sounds (with hypotension and raised JVP = Beck's triad)
- Pulsus paradoxus (drop in systolic BP by > 10 mmHg during inspiration—exaggeration of normal physiology due to greater dependence of cardiac output on filling pressures)

Investigations

ECG—sinus tachycardia, reduced voltage due to pericardial fluid between myocardium and skin, 'pulsus alternans'—changing axis of ECG as heart swings around in fluid

CXR—increased CTR, globular heart with straight left heart border

Echo—confirms the presence of a pericardial effusion but also allows assessment of the haemodynamic impact (Box 13.1, Fig. 13.2)

Box 13.1 Echocardiographic signs suggesting tamponade

- Collapse/partial collapse of right atrium during systole
- Right ventricular collapse during diastole
- Septal deflection to left during inspiration, and right during exhalation
- Dilated IVC with no respiratory variation
- Exaggerated flow across mitral valve during exhalation and tricuspid valve during inspiration

A—parasternal long axis view); with haemodynamic signs of tamponade. B—RV diastolic collapse (parasternal short axis view. C—exaggerated variation in mitral valve inflow Doppler with inspiration. D—dilated IVC with no respiratory variation).

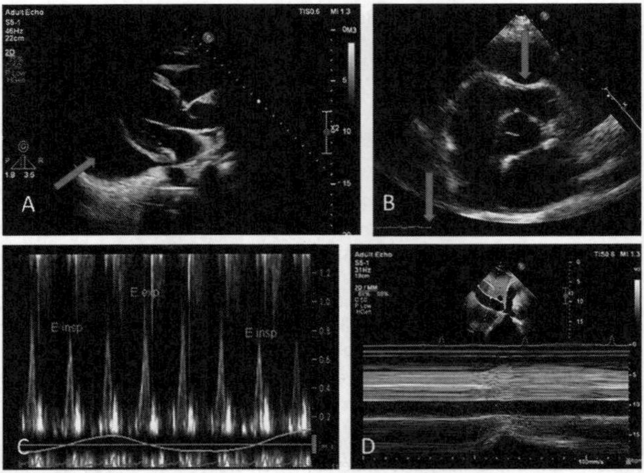

Fig. 13.2 Echo appearances of large pericardial effusion.

Management

- Driven by the clinical state of the patient
- If no signs of haemodynamic compromise, even large pericardial effusions can be managed conservatively, pending investigations for the underlying cause (which may include blood tests and cross-sectional imaging). Diagnostic pericardiocentesis may be required, with fluid analysis for biochemistry, microbiology, and cytology

- In cardiac tamponade, pericardiocentesis should be performed urgently in an appropriate setting, either via the subxiphoid or anterior thoracic approach, usually with placement of a pericardial drain
- Recurrent symptomatic pericardial effusions may require surgical intervention, with a pericardial window

Constrictive pericarditis

Mimics congestive heart failure, but the problem is a thickened, often calcified pericardium, limiting diastolic filling.

Causes

- Most often idiopathic
- Pericarditis, particularly with an infective cause
- After cardiac surgery or radiotherapy

Presentation and clinical signs

- Breathlessness, often with clear lungs
- Associated with high venous pressure (abdominal distension/ascites, peripheral oedema)
- High JVP with prominent *x* and *y* descents, can rise with inspiration (Kussmaul's sign)
- Hypotension
- Loud or palpable S3 due to rapid ventricular filling—pericardial 'knock'

Initial investigations

ECG—non-specific T wave changes, atrial arrhythmias, small complexes

CXR—pericardial calcification, pleural effusions

Cardiac imaging—anatomical changes, plus features indicating enhanced ventricular interdependence and dissociation of intracardiac and intrathoracic pressures

Echo—Pericardial thickening and calcification

- Moderate (rather than severe) biatrial dilatation
- Abnormal ventricular septal motion with diastolic flattening on inspiration
- Rapid early LV filling (high E/A ratio; short deceleration time)
- Exaggerated AV valve flow variation with respiration (like tamponade)
- Dilated IVC and hepatic veins with expiratory diastolic flow reversal (compared to restrictive cardiomyopathy where hepatic flow reversal is inspiratory)
- Fairly normal tissue Doppler values (compared to restrictive cardiomyopathy where reduced)

CT—thickened, calcified pericardium; flat interventricular septum; dilated IVC and hepatic veins (Fig. 13.3)

CMR—thickened pericardium with adherence to adjacent myocardium; septal flattening towards left on inspiration

Cardiac catheterization—often no longer required for diagnosis, but simultaneous measurement of RV and LV pressures shows equal (high) EDP during respiratory cycle

Management

- Investigate and treat underlying cause
- Diuretic therapy
- Surgery (pericardiectomy) may be required for severe and intractable symptoms

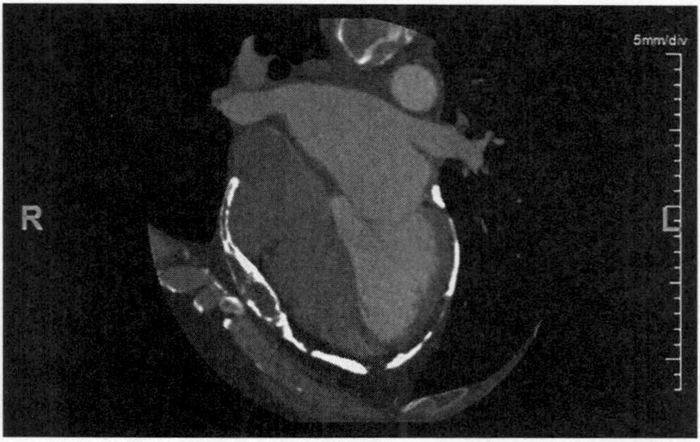

Fig. 13.3 Gated CT image showing heavily calcified (white) pericardium surrounding the heart due to constrictive pericarditis.

Chapter 14

Pulmonary vascular disease

Pulmonary embolism

The annual incidence of PE is 70–80/100,000 with half of cases occurring in hospital. The most common cause is VTE but non-thrombotic causes include air, fat, amniotic fluid, tumour fragments, and septic emboli.

Diagnosis and risk stratification of PE can be difficult and should be based on a combination of clinical assessment ± biomarkers and imaging.

Presentation and signs

- Most patients with PE are breathless (70% of cases) and/or tachypnoeic (respiratory rate > 20/min, 60% of cases)
- Patients may also present with chest pain (50% of cases), cough, syncope, and haemoptysis
- Tachycardia is common
- There may be symptoms or signs of an underlying malignancy. Clinical history and examination recommended
- PE may present with cardiac arrest or shock
- Chronic recurrent PEs may present with signs and symptoms of pulmonary hypertension and progressive right heart failure
- Elevated JVP with prominent a- and v-waves, loud P_2, TR, hypotension, gallop rhythm, pleural rub, peripheral oedema, and cyanosis may occur
- Also see Box 14.1

Box 14.1 Symptoms and signs in suspected PE

Symptoms

• Dyspnoea	70%	
• Chest pain (pleuritic)	52%	
• Chest pain (substernal)	12%	
• Cough	20%	
• Haemoptysis	11%	
• Syncope	19%	

Signs

• Tachypnoea (20/min)		70%
• Tachycardia (> 100/min)	26%	
• Signs of DVT	15%	
• Cyanosis	11%	

Assessment of clinical probability pre-test

Patients should be carefully assessed based on history, physical examination, and known risk factors. Strong risk factors include lower limb fracture, hip or knee replacement, major trauma, previous VTE, spinal cord injury, active cancer, recent myocardial infarction or heart failure hospitalization. Moderate risk factors include chemotherapy, oral contraceptive pill use, central venous lines, and others.

If PE is within the differential diagnosis, the Wells' clinical rule (Box 14.2) can be helpful.

Box 14.2 Wells' rule

Clinical features of DVT	3 points
PE is deemed most likely diagnosis by clinician's judgement	3 points
Heart rate > 100	1.5 points
Immobilization for 3 days or surgery in last 4 weeks	1.5 points
Previous PE or DVT	1.5 points
Haemoptysis	1 point
Malignancy	1 point

Investigations

D-dimer assay

- It is recommended only to consider D-dimer testing following assessment of clinical probability
- If Wells' rule score is four or less, PE can be effectively excluded if D dimer is under the (age-adjusted) threshold
- If PE has been excluded using Wells' rule and D dimer, then imaging is not recommended
- If D dimer is above the age-adjusted threshold and PE is suspected to be cause, imaging with CTPA (CT pulmonary angiography) (or V/Q scan) is recommended
- D-dimer need not be performed in those with a high clinical probability of PE who should proceed to imaging

Other blood tests

- FBC, U&E, CRP, clotting
- Arterial blood gases—hypoxaemia, hypocapnia, mild respiratory alkalosis, metabolic acidosis due to tissue hypoperfusion, though may be normal
- Cardiac troponin may be elevated due to right heart strain but is not of diagnostic value

CXR

- Used to exclude conditions that mimic PE—chest infection, pneumothorax
- May show wedge-shaped peripheral infarcts, pulmonary effusions, pulmonary oligaemia, enlarged proximal pulmonary arteries but insensitive

Diagnostic imaging

- CTPA is the recommended imaging tool
- Isotope lung scanning can be considered following a normal CXR if good-quality facilities and reporting are on site and the patient has no significant concurrent cardiopulmonary disease. Not used routinely to exclude acute PE, but may be preferred where CT contrast allergy exists, or if the patient is breastfeeding
- Venous ultrasonography—in patients with coexisting DVT, leg ultrasound may be considered to confirm VTE

ECG

- ECG cannot reliably rule PE in or out
- The most common finding is sinus tachycardia (see Fig. 14.1)

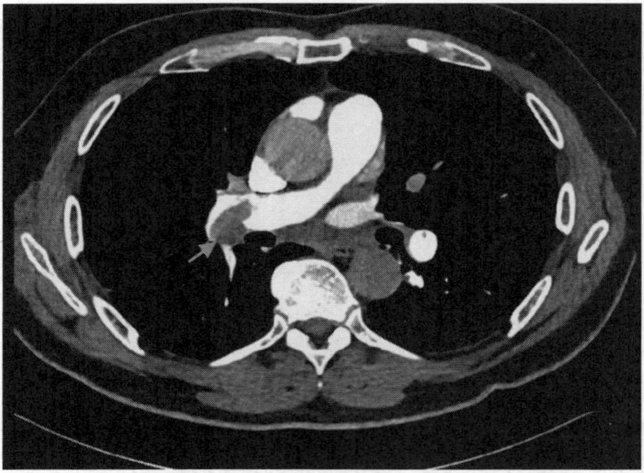

Fig. 14.1 CTPA demonstrating large filling defect (arrowed) in keeping with pulmonary emboli in the right pulmonary artery. See also small thrombus in left pulmonary artery.

- Non-specific ST and T wave changes and atrial arrhythmias are common; incomplete or complete RBBB and RV strain pattern occur
- The classic $S_1Q_3T_3$ pattern is rare

Echocardiography

- Echocardiography cannot reliably rule PE in or out
- Can be abnormal in massive PE (right heart dilatation and global hypokinesia with sparing of apex) and can provide non-invasive information on pulmonary artery pressures
- May provide an alternative diagnosis—aortic dissection, pericardial tamponade, myocardial dysfunction

Risk stratification and initial treatment

PE with haemodynamic instability

Patients with PE and sustained hypotension (SBP < 90 mmHg, or decrease in SBP from baseline of > 40 mmHg) with no other cause such as hypovolaemia or arrhythmia, and evidence of right heart strain are haemodynamically unstable. This group of patients is at high risk of deterioration and cardiac arrest.

- Patients with PE and haemodynamic instability should receive initial resuscitation measures including:
  - Oxygen
  - Analgesia
  - Cautious fluid resuscitation (generally max 1 litre). Excess fluid administration may worsen right ventricular wall stress and cause ischaemia, resulting in reduced cardiac output

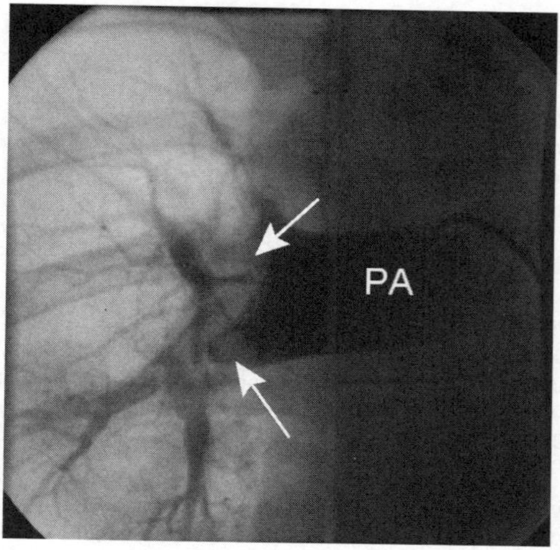

Fig. 14.2 Pulmonary angiography of the right pulmonary artery (PA) demonstrating large filling defects (arrowed) in keeping with massive pulmonary emboli.

  - If no contraindication, systemic thrombolysis should be used (e.g. alteplase IV 10 mg over 2 minutes, further 90 mg over 2 hours)
  - In cardiac arrest due to PE, give alteplase 50 mg stat and continue resuscitation for 30–60 minutes
  - Consider noradrenaline, dobutamine for refractory shock due to RV failure.
- Invasive procedures
  - Right heart catheterization (with potential direct delivery of thrombolysis to the pulmonary circulation ± mechanical disruption of thrombus, or aspiration of thrombus (Fig 14.2)) and surgical pulmonary embolectomy have all been used
  - There is emerging evidence to support the use of percutaneous/ mechanical thrombectomy, however its precise role in PE treatment remains unclear. Larger RCT data are awaited

PE without haemodynamic instability

Patients with PE and without haemodynamic instability should undergo further risk stratification to guide suitability for inpatient versus outpatient treatment. The PESI score or simplified PESI score may be helpful to guide this according to local protocols (Box 14.3).

Anticoagulation

Anticoagulation

- Anticoagulation (DOAC or LMWH) should be commenced before imaging if clinical probability of PE is high or intermediate, and imaging cannot be performed within 1 hour

Box 14.3 Simplified PESI score

Age > 80 years	1 point
History of cancer	1 point
History of cardiopulmonary disease	1 point
Systolic BP < 90 mmHg	1 point
Heart rate >110 bpm	1 point
O_2 saturation < 90%	1 point

Duration and choice of therapy

- Patients with PE should generally be treated with anticoagulation with a DOAC for at least 3 months. For a first proximal DVT or a PE associated with transient risk factors treatment will usually stop at 3 months
- Long-term treatment will be considered for recurrent thrombosis, patients with an ongoing risk factor, or unprovoked/minimally proximal DVT or PE
- LMWH may be used in place of DOAC in pregnancy
- DOAC therapy can be used in most cancer-associated VTE

Further reading

British Thoracic Society guidelines for the initial outpatient management of pulmonary embolism. *Thorax* 2018 Jul; 73(Suppl 2).
2019 ESC Guidelines for the diagnosis and management of acute pulmonary embolism. *European Heart Journal* 2019; 41(4): 543–603

Pulmonary hypertension

- Defined haemodynamically at right heart catheterization by mean pulmonary arterial pressure > 20 mmHg,
- Further divided into pre-capillary, isolated post-capillary (IpcPH), and combined post- and pre-capillary pulmonary hypertension (CpcPH) depending on the pulmonary arterial wedge pressure (PAWP) and pulmonary vascular resistance (PVR):
  - Pre-capillary: PAWP ≤ 15 mmHg, PVR > 2 WU
  - IpcPH: PAWP >15 mmHg, PVR ≤ 2 WU
  - CpcPH: PAWP >15 mmHg, PVR > 2 WU
- Classified by the World Health Organization into 5 groups according to similar pathobiological features, haemodynamic characteristics, and response to treatment
- Affects up to 1% of global population. Worldwide, most cases of pulmonary hypertension are due to left heart disease (Group 2) or lung disease (Group 3)
- Pulmonary arterial hypertension (PAH; Group 1) refers to a rare group of conditions characterized by a progressive vasculopathy and include idiopathic/heritable PAH, as well as PAH associated with other conditions such as connective tissue disease, congenital heart disease, and portal hypertension, amongst others. Many of these patients present with severe pre-capillary pulmonary hypertension

Presentation

- Breathlessness is the usual presenting symptom although patients with late/severe disease may present with exertional syncope (due to fixed or reduced cardiac output), symptoms of right heart failure (peripheral oedema), or angina (from RV ischaemia)
- Angina can also be due to dynamic compression of the left main stem coronary artery from an enlarged pulmonary artery
- Signs include:
  - Elevated JVP with a large a wave—large v wave if severe TR
  - Low volume pulse
  - RV heave—sternal heave.
  - Loud pulmonary component of the S_2
  - Split S_2—widens as RV fails or with RBBB
  - Systolic murmur—TR
  - Diastolic murmur—PR
  - Central and peripheral cyanosis
  - Pulsatile liver, peripheral oedema, ascites
  - Signs of associated disease, e.g. sclerodactyly and telangiectasia in systemic sclerosis

Investigations

- *ECG*—RV hypertrophy (➔ p.214) is highly specific but has a low sensitivity. RBBB with anterior ST abnormalities can occur. Prominent P waves (P pulmonale) suggest right atrial enlargement. See Fig. 14.3
- *CXR*—enlargement of the pulmonary artery and its major branches. Tapering of peripheral arteries. Enlarged RA and RV. Underlying disorder may be apparent

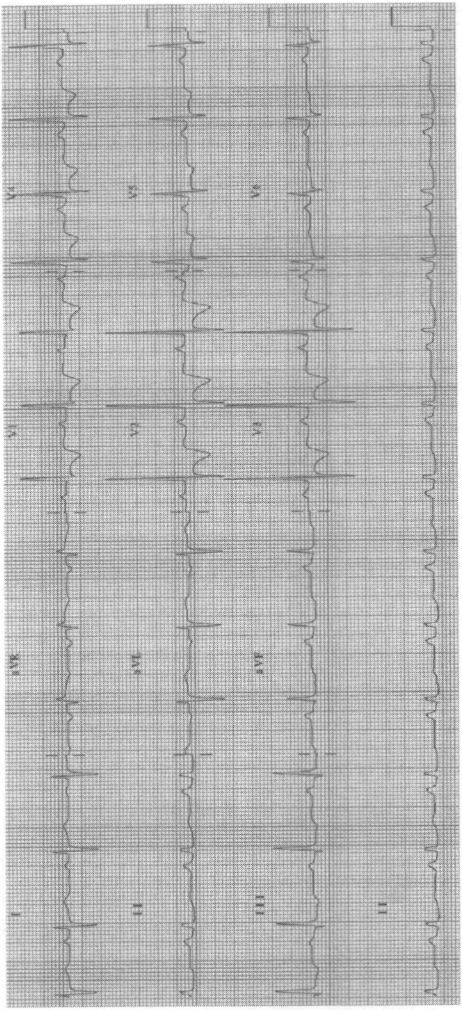

Fig. 14.3 ECG in severe pre-capillary pulmonary hypertension. RV hypertrophy is demonstrated by right axis deviation, large R waves with T-wave inversion in leads V1–V3, and a prominent p wave (p pulmonale).

- *Bloods*—FBC, U&E, LFTs, arterial blood gases, autoimmune profile
- *Echocardiography*—enlarged RV with septal flattening. Doppler estimate of pulmonary artery systolic pressure. Patients with significant and long-standing pulmonary hypertension often have a dilated and impaired RV
- Thorough clinical assessment is required when determining the role for further investigations. Patients with evidence of mild pulmonary hypertension who have coexisting lung disease or LV systolic/diastolic dysfunction usually do not require extensive investigation
- Depending on the clinical picture, further specialist investigations may include a combination of:
  - PFTs including gas transfer
  - Exercise testing (walk test, cardiopulmonary exercise testing)
  - Cross-sectional imaging (high resolution CT scan, CT pulmonary angiography, dual energy CT pulmonary angiography)
  - Lung perfusion scintigraphy/VQ scan
  - Cardiac MRI
  - Abdominal ultrasound to assess portal flow
  - Hepatitis and HIV serology
  - Sleep studies

Right heart catheterization should be performed in specialist centres and should not delay referral for specialist assessment. Dynamic assessment of PAWP with a fluid challenge should be considered in patients with risk factors for left heart disease.

Management

- A high index of suspicion is required to make a diagnosis of pulmonary arterial hypertension. Patients often suffer with symptoms for years and see many physicians before receiving a diagnosis
- Prompt referral to a specialist centre is indicated for patients with PH where Group 1 or Group 4 disease is suspected, or where the cause of PH is uncertain
- Right heart catheterization should be performed in a PH centre to ensure reliable haemodynamics are recorded
- The management of patients presenting *de novo* with pulmonary hypertension includes appropriate use of oxygen to correct hypoxaemia, diuretic therapy, undertaking relevant investigations, and discussion with specialist centres
- Patients are risk-stratified at baseline and at follow-up using a multi-parameter assessment of haemodynamics, exercise capacity, right ventricular function and symptom burden to determine the most appropriate treatment regimen
- Specialist advice is important, both for long-term management and for patients known to have pulmonary hypertension who present unwell. This is a difficult condition to treat for the non-expert

Long-term management typically includes:

- Pulmonary vasodilator therapy (see below)
- Exercise-based rehabilitation in stable patients
- Oxygen therapy:
  - As well as having a short-term acute symptomatic benefit, long-term oxygen therapy (at least 15 hours a day) improves survival in

chronically hypoxaemic patients (PaO_2 of < 7.3 kPa) although specific evidence in patients with PH is limited

- Diuretics:
  - Use loop diuretics such as furosemide 40–80 mg orally or IV in the acutely unwell/with anasarca
  - Spironolactone is commonly used as an adjunct
  - Particularly useful in RV volume overload
  - Excess volume depletion can lead to a decline in cardiac output
  - Watch renal function and K^+ levels

Further reading

2022 ESC/ERS Guidelines for the diagnosis and treatment of pulmonary hypertension: Developed by the task force for the diagnosis and treatment of pulmonary hypertension of the European Society of Cardiology (ESC) and the European Respiratory Society (ERS). *European Heart Journal* 2022; 43(38): 3618–731.

Systemic emboli

Clinical Features

Systemic embolism of thrombus or vegetation leads to signs and symptoms of obstruction of a coronary, cerebral, or peripheral artery.

Causes

- Left atrial thrombus—usually from the atrial appendage
  - AF
  - Mitral stenosis
- Carotid atheroma
- Left ventricular thrombus
  - Post-myocardial infarction
  - Cardiomyopathy
  - LV aneurysm
- Left-sided heart valves
  - Prosthetic (endocarditis, thrombosis)
  - Native (endocarditis)
- Cardiac shunt with paradoxical embolism
  - Atrial septal defect
  - Patent foramen ovale
  - Ventricular septal defect—with raised RV pressure
- Aorta
  - Atheroma
  - Dissection
- Cardiac tumours
  - Myxoma
  - Other 1° and 2° tumours—rare

Presentation

- TIA/stroke—common
- Acute coronary syndrome
- Acute limb ischaemia
- Acute small bowel ischaemia
- Acute renal/splenic infarction

Investigations—tailored according to presentation

- FBC (anaemia, platelet count/clumping), U&Es, ESR/CRP, D-dimer
- Coagulation screen
- ECG—AF, MI
- Echocardiography (see below)
- Cerebral and carotid imaging—if presenting with stroke
- Carotid/peripheral artery Doppler ultrasound
- Doppler ultrasound of leg veins—DVT
- CT abdomen/pelvis—if visceral embolism suspected
- CT angiography—if peripheral embolism suspected
- Coronary angiography—if presenting with ACS

Risk of systemic embolism for patients with AF

- AF is a major risk factor for systemic thromboembolism
- If untreated, the risk of ischaemic stroke in AF is increased 5×

Table 15.1 CHA_2DS_2-VA Score

Component	Definition	Points
Chronic heart failure	Symptoms/signs of heart failure, irrespective of EF, or asymptomatic HF with EF ≤ 40%	1
Hypertension	Resting BP > 140/90 mmHg on at least 2 occasions, or current antihypertensive treatment.	1
Age 75 years or above		2
Diabetes mellitus	Type 1 or 2 DM	1
Prior **S**troke, TIA, or arterial thromboembolism		2
Vascular disease	Coronary or peripheral vascular disease	1
Age 65–74 years		1

- Oral anticoagulation (OAC) is recommended for patients with a CHA_2DS_2-VA score of 2 or more, and should be considered in those with a CHA_2DS_2-VA score of 1 (see Table 15.1)
- In addition, OAC is recommended for *all* patients with AF and underlying hypertrophic cardiomyopathy or cardiac amyloidosis
- Patients at high thrombotic risk who are unable to tolerate anticoagulation due to bleeding should be referred for consideration of left atrial appendage occlusion

Management

- Management of the presenting condition may be necessary before investigation of the source of embolism, e.g. acute limb ischaemia
- Commence anticoagulation if a cardiac source of embolism is demonstrated: therapeutic dose LMWH may be useful initially, if investigations are ongoing or definitive management is unclear
- The timing of anticoagulation in patients presenting with embolic stroke should be made in conjunction with a stroke specialist
- Similarly, if urgent surgery is required, liaison with the surgical team is essential before initiation of anticoagulation
- PFO—consider percutaneous device closure
- ASD—percutaneous device closure or surgery

Echocardiography

Echocardiography is useful in the investigation of systemic emboli, to look for reduced LV function (predisposes to thrombus), apical LV thrombus, or an intracardiac shunt (e.g. PFO/ASD).

Indications for TTE

- Unexplained systemic embolism
- Clinical signs of infective endocarditis or myxoma

Indications for TOE

- Non-diagnostic TTE
- Infective endocarditis suspected and not confirmed on TTE
- Suspected prosthetic valve dysfunction
- Suspected PFO or ASD

Saline contrast echocardiography

Can be performed with either TTE or TOE to look for a PFO.

- A small volume of saline (~8 mL) is drawn into a 10 mL syringe, mixed with 0.5 mL air and agitated by passing it through a 3-way tap to another 10 mL syringe and back again, repeatedly for ~1 min
- Rapid injection will opacify the right heart and evaluate whether there is right-to-left shunting
- The study is positive if > 3 bubbles are seen appearing in the LA within 3–6 beats of appearing in the RA (Fig. 15.1)
- The injection should be repeated with the patient performing a Valsalva manoeuvre to increase RA pressure
- Injection of contrast via the femoral vein increases the diagnostic yield, as blood is directed via the Eustachian valve towards the PFO
- If an ASD is detected, TOE/CT/MRI may be required to assess the atrial septum for suitability for percutaneous device closure

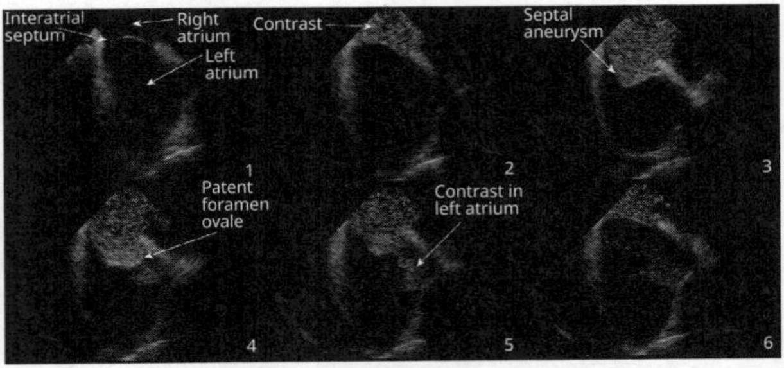

Fig. 15.1 Intracardiac echocardiogram demonstrating passage of agitated saline contrast from the RA through a PFO into the LA.

Paradoxical embolism

Systemic embolism from the venous system across an abnormal communication within the heart (usually an atrial septal defect or patent foramen ovale).

- Approximately 15–20% of the normal population will have a PFO, resulting from the failed closure of the antenatal interatrial communication. A PFO is therefore the most common cause of a right-to-left shunt in adult
- For a PFO to cause systemic embolism, there must be raised RA pressure (permanent or transient, e.g. coughing/straining) and a venous source of thrombus
- As PFOs are highly prevalent in the unselected population, ascribing a causal role to a PFO in a patient presenting with stroke can be challenging
- PFO-associated stroke is more likely in younger patients, with no other identifiable stroke aetiology or vascular risk factors (cryptogenic stroke). This group is most likely to derive benefit from percutaneous device closure of the PFO (see Box 15.1)
- Secundum ASDs are usually amenable to percutaneous closure in the presence of suitable 'rims' for device anchoring, and the absence of significant pulmonary hypertension

Box 15.1 PFO closure in patients with stroke

In the UK, percutaneous device closure of a PFO is offered to patients meeting the following criteria:

- Around age 60 years or younger
- Stroke/TIA, with clinical and imaging evidence to support diagnosis
- PFO with clinically significant shunt or atrial septal aneurysm
- Absence of significant AF that warrants anticoagulation
- Full investigation to exclude vascular disease (including dissection), hypertension or other risk factors
- MDT consider paradoxical embolus to be the most likely cause of stroke

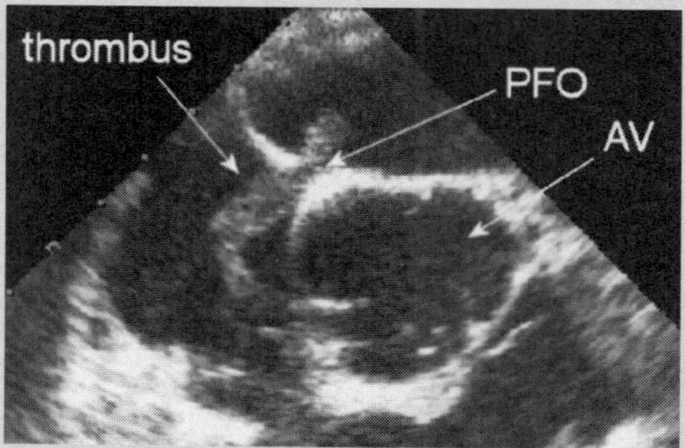

Fig. 15.2 TOE demonstrating a large thrombus trapped in a patent foramen ovale (PFO) in a patient with systemic embolism.

Pregnancy and maternal medicine

Introduction and general principles

Cardiac disease remains the leading cause of indirect deaths in pregnancy.

It affects 0.2–4% of pregnancies and its incidence is increasing as:

(1) women with congenital cardiac disease survive into adulthood

(2) the incidence of acquired heart disease is increasing due to

- obesity
- hypertension
- diabetes
- increasing maternal age

Pregnancy can exacerbate pre-existing cardiac conditions, unmask undiagnosed conditions, or precipitate new conditions.

Therefore, women with known cardiac disease, should be seen in a pre-conception counselling clinic to explain the risks of pregnancy to both mother and foetus, and to discuss management plans including stopping any medication that has adverse effect on the foetus (Box 16.1).

Box 16.1 General principles of cardiac management

- Avoid drugs if possible, or use the fewest drugs in the smallest doses

but

- Do not deny appropriate management because of pregnancy. If the mother is compromised, so is the foetus.
- In particular, do not withhold imaging involving radiation if the woman may have a life-threatening condition, e.g. PE, aortic dissection
- Obtain *early* advice from pregnancy heart team which are part of maternal medicine networks
- The Modified WHO classification is currently the most accurate system of risk assessment (Box 16.2)

Box 16.2 Modified WHO class IV—highest risk of mortality and morbidity

- Pulmonary hypertension
- Severe systemic ventricular dysfunction, LV ejection fraction < 30%, NYHA class III–IV, moderate/severe systemic RV dysfunction
- Previous peripartum cardiomyopathy with any residual left ventricular impairment
- Severe left heart obstruction AS or MS or coarctation of aorta
- Severe aortic dilatation (> 45 mm in Marfan syndrome or other HTAD, > 50 mm in bicuspid aortic valve, Turner syndrome ASI > 25 mm/m^2, tetralogy of Fallot > 50 mm) Vascular Ehlers–Danlos
- Fontan with any complication

However, the majority of deaths occur in women without known pre-existing disease, therefore it is vital to recognize and act upon new symptoms. The management of pregnant women with high risk of complications requires a pregnancy heart team consisting of obstetricians, cardiologists, and anaesthetists as indicated by current guidelines, e.g. those of the European Society of Cardiology.

Normal physiological changes in pregnancy

One of the challenges in diagnosing pregnancy-related heart disease is to distinguish pathological symptoms from the adaptive changes required by pregnancy. Circulating volume, heart rate, stroke volume, and, consequently, cardiac output increases markedly in the first 16 weeks, then plateaus, and then increase further in the weeks before term. Systemic vascular resistance is reduced during pregnancy.

The following symptoms are all consistent with normal pregnancy:

- Fatigue
- SOB
- Palpitation
- Atrial and ventricular premature beats
- Raised JVP
- Pedal oedema
- Sinus tachycardia ~100 bpm
- Full volume, collapsing pulse
- S_3
- Systolic flow murmur

Clinical indicators of pathological states

- Chest pain
- Severe dyspnoea
- Orthopnoea, paroxysmal nocturnal dyspnoea
- Sinus tachycardia > 100 at rest
- AF/atrial flutter
- VT
- Hypotension
- Hypertension
- Pulmonary oedema
- Pleural effusion

Murmurs in pregnancy

Systolic flow murmurs are common during pregnancy due to the increased cardiac output. An 'innocent' murmur should be a typical flow murmur (soft, ejection systolic, second right intercostal space/left sternal edge), and without any other signs of valve disease. Diastolic murmurs, loud murmurs, thrills, and radiation of the murmur are not 'normal' and suggest a significant lesion, which requires echocardiography.

Who to refer for echocardiography

- Patients with a significant murmur that isn't clearly a flow murmur
- Anyone with other signs of valve disease
- Patients with significant breathlessness
- Patients with a history of heart disease
- Abnormal 12-lead ECG

Heart failure in pregnancy

Accounts for around 25% all cardiac deaths in pregnancy. Consider termination if heart failure occurs early in pregnancy.

Causes

- Dilated cardiomyopathy
- Underlying structural conditions, e.g. valvular disease
- Peripartum cardiomyopathy
- Takutsubo cardiomyopathy

Acute management of severe heart failure

- Obtain urgent expert help and seek to arrange transfer to maternal medicine centre
- O_2, bed rest, induction of lung maturation
- Optimize pre-load—diuretics, vasodilators if SBP > 110 mmHg: hydralazine, IV GTN
- Optimization of oxygenation—noninvasive ventilation
- Inotropes/ IABP and urgent delivery—C section
- Anticoagulation with LMWH
- Consider mechanical circulatory support

Management of stabile heart failure

- β-blockers—high dose may require foetal growth monitoring, and heart rate monitoring during delivery
- Referral to pregnancy heart team
- ACE inhibitors contraindicated until delivery (risk of renal agenesis). ARBs, MRAs, ARNIs (There are however special circumstances where the benefits of ACE inhibitors outweigh their risks—expert consideration on a case-by-case basis.)

Peripartum cardiomyopathy

Risk factors: smoking, diabetes, pre-eclampsia, malnutrition, very young/old age, twin pregnancy, hypertension, multiparous, African ethnicity

Clinically indistinguishable from other dilated cardiomyopathies but, by definition, occurs only in the last month of pregnancy or up to 6 months postpartum, *in the absence of any other cardiac pathology*.

LV dysfunction persists in 50% and there is a significant risk of recurrence in subsequent pregnancies, even when LV function has initially returned to normal. If LV function does not return to normal, the risk of death in any subsequent pregnancy is ~20%. Consider bromocriptine to block prolactin release.

Hypertrophic cardiomyopathy

- Generally well tolerated during pregnancy, maternal mortality < 0.5%,
- Some women may experience a deterioration in symptoms of heart failure or arryhthmias
- Pre-pregnancy counselling with genetic counsellors important
- β-blockers—to prevent AF, or for symptoms of outflow tract obstruction, monitor foetal growth with high doses
- Anticoagulation if in AF

Management during delivery

- Maintain good fluid intake (the LV is stiff and responds poorly to dehydration) and avoid excessive fluid shifts as much as possible
- Diuretics, if fluid congestion/heart failure occur
- Epidural anaesthesia can used during labour, but with careful use to avoid hypovolaemia in patients with outflow tract obstruction

Acute myocardial infarction in pregnancy

Acute MI in pregnancy is rare, occurring in 1.7–6.2/100,000 deliveries), however CAD accounts for > 20% of all maternal cardiac death.

Increasing incidence may be due to rising maternal age, obesity, and diabetes but pre-eclampsia, thrombophilia, transfusion, post-partum infection, multiparity, and post-partum haemorrhage all increase the risk.

The aetiology of CAD differs from the general population; the majority of CAD has non-atherosclerotic mechanisms, including pregnancy-related spontaneous coronary artery dissection (P-SCAD) (43%), angiographically normal coronary arteries (18%), and coronary thrombosis (17%). The diagnosis is made using conventional criteria. Troponin I is not affected by normal pregnancy and is the marker of choice for myocardial necrosis in pregnancy.

Acute management

- There are few data to guide treatment. The risk from MI needs to be weighed against the risks of treatment (to both mother and foetus)
- Urgent cardiological assessment is essential
- Aspirin 75 mg OD
- β-blockers
- 1° PCI is the treatment of choice, since the consequences of not treating carry a high risk of both maternal and foetal death. This approach will also allow diagnosis ± treatment of coronary artery dissection. It should be undertaken by an experienced operator due to P-SCAD. Although there are few data on the use of clopidogrel in pregnancy, drug-eluting stents with dual antiplatelet cover have resulted in the successful completion of pregnancies. More potent P2Y12 inhibitors should be used with caution due to high risk of bleeding

Systemic thrombolysis should not be given late in pregnancy because of the risk of premature labour and potentially catastrophic bleeding. However, in the presence of a large anterior acute MI, thrombolysis should be considered if 1° PCI is not available, since the consequence of not treating carries such a high risk of maternal and foetal demise.

Valvular heart disease in pregnancy

Obstructive left-sided valvular disease is poorly tolerated

Valvular stenosis

Severe Aortic or mitral valve stenosis is not well tolerated in pregnancy. Due to the inability to increase cardiac output, which is required. Women are at risk of major decompensation should additional complications occur (e.g. arrhythmias, bleeding).

Aortic stenosis

In pregnancy usually due to a bicuspid aortic valve in the Western world; other parts of the world have a higher incidence of rheumatic valve disease. Patients are usually diagnosed pre-pregnancy. The increased cardiac output required early in pregnancy can lead to problems due to the fixed LV outflow obstruction. Symptoms include SOB, syncope, and chest pain.

Management

Asymptomatic patients can be treated conservatively with low-dose β-blocker.

When symptoms occur with severe AS, despite bed rest and β-blocker consider:

- Delivery (if gestation allows) and then treat the AS
- Palliative balloon valvuloplasty. This should be performed by an experienced operator after thorough assessment of the valve anatomy. Complications include acute severe AR, causing acute maternal decompensation, and the maternal and foetal risks in emergency aortic valve surgery are very high
- Surgical aortic valve replacement—rarely performed, due to risk of miscarriage, but if a women has severe AS, the high maternal complication risk should be managed and surgery should be undertaken

Mitral stenosis

Usually due to rheumatic disease, MS is often undiagnosed until unmasked by pregnancy. Mild or moderate MS is usually well tolerated. The increase in heart rate leads to a reduction in diastolic filling time, and the increase in circulating volume increase LA pressure which in severe mitral stenosis can precipitate acute pulmonary oedema. New or rapid AF will have similar effects.

Treatment (if SOB or heart failure occurs)

- Diuretics (avoid excessive diuresis—risk of hypovolaemia leading to inadequate left atrial pressure)
- β-blockers for rate control to allow time for ventricular filling
- Anticoagulate with heparin—if AF and/or LA dilatation
- Percutaneous (balloon) mitral valvuloplasty by an experienced operator for severe MS, refractory to medical treatment

Valvular regurgitation

MR and AR impose a volume overload on the LV and are generally well tolerated during pregnancy. The decreased afterload is often beneficial in reducing the degree of regurgitation. When symptoms occur, diuretics are the mainstay of treatment. ACE inhibitors should be avoided.

Antibiotic prophylaxis during labour

Antibiotic prophylaxis for valve disease during labour (to prevent infective endocarditis) is no longer recommended.

Mechanical prosthetic valves

In women with mechanical prosthetic valves, pregnancy is associated with a very high risk of complications—WHO risk classification III. Studies reported a favourable outcome for mother and baby in only 28% of cases. The main risks are related to the need for anticoagulation therapy (valve thrombosis and haemorrhagic complications), and pregnancy being a prothrombotic state. Warfarin crosses the placenta and causes an embryopathy in around 10% of foetuses and has a high miscarriage rate. Additional risks are related to ventricular and valvular dysfunction. These women need careful preconception counselling and should be cared for during pregnancy by the pregnancy heart team. See Anticoagulation, p.237.

Arrhythmias in pregnancy

Hormonal and haemodynamic changes may predispose pregnant women to arrhythmias and may also render clinically silent paroxysmal tachycardias symptomatic. Acute treatment of the haemodynamically compromised patient should be the same as if non-pregnant. Note that DC cardioversion is safe in pregnancy (see Box 16.3).

Oral therapy (e.g. β-blockers) may be used to prevent recurrence during pregnancy if arrhythmias result in significant compromise.

Re-entry tachycardias (i.e. SVT)

Treat as for non-pregnant (➲ p.143):

- Vagal manoeuvres
- Adenosine, verapamil, and flecainide have been used successfully
- DC cardioversion for severe haemodynamic compromise

Atrial fibrillation/flutter

(See ➲ p.151 for general management.)

- New onset anticoagulate with LMWH if considering DCCV, otherwise as per CHADS2VASC
- Rate control with β-blockers
- Patients will often revert to sinus rhythm spontaneously within 48 hours, and conservative treatment is usually appropriate, i.e. heparin and rate control
- Beta 1 selective blockers or flecainide may be used for pharmacological cardioversion
- Electrical cardioversion if compromised
- Assess for structural cardiac abnormality

Ventricular tachycardia

- DC cardioversion (Box 16.3)
- Requires further evaluation of underlying cause
- Subsequent management depends on underlying disease
- Involve pregnancy heart team

Box 16.3 DC cardioversion in pregnancy

- Place a wedge under the right hip to avoid IVC compression*
- Use lowest energy shock
- Direct the paddles away from foetus
- No reports of iatrogenic foetal VF
- ... *but* check foetal heart rate post-cardioversion

*Procedures or investigations that usually require the patient to be supine should be done in a left lateral position or with the aid of a wedge to support the pelvis and avoid IVC compression, by the gravid uterus, with consequent syncope.

Aortic disease in pregnancy

- Most commonly seen in heritable thoracic aneurysm conditions. Aortic dissection is the major concern

Causes and associations

- Marfan syndrome especially with aortic root > 4.0 cm ~3% risk (Box 16.4), Ehlers–Danlos type 4- very high risk, Loeys–Dietz syndrome. Turner syndrome (assisted conception) or Turner syndrome ~2% risk of dissection in pregnancy
- Aortic coarctation—whether repaired or not
- Bicuspid aortic valve with dilated aortic root. The risk of dissection in pregnancy is only slightly higher than in the general population

Box 16.4 Marfan syndrome in pregnancy

The major risk during pregnancy is aortic dissection (mostly of the ascending aorta)—hormonal and haemodynamic changes combine with the aortic wall changes in Marfan syndrome to increase the risk of new/further aortic dilation and of dissection in already dilated aortic roots. An ascending aortic dissection while pregnant is a catastrophic situation, with very high risk to the mother and foetus from the emergency cardiac surgery required, and should be avoided at all costs. The following is therefore advised:

- Women with Marfan syndrome and a dilated aortic root (> 4.5 cm) are at significant risk of dissection and should be strongly advised against pregnancy, with good provision of suitable contraception. Termination should be offered if pregnancy occurs.
- Women with Marfan syndrome and a non-dilated aortic root should be monitored closely during pregnancy, with very close attention to BP control, and regular imaging of the aortic root with echocardiography/CMR. Further dilation occurs, a difficult situation has arisen, and expert advice should be sought urgently.

General management

- Patients at risk should have pre-conception evaluation of the aorta with echocardiography and MRI
- Patients with previous aortic coarctation repair or other known aortic disease ***must*** have the aorta assessed for re-coarctation or aneurysm formation (ideally with MRI) and monitored further during pregnancy
- Careful monitoring of BP throughout pregnancy is essential
- β-blockers through pregnancy are advised to reduce the risk of root dilation, celiprolol should be used in EDS type IV
- Surgery for a dilated aorta is rarely undertaken because of the risk to the mother and foetus, but may be considered
- If aortic dilatation is present, Caesarean section should be undertaken to minimize haemodynamic stresses

Acute aortic dissection in pregnancy

► See ➲ p.179 for general management. This is an emergency!

Additional factors in pregnancy

- Requires urgent cross-sectional imaging—during supine imaging use a pelvic wedge to prevent IVC obstruction. Do not withhold investigations involving radiation (i.e. CT) because of pregnancy
- BP control should be with β-blockers and hydralazine. Sodium nitroprusside risks foetal toxicity and should not be used
- Type A dissection with viable foetus, transfer to Cardiothoracic centre with obstetric care for emergency Caesarian section and repair of dissection, otherwise emergency repair of dissection first
- Uncomplicated type B dissection is managed with medical treatment with BP control. In complicated cases thoracic aortic endovascular repair has been undertaken successfully

Hypertension in pregnancy

Hypertensive disorders affect around 5–10% of pregnancies.

There are 3 broad types of hypertension (BP > 140 mmHg systolic and/or > 90 mmHg diastolic) in pregnancy:

Pre-existing hypertension—diagnosed prior to or before 20 weeks pregnancy

Control of BP often requires an alteration to treatment and the hypertension may also deteriorate during pregnancy.

- Methyldopa is usually used for BP control—250 mg TDS PO initially, increasing to maxiumum 1 g TDS
- Calcium antagonists as second-line agents, then β-blockers
- ACE inhibitors, and ARBs are contraindicated in pregnancy and should be discontinued prior to conception

Gestational hypertension

Gestational hypertension occurs after 20 weeks and resolves within 42 days. Its treatment is broadly similar to chronic hypertension, though may not require longer-term antihypertensive medication.

Pre-eclampsia

Pre-eclampsia is a gestational hypertension associated with significant proteinuria > 0.3 g/24 h or ACR ≥ 30 mg/mmol. Abrupt onset oedema and proteinuria with raised plasma uric acid distinguish pre-eclampsia from chronic hypertension. Resolution following delivery is the rule.

High risk of pre-eclampsia includes any of the following:

- hypertensive disease during a previous pregnancy
- chronic kidney disease
- autoimmune disease such as systemic lupus erythematosus or antiphospholipid syndrome
- type 1 or type 2 diabetes
- chronic hypertension

Moderate risk of pre-eclampsia includes more than one of the following risk factors:

- first pregnancy
- age 40 years or older
- pregnancy interval of more than 10 years
- BMI of ≥ 35 kg/m^2 at first visit
- family history of pre-eclampsia
- multiple pregnancy

150mg of aspirin given from 12 weeks to 36 weeks is recommended for women at high or moderate risk.

Management

Obtain expert advice.

Severe cases

- Delivery of the foetus, if gestational age allows. This resolves the problem and provides maximum safety for both mother and foetus
- Inpatient treatment for close monitoring of mother and foetus, if delivery not planned
- Hydralazine (5–10 mg IV, repeated after 30 min in severe hypertension or infusion) or labetalol infusion (20 mg/hour, doubled every 30 min to max. 160 mg/hour)
- Avoid nitroprusside because of foetal toxicity
- Magnesium sulphate infusion to prevent convulsions—4 g (16 mmol) in 100 mL 5% dextrose over 10–15 min followed by 1 g/hour; concentration should not exceed 20%

Mild cases

- May be managed at home but with twice-daily monitoring and rapid access to healthcare
- Methyldopa—250 mg TDS PO initially, increasing to max 1 g TDS

Eclampsia (fitting/seizure)

- This is an emergency and needs urgent expert help
- Deliver the foetus—liaise with obstetricians
- Additional 2 g of magnesium sulphate over 10–15 min

Pulmonary embolism in pregnancy

VTE is the second commonest cause of maternal death, and poor management is implicated in many cases. Patients should be anticoagulated with LMWH pending a confirmed diagnosis.

In general, investigation and management is the same as for a non-pregnant patient (see ➲ p.214). Specific issues in pregnant women are indicated here:

Investigations

(See ➲ p.208.)

- Appropriate investigations should not be withheld because of pregnancy. CTPA and perfusion scans carry a low risk to the foetus
- D-dimers may be raised in a normal pregnancy, but normal D-dimers make a PE unlikely

Acute management

(See ➲ p.209.)

- LMWH The recommended therapeutic dose is calculated on early pregnancy body weight (e.g. enoxaparin 1 mg/kg body weight twice daily, dalteparin 100 IU/kg body weight twice daily, or tinzaparin 175 IU/kg), aiming for 4–6 h peak anti-Xa values of 0.6–1.2 IU/mL
- For life-threatening massive PE, consider (after specialist advice) intrapulmonary thrombolysis, catheter (percutaneous) disruption of embolus, or surgical thrombectomy

Anticoagulation in pregnancy

Anticoagulation in pregnancy, particularly for mechanical valves, presents a difficult problem, with little evidence to guide optimal management. All guidelines differ and involve expert consensus

Warfarin risks teratogenicity (first trimester), foetal haemorrhage (especially in third trimester), and foetal loss throughout pregnancy. LMWH is preferred to UFH, because anti-Xa levels can be monitored and it has a longer half-life so levels are more stable. DOACs are not licensed in pregnancy

- The 3 main options are:
  - LMWH plus aspirin throughout pregnancy
  - Warfarin throughout pregnancy, changing to heparin at 36 weeks
  - LMWH plus aspirin in first trimester, changing to warfarin until 36 weeks when heparin is recommenced

Warfarin is superior to LMWH for preventing mechanical valve thrombosis (MVT) in pregnancy and is recommended as optimal therapy for improving maternal outcomes

There is insufficient evidence to recommend that lower doses of warfarin (e.g. less than 5 mg) are safe in terms of adverse foetal outcome.

When using warfarin, non-pregnancy INR targets should be used. The INR should be checked at least weekly if unstable and if stable, at least fortnightly

When switching from VKA to LMWH in pregnancy, the starting dose of LMWH should be higher than the standard therapeutic dose as there appears to be a high rate of MVT in the first trimester during transition (e.g. total 2.5 mg/kg/day for enoxaparin, 250 IU/ kg/day for dalteparin, and 250 IU/kg/day for tinzaparin in divided doses.

Regular monitoring of LMWH using an anti-Xa assay is recommended. A peak anti-Xa target of 1.0–1.4 IU/mL taken 3–4 h following a BD LMWH dose.

The addition of low-dose aspirin (LDA) 75 mg to anticoagulation with LMWH in individuals with mechanical heart valves (MHV) during pregnancy in the absence of a contraindication.

An increase in the dose of aspirin to 150 mg at 12-week gestation can be considered if indicated for prevention of pre-eclampsia, which is reduced at 36 weeks to 75 mg.

MVT requires MDT management in a specialist centre with the use of thrombolysis where appropriate.

There is insufficient evidence to recommend a specific mode of delivery in pregnant individuals with (MHV). An individualized plan for timing and mode of delivery should be agreed in advance, with input from the pregnancy heart team, and involvement and agreement of the pregnant individual and the mortality rate can be as high as 9%.

Anticoagulation in pregnancy

Adult congenital heart disease

Introduction

Global prevalence of congenital heart disease (CHD) is estimated as 9–18 per 1000 live births. In the UK, live birth prevalence is 5–8 per 1000. Due to major advances in diagnosis and treatment, survival to adulthood is excellent (> 90%) in countries with high socio-demographic index. The adult congenital heart disease (ACHD) population is growing and now exceeds the paediatric CHD population. This has important implications for physicians practising in adult medicine.

Common presentations in emergency situations include:

- Arrhythmia
- Heart failure
- Endocarditis

—all potentially with high morbidity and mortality.

The diagnostic and therapeutic approach towards emergencies in ACHD may differ to that for emergencies in acquired cardiac disease.

Specialist expertise may be required early for optimal management.

Atrial septal defect

ASD causes an interatrial shunt, usually from left atrium (LA) to right atrium (RA), due to the higher compliance of the right ventricle (RV), leading to right heart dilatation and increased pulmonary blood flow (Fig. 17.1).

The unoperated patient

Clinical features can result from:

- Increased pulmonary blood flow
- Inability to increase cardiac output adequately because of the systemic-to-pulmonary shunting
- Paradoxical thromboembolism
- Atrial arrhythmias, related to RA dilatation

Presentation

- Many are asymptomatic
- Symptomatic adults usually present with SOB or palpitation, age 20–40
- May present as an emergency with stroke, heart failure or atrial arrhythmias

Signs

- Wide fixed splitting of the second heart sound (S_2)
- Pulmonary ejection murmur due to increased pulmonary blood flow
- Rarely cyanosis, i.e. Eisenmenger syndrome. Occurs at a late stage in large defects if pulmonary hypertension has occurred

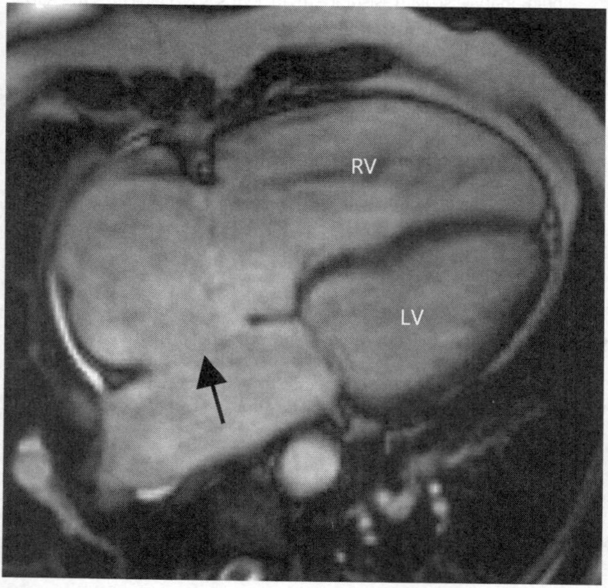

Fig. 17.1 CMR image of an ASD. Note the partial absence of atrial septum (arrowed) and the dilated RV.

Investigations

- *CXR*—cardiomegaly, RA dilatation, prominent pulmonary arteries
- *ECG:*
  - Right axis deviation and incomplete RBBB are typical findings in patients with significant defects
  - Atrial arrhythmia—AF, atrial flutter, SVT
- MRI and TOE imaging is helpful where ASD is suspected but has not been demonstrated on TTE. CT is also useful, particularly for delineating pulmonary veins

Management

- Emergencies are very rare. Acute management of stroke, heart failure, or AF, as in the non-ACHD setting
- An ASD that causes RV enlargement should usually be closed irrespective of symptoms. Closure may be surgical or percutaneous
- Patients with cryptogenic TIA or stroke with either an ASD or PFO may also benefit from elective closure of the defect
- Small ASDs without RV enlargement may not need intervention
- Prior to closure, it is important to assess for:
  1. Pulmonary hypertension—in the presence of a significant left-to-right shunt, a modest elevation in pulmonary artery pressure is expected due to increased pulmonary blood flow (*Pressure = flow × resistance)*. However, if the echo indicates *disproportionately* high pulmonary artery pressure, a cardiac catheter should be performed to assess the pulmonary vascular resistance (PVR). PVR < 3 WU indicates the ASD is safe to close; 3–5 WU requires discussion with specialist centre; > 5 WU is a contraindication to closure.
  2. Elevated left heart filling pressure—where LA pressure is high, closing the ASD may precipitate pulmonary oedema. This can be assessed with cardiac catheter and test balloon occlusion.
  3. Left-sided atrial arrhythmias—device closure of ASD may preclude future transseptal access for left sided ablation.
  4. Anomalous pulmonary veins—these are associated with ASDs and another cause of right heart dilatation; they are best assessed with CT.

Potential closure of an ASD should be considered by a congenital heart disease multidisciplinary team (MDT) meeting.

The operated patient

- Usually, symptom free but can present with atrial arrhythmia or heart failure, especially when the defect has been closed late in life and the pulmonary artery pressure has been elevated prior to closure
- Complete heart block or sinus node dysfunction can occur after closure

Ventricular septal defect

In an uncomplicated VSD (Box 17.1, Fig 17.2), blood shunts left-to-right because the right-sided pulmonary vascular resistance (PVR) is lower than the left-sided systemic vascular resistance (SVR). This leads to pulmonary overcirculation, left heart volume loading, and left heart dilatation.

Box 17.1 Restrictive and non-restrictive VSD

Restrictive VSDs 'restrict' the flow across the defect. They are small (< 1/3 of the aortic root diameter), and there is a high pressure gradient between the LV and RV. RV pressures and PVR are normal.

Moderately restrictive VSDs are about half the size of the aortic root, with moderate to severe shunting early in the disease process. RV pressures are increased, but not to systemic levels. PVR can be raised, and the LA and LV can be dilated due to volume overload.

Non-restrictive VSDs are large, resulting in equal LV and RV pressures. The pulmonary circulation is subject to increased blood flow at systemic pressure, leading to pulmonary vascular remodelling and increased PVR. This reduces the left-to-right shunt and, if uncorrected, eventually leads to shunt reversal (right-to-left) and Eisenmenger syndrome.

The unoperated patient

- Large VSDs with haemodynamically significant left-to-right shunt typically present in childhood with:
  1. Left heart failure due to volume loading of the LV.
  2. As the pulmonary vasculature is subject to increased pulmonary blood flow at high pressure, the PVR rises. This causes reduction in left-to-right shunt.
  3. If uncorrected, the shunt eventually reverses (right-to-left) resulting in Eisenmenger syndrome and cyanosis.

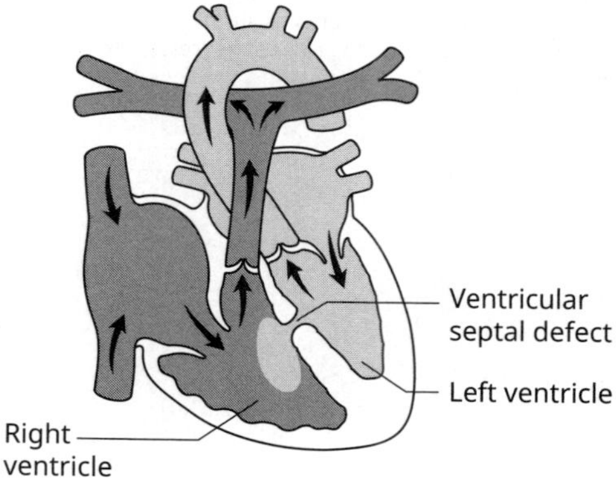

Fig. 17.2 Schematic diagram of a VSD.

- Even small VSDs can also cause the following:
  1. Aortic regurgitation, due to the potential proximity of the defect to the aortic valve.
  2. Double chambered right ventricle (sub pulmonary stenosis), due to muscle bundle hypertrophy in the RV outflow tract.

Acute presentation

Endocarditis, atrial and ventricular arrhythmias, heart failure.

Signs

- Coarse pansystolic heart murmur at left sternal border (as a rule of thumb, 'the louder the VSD murmur, the smaller the defect')
- LV ± RV heave
- Cyanosis if Eisenmenger syndrome has developed

Investigations

- *CXR*—normal (small defect); cardiomegaly, increased pulmonary markings (moderate defect); oligemic lung fields, enlarged proximal pulmonary arteries (large defect with Eisenmenger syndrome)
- *ECG*—broad P wave, signs of LV enlargement or RV hypertrophy (Eisenmenger syndrome), arrhythmia

Management

- Acute problems managed as in the non-ACHD setting
- VSDs with left heart volume loading should be closed to prevent the development of irreversible pulmonary vascular disease
- VSDs (even small ones) with progressive aortic regurgitation and VSDs with recurrent endocarditis should be considered for closure
- Closure is contraindicated in patients with Eisenmenger syndrome and severe pulmonary arterial hypertension

The operated patient

- Usually symptom-free but can present with atrial or ventricular arrhythmias or heart failure, especially when the defect has been closed late in life and the pulmonary artery pressure has been elevated
- Complete heart block can occur after closure
- Pulmonary vascular disease can progress, regress, or remain stable postoperatively

Atrioventricular septal defect

An AVSD is a deficiency of myocardial tissue at the atrioventricular (AV) junction, resulting in a *common AV junction* (Fig. 17.3). The term AVSD covers a spectrum of anomalies:

- There may be a common AV orifice or separate AV orifices
- There may be an ASD (ostium primum) or a VSD (inlet-type) or both
- The AV valves are abnormal and may be regurgitant
- AVSDs occur in 35% of patients with Down syndrome

Physiological consequences

- Physiology will be mainly determined by the degree of shunting across the ASD ± VSD; the presence or absence of pulmonary hypertension and the degree of AV valve regurgitation
- Heart failure, atrial arrhythmias, and AV conduction disease may occur

The operated patient

- Potential problems include left or right AV valve regurgitation or stenosis, subaortic stenosis, and complete AV block

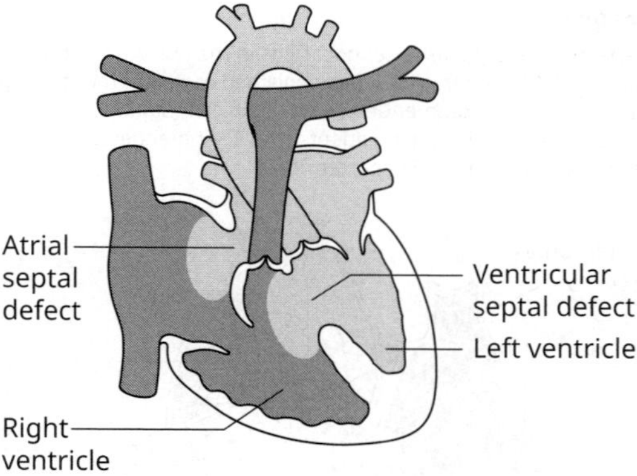

Fig. 17.3 Diagram of an AVSD.

Patent ductus arteriosus

- A PDA represents a persistent communication between the descending aorta and the proximal left pulmonary artery (Fig. 17.4)
- Blood shunts left-to-right (aorta to PA) because the right-sided pulmonary vascular resistance is lower than the left-sided systemic vascular resistance. This leads to pulmonary over-circulation, left heart volume loading and left heart dilatation
- If uncorrected, large PDAs result in pulmonary vascular disease and ultimately Eisenmenger syndrome with right-to-left shunt across the PDA into the *descending* aorta. This results in differential cyanosis—reduced lower body oxygen saturations with maintained upper body saturations
- Small ducts cause a murmur without haemodynamic effects

Signs

Continuous (systolic and diastolic) murmur at upper left sternal border; long ejection systolic murmur with small PDAs.

Acute presentation

Rare—endarteritis (like endocarditis) is the main cause.

Management

- Endarteritis managed as for endocarditis in the non-ACHD setting
- Closure of PDA is indicated if left heart enlarged or when a murmur is present
- Device closure is recommended when technically suitable
- Closure is contraindicated in patients with Eisenmenger syndrome and severe pulmonary arterial hypertension

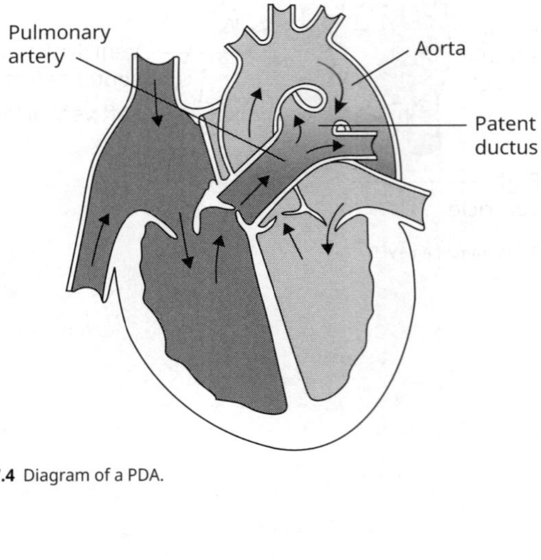

Fig. 17.4 Diagram of a PDA.

Aortic coarctation

Coarctation is a narrowing of the aorta at the isthmus (just distal to the left subclavian artery). (Fig. 17.5). If severe, the lower body relies on collateral vessels via the intercostal arteries for perfusion. Complete occlusion is also possible ('interruption').

Important associations with coarctation include bicuspid aortic valve (85%), left heart obstructive lesions, syndromes (Turner syndrome, 22q11), hypertension and intracranial aneurysms.

The unoperated patient

Risks

- Upper body hypertension
- Heart failure from long-standing LV pressure load
- Aortic rupture or dissection
- Infective endocarditis
- Stroke from an associated ruptured berry aneurysm + hypertension
- Premature coronary artery disease

Symptoms and signs

- Headache, nosebleeds, claudication, cold feet
- Upper limb hypertension and differential arm–leg pulses. BP measurement in the right arm and a leg is necessary in all new patients with hypertension. A pressure difference of ^{3} 20 mmHg may suggest coarctation
- Continuous murmur in the interscapular region

Investigations

- *ECG*—LV hypertrophy
- *CXR*—the '3 sign' caused by narrowing of the aorta at the site of coarctation with dilatation of the vessel before and after the coarctation; 'rib notching' caused by erosions of the inferior edge of the ribs by enlarged intercostal arteries
- *Echo*—look for persistent diastolic antegrade flow in descending aorta, associated abnormalities
- *CT, MRI*—good visualization of location and severity, assess for aneurysm, collaterals

Management

- Acute consequences managed as in the non-ACHD setting
- Haemoptysis requires urgent aortic imaging with CT or MRI and referral to a tertiary centre as it may herald aortic dissection and/or rupture of a para-coarctation pseudoaneurysm
- Surgical repair or stenting of the stenosis may be indicated if significant gradient across coarctation (> 20 mmHg) and upper limb hypertension. Stenting is preferred treatment in adults where technically feasible

The operated patient

- Recoarctation and aneurysm formation (often intercostal) at the site of repair are not uncommon; aneurysm rupture presents acutely
- Other aortic wall complications are frequent
- Hypertension can persist or develop in adulthood and needs to be treated aggressively because of the risk of atherosclerosis

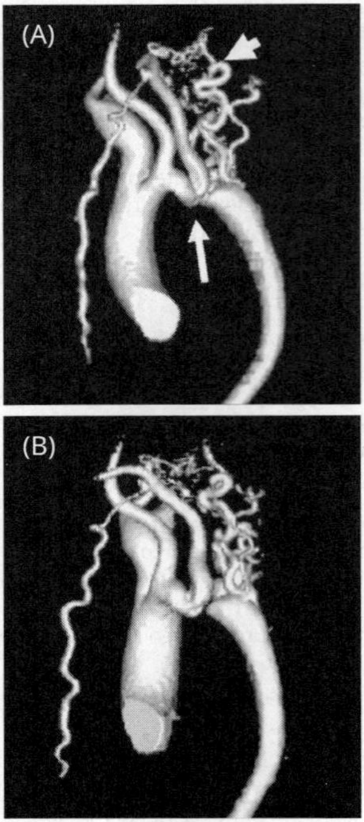

Fig. 17.5 Magnetic resonance angiogram of aortic coarctation.
Top: AP view showing site of coarctation (long arrow), enlarged head and neck vessels and extensive collateral circulation to the descending aorta (short arrow)
Bottom: slightly rotated view showing the nature of coarctation.

Transposition of the great arteries

The unoperated patient

The aorta arises from the RV and the pulmonary artery arises from the LV (Fig. 17.6). Instead of functioning in series, systemic circulation and pulmonary circulation function in parallel ('pink' blood circulating between left heart and lungs; 'blue' blood circulating between right heart and the body).

After birth, mixing of the systemic and pulmonary circulation is essential for survival. This can be achieved using prostaglandin (to maintain ductal patency) and balloon atrial septostomy (to allow mixing between the atria) before proceeding to surgical repair.

Surgical options

Atrial switch operation (Mustard and Senning procedures)

- Blood is redirected at the atrial level using baffles
- Redirection of 'pink' blood: pulmonary veins > TV > systemic RV > aorta
- Redirection of 'blue' blood: SVC/IVC > MV > subpulmonary LV > pulmonary artery
- Achieves 'physiological correction', but multiple problems occur (morphological RV now functioning as systemic pump, arrhythmias)
- These procedures were superseded by arterial switch in 1980s

Arterial switch operation

- Blood is redirected at arterial level by switching aorta and pulmonary artery to anatomically correct positions
- 'Pink' blood: pulmonary veins > MV > systemic LV > aorta
- 'Blue' blood: SVC/IVC > TV > subpulmonary RV > pulmonary artery

The patient after arterial switch operation

- Arrhythmias are less common compared with atrial switch patients and ventricular function is usually well conserved
- Suture lines in the pulmonary trunk can cause stenosis
- Peripheral pulmonary artery stenosis can be caused by the position of the pulmonary bifurcation anterior to the ascending aorta
- Progressive dilatation of the aortic root (former pulmonary root) can cause neo-aortic valve regurgitation
- Coronary artery reimplantation may result in ostial coronary stenosis and myocardial ischaemia

Signs

- Ejection systolic heart murmur from pulmonary artery stenosis
- Diastolic heart murmur from AR

Investigation

ECG—typically normal, less often signs of myocardial ischaemia and RV hypertrophy

Management

Assessment for pulmonary arterial stenoses, AR, and coronary stenoses, which may warrant intervention.

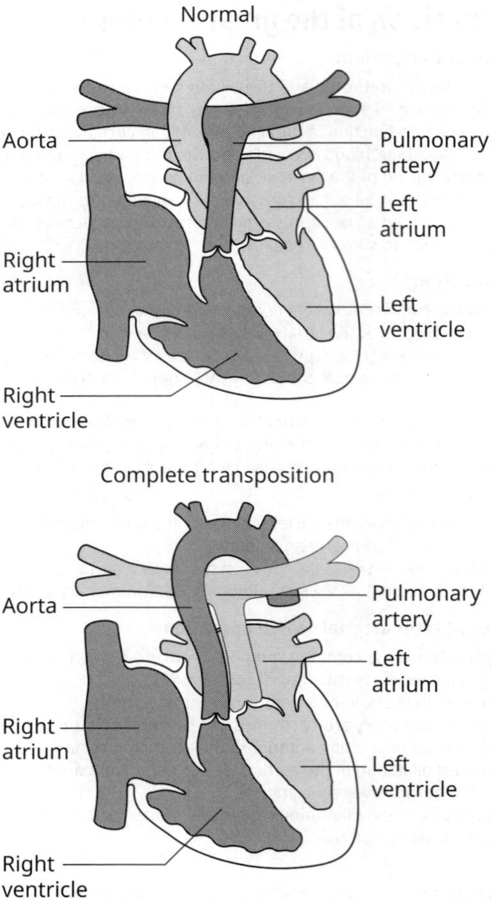

Fig. 17.6 Diagram illustrating TGA.

The patient after atrial switch operation

Problems include:

- Significant morbidity from arrhythmia related to extensive atrial surgery: bradyarrhythmias (sinus node dysfunction, slow junctional escape rhythm) and tachyarrhythmias (atrial flutter and AF)
- Systemic RV dysfunction leading to heart failure (the morphological RV struggles to support systemic circulation)

- Regurgitation of the systemic tricuspid valve
- Baffle stenoses (causing systemic or pulmonary venous congestion) and baffle leaks (causing volume loading of the subpulmonary LV ± paradoxical emboli)
- Pulmonary hypertension, usually post-capillary due to systemic RV dysfunction

Signs

- Systolic heart murmur from TR
- Heart failure
- Peripheral oedema and ascites from systemic venous congestion

Investigations

- *ECG*—sinus bradycardia or junctional escape rhythm, right axis deviation, RV hypertrophy, atrial arrhythmias
- *CXR*—cardiomegaly, pulmonary congestion, narrow vascular pedicle

Management

- Specialist ACHD input required due to the complexity of arrhythmia management, including pacing, and the difficulty in assessing RV function
- Thorough assessment of the RV, TV, atrial baffles, and heart rhythm is paramount
- At present there is lack of evidence for prognostic benefit of conventional heart failure medications in atrial switch patients
- Management of heart failure is empirical—loop diuretics and mineralocorticoid receptor antagonists form the mainstay of treatment; conventional heart failure medications may be used in symptomatic patients
- CRT may be offered if technically feasible
- Percutaneous treatments for baffle lesions may be offered (balloon dilatation/stenting for obstruction; device closure for leaks)
- Surgical treatment options include TV repair/replacement or even conversion to the arterial switch operation for selected patients
- The end of the therapeutic spectrum is heart transplantation
- Atrial arrhythmias are often poorly tolerated and urgent DC cardioversion should be considered
- Heart rate lowering medications should be used cautiously in view of the propensity to bradyarrhythmias
- Pacing is performed in specialist centres as lead placement can be challenging

Congenitally corrected transposition of the great arteries

In ccTGA the ventricles are 'inverted' (Fig. 17.7). Systemic venous return ('blue' blood) enters the RA, which connects to the subpulmonary LV, which connects to the pulmonary artery. Pulmonary venous return ('pink' blood) enters the LA, which connects to the systemic RV, which connects to the aorta. The circulation is therefore 'physiologically corrected' but the morphological RV is supporting the systemic circulation.

ccTGA is often associated with other defects, e.g. abnormalities and regurgitation of the systemic TV, VSD, PS/sub PS, and complete heart block. ccTGA can occur with dextrocardia.

The unoperated patient

- Progressive systemic RV dysfunction is common (the morphological RV struggles to support systemic circulation)
- Progressive regurgitation of the systemic TV may occur
- Risk of bradyarrhythmias (complete AV block) and tachyarrhythmias (atrial arrhythmia or SVT 2° to WPW syndrome)
- Patients with a VSD and PS can be cyanotic

The operated patient

Patients may have been operated on for their associated lesions, for example:

- VSD closure
- Implantation of LV to pulmonary artery conduit to relieve sub PS
- Replacement of the systemic TV

A 'corrective procedure' would be the 'double switch operation' (combination of an atrial and arterial switch operation); this is rarely performed in adults.

Signs

Systolic murmur—VSD, PS, or TR may be difficult to differentiate.

Investigations

- *ECG*—arrhythmia (complete AV block, atrial arrhythmia), Q waves in V1 and V2, and absent Q wave in V5 and V6
- *CXR*—dextrocardia (20% of patients), cardiomegaly

Management

- Currently there is lack of evidence to support conventional heart failure treatments in systemic RV failure but diuretics may provide symptom relief
- Symptomatic bradycardia or chronotropic incompetence warrant pacemaker implantation; CRT should be considered
- Atrial arrhythmias are common after atrial surgery or with severe TR. They are not well tolerated in the setting of a systemic RV, especially with RV dysfunction and TR. Urgent DCCV should be considered
- TR should be treated surgically (i.e. valve repair/replacement) before ventricular dysfunction becomes irreversible

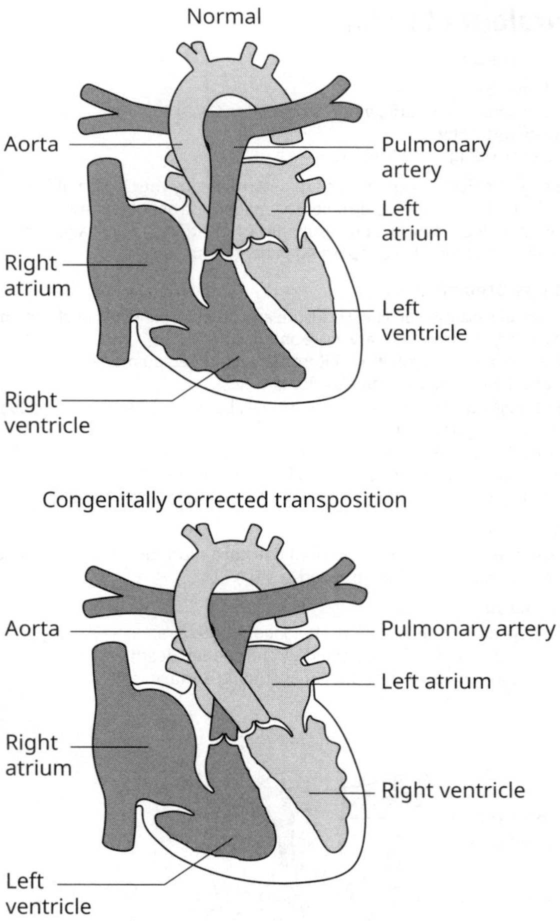

Fig. 17.7 Diagram illustrating ccTGA.

Tetralogy of Fallot

ToF consists of:

- A large VSD
- Right ventricular outflow tract obstruction (RVOTO)
- RV hypertrophy
- An over-riding aorta (Fig. 17.8)

The physiological consequences are determined by the degree of RVOT obstruction, which in turn determines the magnitude of pulmonary blood flow. Significant RVOT obstruction results in a right-to-left shunt and cyanosis. Survival to adulthood in unoperated patients with ToF is rare.

The operated patient

- Surgical repair includes VSD closure and relief of the RVOT obstruction ± patching of the pulmonary valve annulus
- The commonest problem is PR from the enlarged pulmonary outflow tract, but (re)stenosis can also occur
- The majority of patients tolerate PR well, but severe PR eventually leads to RV enlargement and dysfunction ± TR
- LV dysfunction and aortic dilatation may also occur
- Repaired TOF is associated with VT and sudden death
- Atrial arrhythmias occur, especially if RA enlargement is present

Signs

Parasternal RV heave (RV dilatation), diastolic murmur (PR or AR), systolic murmur (residual RVOT obstruction or VSD).

Investigations

- *ECG*—complete RBBB, QRS prolongation (QRS duration >180 ms is a prognostic marker for sustained VT and sudden death)
- *CXR*—cardiomegaly, dilatation of ascending aorta

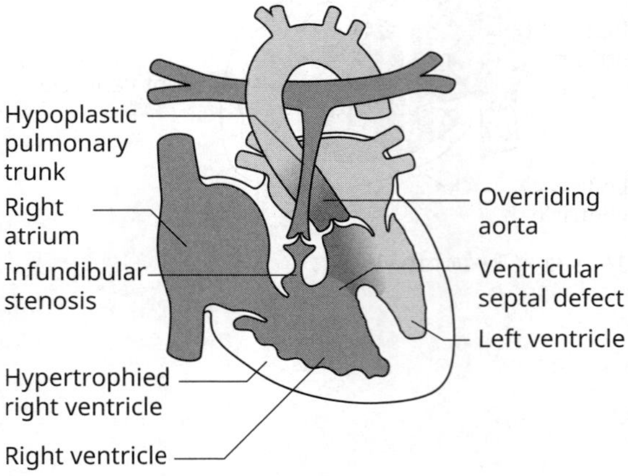

Fig. 17.8 Diagram illustrating ToF.

Management

- Most patients are minimally symptomatic
- Patients with RV dysfunction ± severe dilation should be considered for pulmonary valve replacement (PVR)
- Percutaneous PVR should be offered if technically feasible in patients with RVOT conduits and in selected patients with native outflow tracts
- There is increased risk of endocarditis with percutaneous PVR
- The development of arrhythmias (VT and atrial flutter/AF) warrants both full electrophysiologic assessment and thorough review of the haemodynamics
- ICD implantation should be considered in patients with multiple risk factors for SCD, although criteria for primary prevention ICDs in this group are not yet well defined

The single ventricle

The term 'single ventricle' refers to hearts which are incapable of supporting biventricular circulation because:

- One ventricle is anatomically and/or functionally deficient, or
- There are other factors that preclude biventricular repair (e.g. a very large septal defect)

The single ventricle receives both systemic and pulmonary venous blood and pumps blood into both the pulmonary artery and the aorta (Fig. 17.9). This results in volume loading of the single ventricle and cyanosis.

Clinical presentation is determined by the amount of pulmonary blood flow (PBF) and the presence of associated lesions:

- In the absence of any pulmonary outflow tract obstruction, there will be excess PBF, eventually resulting in pulmonary hypertension, shunt reversal and Eisenmenger syndrome
- In the presence of severe pulmonary outflow tract obstruction, there will be inadequate PBF and severe cyanosis
- In some scenarios there will be 'just the right amount' of pulmonary outflow tract obstruction, which permits sufficient PBF, but prevents excess PBF and pulmonary hypertension. This is called 'balanced circulation'

Surgery in patients with single ventricles is palliative and aims to secure adequate pulmonary and systemic blood flow and maintain systemic ventricular function.

Surgery for single ventricles

- In the absence of pulmonary outflow tract obstruction, pulmonary artery banding is performed to protect the lungs from developing pulmonary hypertension
- In the presence of severe pulmonary outflow tract obstruction, aortopulmonary shunts are performed in early infancy to increase PBF. As the single ventricle continues to pump blood into both the aorta and pulmonary arteries, volume overload remains a problem
- Systemic venous-to-pulmonary artery connections such as the Glenn shunt (Fig 17.11) or the Fontan operation (Fig 17.10) are subsequently performed as definitive palliations to improve PBF and separate the pulmonary from the systemic circulation while unloading the systemic ventricle

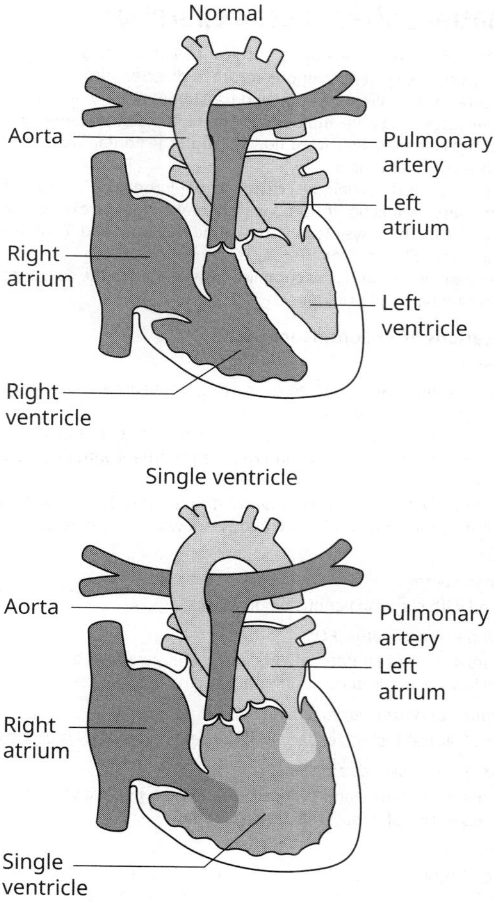

Fig. 17.9 Diagram showing a normal (2-ventricle) heart and a heart with effectively a single ventricle.

The patient after Fontan operation

The Fontan procedure is a staged surgical palliation for a single ventricle heart, in which the systemic venous return is diverted directly into the pulmonary arteries (i.e. without employing a subpulmonary ventricle). Blood flow to the lungs is passive and depends on high systemic venous pressure, low atrial pressure, unobstructed flow through the Fontan pathways/lungs, and good ventricular function.

Different surgical techniques exist: atriopulmonary (AP) Fontan; total cavopulmonary connection ('TCPC') with lateral tunnel or extracardiac conduit. (Fig 17.10). The physiology is the same however and 'Fontan' can be used as an umbrella term for all.

Fontan patients are at risk of complications related to the surgery and the abnormal circulatory physiology.

Complications after Fontan operation

Arrhythmias

- Atrial flutter/fibrillation related to scarring from surgery, or to atrial distension from high venous pressure
- Atrial arrhythmias in Fontan patients can precipitate profound haemodynamic deterioration and require treatment with urgent DCCV (see below)
- Sinus node dysfunction and bradyarrhythmias may occur. Transvenous pacing may not be possible (SVC and IVC now connected to pulmonary artery)

Thromboembolism

Associated with sluggish venous blood flow.

Protein-losing enteropathy (PLE)

PLE occurs in 10% of Fontan patients and is characterized by intestinal protein loss, low serum protein, peripheral oedema, and ascites.

Deterioration of ventricular function

This is the 'natural' history, especially if the ventricle is of RV morphology.

Fontan-associated liver disease (FALD)

Development of fibrosis and cirrhosis due to high hepatic venous pressure and increased risk of hepatocellular carcinoma.

Cyanosis

From persistent right-to-left shunting through a fenestration (small hole made in Fontan pathway at time of surgery) and/or collaterals.

Signs

- A patient with a 'good' Fontan has no murmurs and a single S_2 (systolic murmurs can indicate AV valve incompetence)
- Peripheral oedema—heart failure or PLE

Investigations

- *ECG*—arrhythmia
- *CXR*—cardiomegaly, atrial enlargement
- *Bloods*—abnormal LFTs, low platelets, raised AFP indicate FALD. Low protein/albumin suggestive of PLE

Management

- Fontan patients are one of the most challenging group of patients in cardiology and require close follow-up by tertiary centre specialists
- Treatment aims to maintain optimal pulmonary and systemic circulation and to preserve ventricular function
- Avoid dehydration —patients are very susceptible
- Currently there is lack of evidence regarding anticoagulation in Fontan patients. Some centres anticoagulate all Fontan patients. Others only anticoagulate patients at highest risk of thrombosis (AP Fontan, atrial arrhythmias, previous thrombosis, or patent fenestration) and use aspirin for lower-risk patients

Management of atrial arrhythmias in Fontan

- Atrial arrhythmias in a Fontan are an emergency
- Diagnosis may be challenging. A high index of suspicion is required in all Fontan patients; old ECGs are invaluable
- Treatment is urgent DCCV
- Anti-arrhythmic drugs are generally not recommended as they can precipitate bradyarrhythmias and transvenous pacing may not be possible. Be prepared to pace externally if necessary. Seek specialist help
- Patients should be anticoagulated (LMWH if not already on warfarin or NOAC)
- Must receive IV fluids whilst NBM to avoid dehydration
- Positive pressure ventilation should be avoided
- Recommend slow administration of anaesthetic (low cardiac output)
- Advice should be sought from tertiary centre specialist regarding ongoing management

The cyanotic patient

Cyanosis is common in ACHD and occurs due to right-to-left shunting. The resulting hypoxaemia leads to adaptive mechanisms to increase oxygen delivery to the tissues. These include a rightward shift in the oxyhaemoglobin binding curve and increased haemoglobin (Hb) concentration (2° erythrocytosis).

Symptoms related to hypoxia include SOB, chest pain, and symptoms arising from the multiorgan consequences of cyanosis.

Multi-organ consequences of cyanosis

Haematological

- 2° erythrocytosis and increased blood viscosity
- Iron deficiency (high demand, dietary, or induced by inappropriate venesections); often missed as MCV and Hb can be 'normal' (cyanotic patients should have an Hb well above the upper limit of normal). Look for low serum ferritin in a stable patient and/or reduced transferrin saturation (< 20%) to establish if iron deficiency is present. Treat with iron supplementation
- Haemostatic abnormalities with increased risk of bleeding *and* thrombosis (thrombocytopenia, abnormal platelet function, abnormal clotting factors. stasis, presence of thrombogenic material, arrhythmia)

Neurological

- Brain injury from thromboembolic events (paradoxical embolism, arrhythmia), haemorrhage, abscesses

Renal

- Hypoxaemia-induced glomerulopathy—haematuria, proteinuria

Other

- Gout
- Osteoarthropathy
- Cholelithiasis (increased uric acid and unconjugated bilirubin)

Management

Venesection in cyanosed patients

- Venesection is hardly ever needed as it compromises the patient's ability to carry oxygen to the tissue
- A trial of venesection may only be considered with tertiary input when severe symptoms of 'hyperviscosity syndrome' (headache, dizziness, fatigue, visual disturbances, tinnitus, and myalgia) are present in the setting of extreme erythrocytosis (Hct > 65%) after 'correcting' dehydration and iron deficiency (symptoms of the latter mimic symptoms of 'hyperviscosity syndrome'). Seek specialist advice first

Venesection procedure

- Slow removal of 400–500 ml blood, with simultaneous IV administration of 750 ml isotonic saline
- Use IV 'air filters'—to reduce the risk of systemic air embolus
- BP and heart rate monitoring are required

Iron deficiency

- Needs oral or IV iron supplements; aim for transferrin saturation > 20%

Anticoagulation

- No general consensus on routine anticoagulation
- Anticoagulation indicated for atrial arrhythmias
- Caution when measuring clotting—if Hct > 55% , need to use adjusted citrate tubes to measure PT/APTT (otherwise PT/APTT may be falsely elevated)

Eisenmenger syndrome

Eisenmenger syndrome is a pathophysiological condition resulting from CHD. Uncorrected left-to-right shunting and progressive pulmonary hypertension eventually leads to reversal of the shunt and cyanosis when right-sided pressure exceeds systemic pressure. VSD, AVSD, and large PDAs are responsible for 80% of cases. Eisenmenger patients exhibit signs and symptoms related to chronic cyanosis and are at risk of complications related to pulmonary hypertension.

Signs

- Cyanosis
- Loud S_2
- No murmur from original lesion

Investigations

- *ECG*—RV hypertrophy
- *CXR*—oligaemic lung fields, enlarged proximal pulmonary arteries

Acute presentation

- Progressive heart failure
- Atrial arrhythmias
- Angina
- Syncope and SCD
- Haemoptysis due to thrombotic event or intrapulmonary haemorrhage
- Pulmonary artery thrombosis—usually *in situ* thrombosis and not thromboembolic

Management

Also see Box 17.2.

Haemoptysis/intrapulmonary bleeding

- Bed rest
- Volume resuscitation
- CXR and CT scan to determine source and extent of haemorrhage
- Bloods—repeat FBC if continuous bleeding is suspected; remember that a 'normal' Hb is *not normal* in cyanotic patients. Remember to use adjusted citrate tubes for clotting sample if Hct > 55%
- Consider tranexamic acid
- Antibiotics
- Consider embolization of culprit vessels identified by angiography

Anticoagulation

- No general consensus on routine anticoagulation
- Risks of bleeding vs risks of thrombosis need to be carefully weighed up. Consider anticoagulation for atrial arrhythmias ± thromboembolic events

Treatment of pulmonary hypertension

Advanced therapies such as prostacyclin analogues, endothelin antagonists like bosentan (a dual endothelin antagonist), and phosphodiesterase inhibitors have been shown to reduce pulmonary vascular resistance and improve symptoms in patients with Eisenmenger syndrome, similarly to patients with idiopathic pulmonary hypertension. Stable patients with functional class > II should therefore be considered for advanced therapy once iron deficiency—if present—is corrected. Seek specialist advice.

Long-term oxygen is not routinely recommended, as there are alternative oral therapies and it restricts the patient from physical activity, which should be encouraged.

Box 17.2 Rules in the care of Eisenmenger and other cyanotic patients

- Avoid dehydration
- Maintain sinus rhythm
- Use air filters for IV lines to prevent air embolism
- Avoid nephrotoxics
- Treat iron deficiency
- Consult with ACHD specialist prior to any non-cardiac surgical/interventional procedure
- Postoperative care in ICU
- Good contraceptive advice and avoidance of pregnancy
- Avoid strenuous exercise and competitive sports, but encourage low-grade regular physical activity
- Annual immunization against influenza and pneumococcal infections
- Prompt antibiotic treatment for respiratory tract infections
- Antibiotic prophylaxis for invasive dental work

Arrhythmias

Arrhythmias are common in ACHD, occurring as a result of the original lesion, surgical treatment, or residual haemodynamic lesions. Arrhythmias in these patients are associated with significant morbidity and mortality and their detection and treatment can be challenging.

Atypical atrial flutter and intra-atrial re-entry tachycardia

Usually caused by atrial dilatation or previous extensive atrial surgery (Fontan, Mustard, Senning). Intra-atrial excitation circuits around electrical barriers such as scars and suture lines cause rapid atrial heart rate or flutter. AV conduction may be normal in relatively young adults, allowing for a fast 1:1 conduction and a fast ventricular rate with haemodynamic compromise.

Treatment

- Chemical cardioversion is not often successful. Consider urgent (same day) electrical cardioversion for all subjects, particularly those with Fontan/TCPC, atrial switch, cyanotic heart disease, or severe ventricular impairment. Have a low threshold for TOE to exclude clot
- Administer IV fluids whilst patients NBM to avoid dehydration
- Amiodarone and β-blockade may be used for rate control whilst organizing DCCV but should be used with caution because many of these ACHD patients also have a propensity to bradyarrhythmias and anatomy may preclude transvenous pacing, e.g. Fontan
- Radiofrequency ablation can block the circuits and potentially treat the arrhythmia. Electrophysiologists with special expertise in CHD are required for these demanding procedures

Ventricular tachycardia

VT is commonly associated with previous ventricular surgery or long-standing abnormal ventricular load:

- Previous VSD closure
- ToF repair—prolonged QRS duration is a risk marker
- PR and RV enlargement
- Single ventricles
- Mustard or Senning repairs; Rastelli operation
- ccTGA
- Eisenmenger syndrome

Treatment

- Identifying and treating the culprit haemodynamic lesion is an integral part of arrhythmia management
- Standard indications for secondary prevention ICD implantation can be applied to the CHD population
- ACHD patients with biventricular physiology, LVEF < 35%, and symptomatic HF should be considered for primary prevention ICD
- Other indications for primary prevention ICD implantation in the CHD population are currently not well defined

General considerations for the treatment of arrhythmias

- Obtain as much information on the patient as possible
- Assess the patient thoroughly for signs of heart failure and infection

- Obtain a 12-lead ECG and compare with previous ECGs (ACHD patients often have a broad QRS complex)
- Amiodarone and β-blockers, including sotalol, are the most commonly used drugs. Negative inotropes are poorly tolerated especially in patients with single ventricle physiology
- Low threshold for DCCV
- Seek expert advice early

Syncope

Syncope is always a matter of concern in patients with ACHD, especially if they are cyanosed or have pulmonary hypertension. See Box 17.3 for causes.

Box 17.3 Causes of syncope in ACHD

- Tachyarrhythmia—symptoms depend on rate and haemodynamic substrate
- Bradycardia from sinus node dysfunction, AV block
- PE
- Severe pulmonary hypertension
- Severe obstructive lesion—valve stenosis/outflow tract obstruction
- Aortic dissection, rupture
- Myocardial ischaemia
- Hypotension—?drug induced
- Vasovagal

Investigations

12-lead ECG, echocardiography, and Holter monitoring (low threshold for implantable loop recorder).

If requesting CTPA to exclude PE, consider the anatomy. For Fontan patients, recommend delayed acquisition to ensure homogeneous opacification of pulmonary arteries and avoid a non-diagnostic scan.

Management

Any syncope in a patient with congenital heart disease should initiate thorough electrophysiological and haemodynamic assessment. Seek advice from an ACHD specialist early.

Heart failure

ACHD patients presenting with heart failure need thorough evaluation to look for acute precipitants and assess the underlying lesions.

Common acute precipitants include:

- Arrhythmia
- Infection
- Ischaemia

Patients with ACHD often have very finely balanced haemodynamics with minimal cardiac reserve and even minor changes in their condition can cause severe deterioration.

Underlying lesions presenting with left or 'systemic' heart failure

- Left-sided valve disease—mitral and aortic valve
- TGA after Mustard or Senning repair and ccTGA
- Systemic LV dysfunction in older ToF patients

Underlying lesions presenting with right or 'subpulmonary' heart failure

- Fontan patients
- Pulmonary hypertension/Eisenmenger syndrome
- Right-sided valve disease—tricuspid and pulmonary valve
- Mustard with obstruction of intra-atrial pathways
- Elderly patients with late repair or unrepaired ASD

Medical treatment

Seek expert advice early.

- Look for the cause— medical treatment will not cure anatomic lesions
- Restore sinus rhythm as soon as possible in compromised patients
- Use standard treatment for heart failure including diuretics but be cautious with vasodilator therapy (Table 17.1)
- Consider CRT in patients with systemic ventricular EF < 35%, sinus rhythm, broad QRS and NYHA II-ambulatory IV. Consider also in patients with systemic ventricular EF < 35% who are undergoing new device placement with anticipated requirement for significant ventricular pacing
- There are many barriers to transplant in ACHD patients (previous sternotomies, HLA sensitization, increased risk of pulmonary hypertension). Early survival post-transplant is worse compared with non-CHD patients, but long-term survival post-transplant is superior for ACHD patients. Organ shortage remains a limiting factor

Table 17.1 Heart failure treatment—considerations for ACHD patients

	Pros	Cons
Loop diuretics	Effective Improve symptoms	Rapidly reduces preload Caution in Fontan patients
Spironolactone	Effective Improves symptoms	
ACE inhibitors	Effective to reduce hypertension Unknown long-term benefits on heart function	Little evidence to improve heart function. Contraindicated in pregnancy Caution if: Preload dependant. Obstructive lesion present Renal dysfunction Pulmonary hypertension
β-blocker	Antiarrhythmic Good for heart rate control	Caution in bradycardia
Digoxin	Rate control in atrial flutter	

Data from with Gatzoulis MA *et al.* (eds), *Adult Congenital Heart Disease: A Practical Guide*, 2005. Oxford: BMJ Books, Blackwell Publishing Group.

Glossary of common surgical procedures

Arterial switch operation or Jatene procedure

Operation for TGA patients. Switch of the great arteries to bring the aorta to the former pulmonary artery position and the pulmonary artery to the former aortic position. The coronary arteries have to be transposed from the aortic root to the former pulmonary artery root (neo aorta). Ultimately, the LV will perfuse the aorta and the RV will perfuse the pulmonary artery.

Bentall operation

Replacement of the ascending aorta and aortic valve with a composite graft (conduit) and valve and reimplantation of the coronary arteries into the conduit.

Brock procedure

Palliative procedure for ToF patients. Closed resection of RV musculature from the outflow tract using a biopsy-like instrument and dilatation (valvotomy) of the pulmonary valve.

Classic Blalock–Taussig shunt

Subclavian artery to ipsilateral pulmonary artery anastomosis—direct end-to-side junction.

Modified Blalock–Taussig shunt

Subclavian artery to ipsilateral pulmonary artery anastomosis using a prosthetic graft.

Damus–Kaye–Stansel operation

Operation connecting aorta and pulmonary artery in a side-to-side fashion to provide unrestricted blood flow from the systemic ventricle to the aorta. For patients with single ventricles, TGA and restrictive VSD/subaortic stenosis.

Fontan operation

Palliative operation for patients with 'single' ventricle physiology (Fig. 17.10). Diversion of the systemic venous return to the lung without interposition of a subpulmonary ventricle. Achieves volume unloading of the 'single' ventricle and ideally normalization of the arterial oxygen saturation.

Multiple variations of the procedure exist regarding the type of connection between the systemic veins and the pulmonary arteries (Fig. 17.10):

- *Classic Fontan:* connection between RA and pulmonary artery
- *Extracardiac Fontan:* IVC connected to pulmonary artery via an extracardiac conduit combined with a Glenn shunt
- *Bjoerk or RA–RV Fontan:* valved conduit between the RA and the RV
- *Total cavopulmonary connection (TCPC):* IVC connected to pulmonary artery via an intra-atrial tunnel (also called lateral tunnel), combined with a Glenn shunt to the SVC

A) Atriopulmonary Fontan. B) Total cavopulmonary connection (TCPC, lateral tunnel). C) TCPC (*extracardiac conduit).

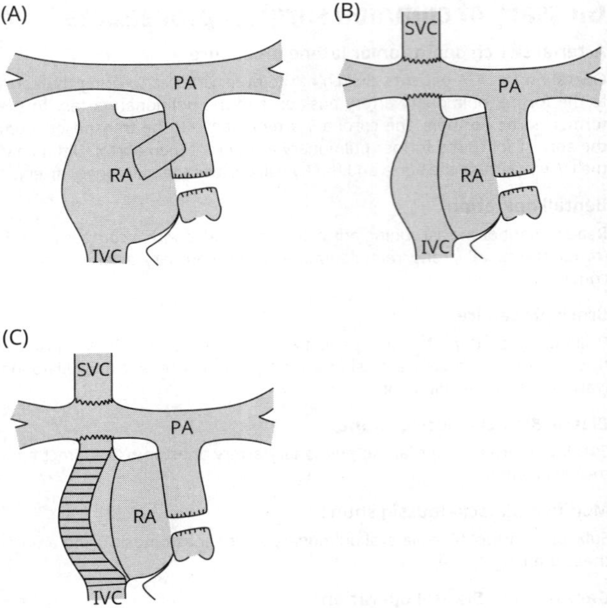

Fig. 17.10 Diagrams illustrating various types of Fontan operation.

Glenn shunt

SVC to pulmonary artery anastomosis (Fig. 17.11).

- *Classical Glenn shunt:* anastomosis of the SVC to the distal right pulmonary artery with ligation of the SVC below the anastomosis and division of the proximal right pulmonary artery from the pulmonary bifurcation
- *Bidirectional Glenn shunt:* anastomosis of the SVC to the undivided pulmonary artery

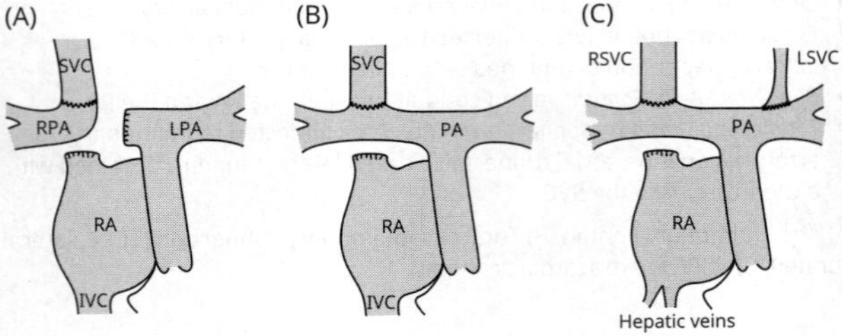

Fig. 17.11 Diagrams illustrating various types of Glenn shunt. A) Classical Glenn. B) Bidirectional Glenn. C) Bilateral bidirectional Glenn.

Konno operation

Complex repair and reconstruction of the LVOT for patients with tunnel-like subvalvar LVOT obstruction. The operation involves enlargement of the outflow tract by inserting a patch in the interventricular septum and aortic valve replacement as well as enlargement of the aortic annulus and the ascending aorta.

Lecompte manoeuvre

Manoeuvre that brings the pulmonary artery in a position anterior to the ascending aorta (part of the arterial switch operation or Jatene procedure).

Mustard operation

Atrial switch operation for patients with TGA—redirection of the venous blood to the contralateral ventricle using pericardial or synthetic patches.

Norwood operation

Initial palliative procedure for the treatment of hypoplastic left heart syndrome with aortic atresia and hypoplasia of the ascending aorta. Operation involves the reconstruction of 'neo-ascending' aorta using the pulmonary valve and trunk and the creation of an aortopulmonary shunt (usually modified BT shunt).

Potts anastomosis shunt

Descending aorta to left pulmonary artery anastomosis.

Rastelli operation

Operation for patients with TGA, VSD, and PS—closure of the VSD in a way that the patch recommits the LVOT to the aorta. The RV is connected to the main pulmonary artery using a valved conduit.

Ross operation

Aortic valve replacement by transplantation of the patient's pulmonary valve into aortic position (pulmonary autograft) and by replacing the pulmonary valve using a homograft valve. Major advantages:

- Potential of the 'neo-aortic' valve (former pulmonary valve) to grow in children
- No need for anticoagulation

Senning operation

Atrial switch operation for patients with TGA, redirection of the venous blood to the contralateral ventricle using the atrial wall and the septum.

Waterston shunt

Ascending aorta to right pulmonary artery anastomosis.

Further Reading

2020 ESC Guidelines for management of adult congenital heart disease *European Heart Journal* 2021; 42(6): 563–645.

Michael A. Gatzoulis, Margarita Brida, Gary Webb, and Piers E.F. Daubeney (eds), *Diagnosis and Management of Adult Congenital Heart Disease*, 4th edn. . Elsevier, 2014.

Chapter 18

Perioperative care

Perioperative issues

Cardiovascular complications of anaesthesia and surgery are common in patients suffering from ischaemic heart disease, LV dysfunction, arterial hypertension, and valvular heart disease.

Size of the problem

Large numbers of patients undergo non-cardiac surgery (NCS) throughout the world. The proportion of those with risk factors for cardiac disease is high and increasing. NCS is offered to older and more multi-morbid patients as surgical techniques and anaesthesia have improved. Nevertheless cardiac complications dominate and concern regarding them, whether exaggerated or not, generates significant perioperative discussion. The high number of cardiovascular complications reflects the nature of surgery: a stress test that cannot easily be stopped once the operation has started.

Pre-operative risk assessment is therefore an important element of informed consent and also influences the strategy for anaesthesia and perioperative care. Collaboration between surgeons, anaesthetists, and physicians—especially cardiologists—is essential to ensure optimal management.

Preoperative assessment

Medical opinion is sought on diagnosis, clinical status, and the appropriateness of the patient's current treatment. The medical opinion may conclude that further evaluation is required and/or recommend specific treatments, e.g. coronary revascularization or pacing, prior to surgery.

Guided by this medical opinion, the peri-op physician and anaesthetist can determine the patient's fitness for anaesthesia and surgery and develop a strategy for anaesthesia and postoperative care. This includes the extent of cardiovascular monitoring and the best location for postoperative care, e.g. ICU or HDU. *Informed consent* will require consideration of the risks as well as the benefits of the procedure, and may ultimately result in surgery not being offered.

Predictors of risk

The risk of perioperative cardiac complications relates to both the clinical status of the patient and the nature of the proposed surgery. The following stratification of predictors is based on the European Society of Cardiology 2022 guidelines. Clearly, the highest risk occurs when a patient with a 'major' clinical risk factor(s) undergoes a 'major' risk surgical procedure.

Predictors related to the patient

Chronic

- Age > 75 years
- Coronary artery disease
- Heart failure
- Severe aortic stenosis
- Peripheral arterial disease
- Cerebrovascular disease
- Renal insufficiency
- Diabetes
- Anaemia

(Sub) -acute

- Acute coronary syndrome
- Acute aortic syndrome
- Acute stroke
- Acute trauma (e.g. hip fracture)

Procedure and post-op-related factors

- Urgency of the procedure
- Hypotension
- Hypercoagulability
- Bleeding
- Inflammation
- Tachycardia
- Hypothermia
- Sympathetic nervous system stimulation
- Pain
- Hypoxaemia

Predictors related to surgery

Major (reported cardiac risk > 5%)

- Adrenal surgery
- Aortic and other major vascular surgery
- Carotid (symptomatic)
- Duodenal-pancreatic surgery
- Liver resection, bile duct surgery
- Open limb revascularization
- Pneumonectomy
- Pulmonary or liver transplant
- Perforated bowel repair
- Open cystectomy

Intermediate (reported cardiac risk generally < 5%)

- Carotid endarterectomy (asymptomatic)
- Head and neck surgery
- Intraperitoneal and intrathoracic surgery
- Neurological or orthopaedic surgery
- Prostate surgery
- Renal transplant
- Urological or gynaecological surgery

Low risk

- Breast surgery
- Cataract and other eye surgery
- Dental surgery
- Endocrine—thyroid
- Endoscopic procedures
- Superficial procedures

In addition, special consideration should be given to the following

- Cardiovascular effect of aortic cross-clamping and de-clamping
- Gut handling leading to the release of inflammatory mediators
- Surgery likely to impair postoperative respiratory function
- Positioning of the patient on the operating table (often for minimally invasive surgery), e.g. steep head-down position with or without leg elevation

Predictors related to the type of anaesthetic

Spinal or epidural anaesthesia

- *Perceived* to be safer for cardiac patients than GA
- ***But*** no scientific evidence of reduced cardiac risk
- ***And*** severe hypotension can result from autonomic blockade, so may actually be worse!
- Where spinal or epidural anaesthesia offers major advantages, monitoring needs to be extensive because of the possibility of hypotension

Local and regional anaesthesia (regional nerve blocks)

Associated with a relatively low risk of postoperative cardiac events.

General considerations

Cardiac disease is not always clinically obvious, particularly where function is limited, e.g. by respiratory disease, lower limb arthropathy, or peripheral vascular disease

Emergencies

Where potentially life-saving emergency surgery is required (e.g. ruptured aortic aneurysm, major trauma), identify and treat cardiac complications where possible, with a view to further cardiac evaluation postoperatively.

Elective/semi-urgent cases

- In the non-emergency setting, patients with 'major' clinical risk factors may require further investigation and/or treatment
  - An urgent multidisciplinary approach is required if surgery is time sensitive, e.g. cancer
- If not low-risk surgery, then these patients require an assessment of functional capacity, ECG, and biomarkers
  - The ability to walk up a flight of stairs unaided is approximately 4 METS and a reasonable discriminator of fitness
  - Cardiology consultation in those with known CAD is also recommended
  - A review of prior CT imaging may identify excess arterial calcification which is a useful marker of plaque burden
- For 'major' risk procedures and/or where functional capacity is low, non-invasive functional investigation may be required, depending on the individual situation, for example:
  - Echocardiography—to check LV function/valves/pulmonary pressures
  - Stress echocardiography—using exercise or dobutamine
  - Myocardial perfusion scan (SPECT) to investigate potential coronary disease and functional capacity
  - Cardio-pulmonary exercise testing to assess VO_2 max and anaerobic threshold

► Significant reversible myocardial ischaemia increases the risk of cardiac events after major surgery and further evaluation/treatment may be indicated after due consideration.

Cardiovascular drugs

- Most cardiovascular drugs can be safely administered throughout the perioperative period
- ACE inhibitors and angiotensin receptor antagonists may have to be omitted on the morning of surgery to reduce the risk of hypotension
- Antiplatelets can usually be stopped safely if more than one year post revascularization
- β-blockers are generally not omitted prior to NCS
- Statins have evidence suggesting protection in NCS. The dose should be optimized pre-op

Coronary artery disease

Coronary disease is the most frequent cause of cardiac complications from anaesthesia and surgery. In susceptible individuals, coronary events may be precipitated by haemodynamic perturbations (tachycardia, hypotension, hypertension), perioperative hypoxaemia (especially nocturnal hypoxaemia after abdominal surgery), altered coagulation, postoperative anaemia, or perioperative release of inflammatory cytokines causing disruption of vulnerable coronary plaques.

Angina

- Controlled angina increases the risk of anaesthesia and surgery but this increase is generally acceptable
- Unstable and recent onset angina should be investigated preoperatively as perioperative morbidity and mortality are increased

Prior MI

- The time between the MI and proposed elective surgery is important. An interval of at least 3–6 months is generally advocated. A delay of 6 weeks can be acceptable in uncomplicated MI, especially if there is no subsequent ischaemia on a stress test, and relatively preserved LV function
- As myocardial function is a major determinant of risk, patients with reduced LV function remain at increased risk irrespective of the time that has elapsed since the MI

Prior CABG

Asymptomatic patients following successful CABG are at low risk for perioperative cardiac events providing ventricular function is good and they remain asymptomatic.

Prior PCI

While CABG offers some protection, there is no such evidence for PCI. There is evidence that perioperative risk is *greater* in the first 1–3 months following PCI, though whether this reflects a higher risk population or an effect of the procedure is unclear.

Antiplatelet therapy

- To minimize the risk of stent thrombosis (from the exposed metal struts), patients usually receive aspirin and another anti-platelet medicines (clopidogrel, ticagrelor, or prasugrel) for up to 12 months for drug-eluting stents, although newer generation stents require 6–12 weeks of dual anti-platelet drugs
- The pronounced antiplatelet effect of these drugs poses a risk of perioperative haemorrhage, so it is preferable to defer surgery until a week after patients no longer need dual antiplatelet therapy
- If surgery cannot be delayed, the decision on the withdrawal or maintenance of dual antiplatelet therapy requires a discussion involving surgeon, cardiologist, anaesthetist, and haematologist. Surgery in closed cavities generally requires the withdrawal of dual antiplatelet therapy with the attending risk of stent thrombosis

- Maintaining single antiplatelet aspirin throughout the peri-operative phase is recommended in post-PCI/CABG patients
- In emergency situations, excessive bleeding may require the administration of platelets

Box 18.1 The need for coronary revascularization

Coronary revascularization (either CABG or PCI) may be necessary in selected patients to decrease the risk of cardiac complications from anaesthesia and surgery. Current guidelines recommend that coronary revascularization should be performed prior to non-cardiac surgery if it is indicated for conventional indications, e.g. angina (irrespective of planned non-cardiac surgery). If coronary revascularization is not warranted for conventional clinical indications, it should only be considered before high-risk surgery (particularly major vascular surgery).

The evidence for protection is weak; however, there is observational data to suggest that patients who have undergone successful CABG are protected against perioperative cardiac events if their cardiac function is good and there is no recurrence of symptoms. By contrast, the incidence of perioperative cardiac complications does not appear to be reduced by PCI.

Cardiac failure/reduced LV function

Both objective cardiac function and the patient's functional capacity are useful for predicting operative risk (see ➲ NYHA classification, p.77, Table 8.1). The ability to climb 1 flight of stairs with some load (or equivalent) is considered adequate reserve for most surgeries. Heart failure management should be optimized before surgery.

Objective testing that may be required

- Echocardiography
- Nuclear testing (MUGA or MPS SPECT scan)
- CMR

Optimization of heart failure therapy

- Avoid symptomatic hypotension pre-op
- Avoid acute cessation of HF therapy especially β-blockade
- Avoid over diuresis perioperatively
- Optimize hypoxaemia, especially if nocturnal
- Involve specialist HF team (if at all possible)

Arterial hypertension

- Hypertension confers a modest increase in the risk of cardiovascular complications, irrespective of the admission BP
- Presence of target organ involvement is more important than the level of BP for predicting events
- Defer surgery and treat hypertension if systolic pressure > 180 mmHg and/or diastolic > 110 mmHg. A delay of 4–6 weeks is necessary to improve autoregulation of blood flow, particularly in the brain
- Acutely dropping the BP with IV therapy is unhelpful unless there is evidence of acute dissection

Box 18.2 Prophylactic perioperative β-blockade

Patients on chronic β-blocker therapy should continue on β-blockers for an established indication (e.g. angina, hypertension, congestive heart failure, arrhythmia) throughout the perioperative period.

Though acute (within a few days of surgery), β-blockade has been widely advocated for the prophylaxis of perioperative cardiac events, evidence of their efficacy was inconclusive. The largest, randomized controlled trial of acute perioperative β-blockade (the POISE study)[1] has shown that while the risk of cardiac death and MI is reduced, there is an increase in all-cause mortality and in strokes. This balance of risks requires decisions based on the circumstances of individual patients

Where β-blockers are considered advantageous, treatment should be started days or weeks before elective surgery and the dose titrated to obtain a resting heart rate of ~60–70 bpm with strict protocols for rate and BP control.

1. Devereaux PJ et al. Effects of extended-release metoprolol succinate in patients undergoing non-cardiac surgery (POISE trial): a randomised controlled trial. *Lancet* 2008; 371: 1839–47.

Valvular heart disease

See also ➲ Chapter 8.

Aortic stenosis

Severe AS represents the most serious threat. The fixed obstruction to cardiac output permits very little adaptation where increased output is required. Peripheral vasodilatation, e.g. from regional anaesthesia or hypotension from haemorrhage cannot be matched by an adequate increase in cardiac output. The consequent fall in BP can lead to coronary hypoperfusion, reduced myocardial function, and further hypotension. This is a potentially fatal downward spiral. Although AS cannot be alleviated easily, knowledge of the severity can inform the patient and doctor of the risks and help determine the required monitoring.

Even in *moderate AS*, stiffness of the LV reduces the tolerance of variability of filling conditions. In fluid overload, the LA pressure will increase sharply, provoking pulmonary oedema, while low filling pressure (hypovolaemia) or low diastolic filling time (high ventricular rates) will decrease cardiac output. Where symptoms or physical signs suggest AS, a preoperative echocardiogram should be considered.

Nevertheless, severe AS with good LV function is usually not a contraindication to low or moderate risk surgery, even with the availability of TAVI.

Mitral stenosis

- Maintain slow heart rate—the onset of AF or loss of rate control in the perioperative period will decrease diastolic filling and cause a fall in cardiac output. This can provoke an abrupt deterioration ±pulmonary oedema
- Careful fluid balance—underfilling may cause an inordinate reduction in output while overfilling may cause pulmonary oedema
- Consider invasive monitoring

Mitral and aortic regurgitation

- In general, both are well tolerated
- Require careful fluid management
- May benefit from afterload reduction, e.g. with nitrates/ACE inhibitors

Valve intervention

In some cases, it may be appropriate to alleviate valve lesions prior to non-cardiac surgery, though a full discussion of indications are given in ➲ Chapter 8. The decision must consider the risks of prosthetic valve thrombosis and endocarditis (Box 18.3) related to future surgery.

Anticoagulation

(Also see ➲ p.110.)

- Metallic prosthetic valves—anticoagulation is discontinued before most operations. Warfarin is replaced by low molecular weight heparin until shortly before surgery to provide perioperative anticoagulation if there is a high risk of valvar thrombosis
- In emergencies, anticoagulation with warfarin can be transiently reversed by administration of FFP, which provides clotting factors

- ► Be very wary of giving vitamin K since this will prevent anticoagulation with warfarin for a prolonged period. With expert guidance, small doses of vitamin K (phytomenadione, e.g. 1 mg), can be administered

Box 18.3 Endocarditis avoidance

Abnormal heart valves, prosthetic mechanical valves, or biological valves are at ↑risk for infective endocarditis from organisms introduced at the time of surgery.

Antibiotic prophylaxis

This is a controversial topic—there is little evidence for its effectiveness, and the ↑risk from surgery is small compared to the background risk from everyday activities such as tooth-brushing. A fuller discussion on this can be found in Chapter 10 on Infective endocarditis (➲ Prophylaxis, p.130).

Vascular access

- Keep vascular access to the minimum necessary
- Take precautions to avoid infections at insertion
- Observe the skin around lines for signs of infection and revise lines regularly
- Seek to remove all vascular catheters as soon as they are no longer needed

Arrhythmias/pacing

- Most arrhythmias should be stabilized prior to surgery
- Controlled chronic AF (rate < 110 bpm) is rarely a significant problem
- During anaesthesia and surgery, arrhythmias occur frequently and require treatment only if haemodynamic compromise occurs
- See ➲Chapter 11 for specific details of management

Preoperative pacemaker insertion

In general, the indications for preoperative pacemaker insertion, including temporary pacemaker insertion, are the same as those for the non-surgical setting (see ➲ p.133, Box 11.1). These include complete heart block, Mobitz type II block, and symptomatic bradycardia. There are thus almost no circumstances where pacing is required purely for surgery,

Pacemakers and implantable defibrillators during surgery

►Establish the type of pacemaker or defibrillator, the indications for implantation, and the functional settings from the patient's pacemaker identification card or from the centre where it was implanted.

►With modern complex pacemakers/defibrillators it is no longer advisable to blindly return the pacemaker to its simplest mode of operation by fixing a magnet over it.

Electromagnetic interference (EMI)

Pacemakers and defibrillators are susceptible to interference, and in the operating theatre, diathermy equipment is the major concern. EMI may affect the device by direct electrical interference during diathermy or by exposure to an electromagnetic field (with the device lead acting as an aerial).

- Potential effects:
  - Inappropriate inhibition or triggering of paced output
  - Asynchronous pacing
  - Reprogramming—usually into a back-up mode
  - Damage to circuitry, or triggering of defibrillator discharge
  - Defibrillators may interpret electrocautery as VF and deliver a shock
- Bipolar leads, generally used in contemporary pacing systems, are much less sensitive to EMI than unipolar leads
- Electrocautery is usually applied in unipolar configuration between the handheld instrument (cathode) and the anode attached to the patient's skin
- ► Diathermy should be avoided near the pacemaker/ICD generator
- ► Bipolar diathermy should be used wherever possible

Post-cardiac surgery problems

This section is intended as a practical guide to situations commonly experienced after cardiac surgery.

The hypotensive patient

Read the operation note and anaesthetic chart.

Was the operation straightforward? The surgeon will have noted any difficulties, e.g. were small calibre coronary arteries prejudice graft patency, or were there problems with haemostasis. What was the preoperative assessment of LV function?

Blood pressure

Note the BP and pulse trends. Was there an abrupt change suggestive of an acute 'event' or has the change been gradual? Compare with preoperative values. Determine peripheral perfusion. Is the patient cold and 'shut down' or peripherally vasodilated? What is the urine output?

Filling

Is the patient adequately filled? One size does not fit all in this respect. Patients with LV hypertrophy but good LV systolic function (e.g. after aortic valve replacement) are likely to require higher filling pressures. In patients with significant TR (e.g. after mitral valve replacement), filling will be difficult to gauge from the venous pressure. Remember that early after surgery, you are likely to have the benefit of a CVP line—see ➲ p.357.

ECG

Does the ECG show evidence of myocardial ischaemia? Has the rhythm changed? AF is common postoperatively. New-onset or fast AF may be sufficient to compromise BP in susceptible patients.

Pericardial drains

Are the pericardial drains working? Has the rate of drainage changed (new bleeding, drain occlusion)? Hypotension with tachycardia, and elevated CVP may indicate pericardial tamponade. This can occur rapidly and may be caused by a relatively small volume of pericardial blood. Postoperatively, this may be caused by localized effects on a single chamber.

►An urgent echocardiogram should be obtained. In extreme cases, sudden haemodynamic collapse necessitates emergency exploration and direct drainage with the chest reopened.

- When hypotension persists despite correction of the reversible causes, further evaluation with echocardiography may be indicated. New wall motion abnormalities suggest perioperative infarction or 'stunning'
- Consider support with inotropic drugs ± IABP. These are considered in greater detail elsewhere (➲ p.19, 369)

Atrial fibrillation post-cardiac surgery

- Occurs in approximately 25% of patients
- More frequent in elderly patients and those with a prior history of AF
- Likely to return spontaneously to sinus rhythm unless AF was present preoperatively

Actions

- Markedly compromised patients need DC cardioversion
- Correct hypokalaemia: keep K^+ above 4.5 mmol/L
- Control rate with amiodarone or digoxin. β-blockers/calcium-channel blockers can be used if the underlying cardiac function is good
- IV amiodarone (central line) may hasten reversion to sinus rhythm. In selected patients, continuation with oral therapy may be indicated
- Anticoagulation is needed if persistent (heparin → warfarin)
- Arrange outpatient review of continuing need for antiarrhythmic therapy ± cardioversion

AV conduction block

- Most likely after aortic valve surgery because of the valve's proximity to the AV node
- Pacing is necessary using epicardial pacing electrodes implanted at surgery or a temporary transvenous system
- Permanent pacemaker implantation is sometimes required. Predicted by preoperative features—AV block, LBBB, root abscess, calcified aortic annulus, AR, and prior MI. See ➲ p.133, Box 11.1 for indications

Post-pericardiotomy syndrome

- Inflammatory (possibly autoimmune) pericarditis that occurs > 1 week after cardiac surgery where the pericardium has been opened
- Often associated with fever, pericarditic pain, and malaise
- The associated effusion may be serous or serosanguinous. It can be large and can lead to tamponade
- The diagnosis is clinical. Echocardiography is helpful in helping to determine the size, distribution, percutaneous accessibility, and haemodynamic significance of any effusion
- Usually self-limiting, but may recur
- ►Treat with NSAIDs

Further reading

Halvorsen S *et al*. 2022 ESC Guidelines on cardiovascular assessment and management of patients undergoing non-cardiac surgery: Developed by the task force for cardiovascular assessment and management of patients undergoing non-cardiac surgery of the European Society of Cardiology (ESC) Endorsed by the European Society of Anaesthesiology and Intensive Care (ESAIC). *European Heart Journal* 2022 43(39): 3826–924. https://doi.org/10.1093/eurheartj/ehac270

Cardiac drugs: effects and cardiotoxicity

General approach to cardiotoxicity

Cardiovascular side effects can occur with both cardiac and non-cardiac medication. In particular, side effects secondary to recreational drug use are becoming more prevalent. Patient history may be unreliable and any witnesses should be sought.

This chapter should be used as a brief guide—detailed information is available, particularly on drug doses (see 'Sources of information').

Specialist advice should be sought for overdoses in children.

General management principles

- Resuscitate the patient
- Consider the prevention of drug absorption:
  - Activated charcoal (50 g orally) will absorb many drugs if given < 1 hour after ingestion
  - Gastric lavage can be considered if a substantial overdose has been ingested < 1 hour previously. The evidence for benefit is weak however, and it is performed less commonly now
- Supportive care—e.g. airway maintenance, acid–base and electrolyte balance, treat seizures—is important
- Any unstable (haemodynamically compromising) arrhythmias (VT, fast SVT > 180/min) are better dealt with by cardioversion than drugs

Sources of information

- TOXBASE: www.toxbase.org
- UK National Poisons Information Service: 0870 600 6266
- British National Formulary: bnf.nice.org.uk

β-blockers

Main indications

- Coronary artery disease—angina, cardioprotection post-MI
- Cardiac arrhythmias
- Hypertension
- Heart failure with reduced ejection fraction
- *Other*: aortic dissection, aortic root dilatation (i.e. Marfan's), HCM, phaeochromocytoma—with α-blocker

Mechanism of action

- Block action of endogenous catecholamines
- Negative chronotropic and inotropic effect
- Reduce renin release—via renal β1-adrenergic receptors
- Depressed conduction through sinoatrial and AV nodes
- Antisympathetic central effect
- Reduce cardiac workload, cardiac output, and salt/water retention

Contraindications

- Decompensated heart failure
- Cardiogenic shock
- Acute bronchospasm or severe asthma
- Bradyarrhythmias
- Sick sinus syndrome, 2nd- and 3rd-degree AV block
- Long QT syndrome and torsade de pointes (sotalol)
- Severe peripheral vascular disease
- * Caution in AR, COPD, congestive cardiac failure with ongoing fluid overload, rate-slowing calcium-channel blockers

Side effects

- *Cardiac*—hypotension, bradycardia, AV block, heart failure
- *Vascular*—cold extremities, Raynaud's, peripheral vasoconstriction
- *Respiratory*—dyspnoea, bronchospasm
- *GI*—diarrhoea
- *CNS*—headache, paraesthesia, visual disturbance, insomnia, hallucinations, depression, psychoses
- *Other*—fatigue, erectile/sexual dysfunction, thrombocytopaenia purpura, psoriasis exacerbations

Dosing

- *Atenolol*—25–50 mg PO daily, max 100 mg/day
- *Bisoprolol*—1.25 mg PO daily (heart failure); 2.5–5 mg (IHD/HT); max 10 mg/day
- *Metoprolol*—25–50 mg BD/TDS PO, max 400 mg/day; 5 mg IV every 5 min up to 15 mg in acute MI or tachyarrhythmias
- *Sotalol*—40–80 mg BD PO, may increase to 160 mg BD
- *Carvedilol*—3.125–6.25 mg BD PO to start, max 50 mg/day
- Propranolol—20–40 mg BD PO, max 320 mg/day

β-blocker toxicity

Clinical features

- Light-headedness, dizziness, syncope
- Bradycardia
- Hypotension
- Heart failure
- Cardiogenic shock
- Hypoglycaemia
- Drowsiness, confusion, seizures
- Cardiorespiratory arrest, due to asystole or VF—rare
- Bronchospasm—uncommon
- Sotalol—may cause QT prolongation and torsade de pointes
- Toxicity is exacerbated in patients in patients taking negatively inotropic CCBs and those with pre-existing LV dysfunction

Investigations

ECG—AV block, intraventricular conduction defects (RBBB, LBBB), ventricular extrasystoles, asystole

Management

- Consider activated charcoal (or lavage for large overdoses) if < 1h
- Observe for at least 6h (12h if slow-release preparation)
- IV fluids
- Atropine
  For bradycardia and hypotension
  Dose: 3 mg IV bolus
- Glucagon
  For severe bradycardia and/or hypotension unresponsive to atropine
  Dose: 2–10 mg IV bolus ± IV infusion (1–5 mg/hour) if required
  Can cause vomiting, so antiemetic sometimes required
- Pacing
  Temporary transvenous or external pacing should be considered if atropine and glucagon are ineffective
- Salbutamol
  For bronchospasm
  Dose: 5–10 mg nebulized
- Dextrose
  For hypoglycaemia
  Dose: give 25 mL of 50% dextrose. Monitor blood glucose closely.
- Inotropes
  In severe cases, may be needed to maintain cardiac output
  Dobutamine (2.5–10 mcg/kg/min) or isoprenaline (5–10 mcg/min)

Calcium-channel blockers

Calcium-channel blocker classes

Dihydropyridine (DHP) group

- Amlodipine, felodipine, nifedipine, lercanidipine
- Vasodilation but no negative ino- or chronotropic effects

Non-dihydropyridine (non-DHP) group

- Diltiazem, verapamil
- Vasodilation *and* negative ino- and chronotropic effects (the latter are lower in diltiazem, higher in verapamil)

Main indications

- Coronary artery disease—angina
- Coronary artery spasm
- Cardiac arrhythmias—non-DHP group
- Hypertension
- Peripheral vasoconstriction (e.g. Raynaud's)—esp. nifedipine

Mechanism of action

- Blockade of cardiovascular L-type Ca^{2+} channels
- Peripheral vasodilatation—reduced contraction of VSM
- Negative chronotropic and inotropic effect—*verapamil* and *diltiazem*
- Above mechanisms reduce cardiac output and cardiac oxygen demand
- Antidromotropic effect—depressed cardiac conduction

Contraindications (mostly apply to non-DHP group)

- Cardiogenic shock—applies to all
- Decompensated heart failure
- Bradyarrhythmias—sick sinus, 2nd- or 3rd-degree AV block
- Caution in severe AS, WPW, 1st-degree AV block, impaired LV function, concomitant use with other drugs (β-blockers, quinidine), and in renal/ hepatic impairment

Side effects

- *Ankle oedema*—very common in DHP group
- *Cardiac*—palpitation, bradycardia, hypotension, AV block, CCF
- *GI*—nausea/vomiting, dyspepsia, constipation, hepatitis
- *CNS*—headaches, dizziness, insomnia, depression
- *Other*—lethargy, gynaecomastia, flushing, gingival hypertrophy, erectile dysfunction, blood dyscrasias, inhibition of hepatic CYP enzymes

Dosing

- *Amlodipine*—initially 5 mg OD PO up to 10 mg daily
- *Nifedipine*—immediate release: initially 5 mg TDS PO, max 60 mg daily; modified release: 20–30 mg OD PO, max 90 mg daily
- *Felodipine*—initially 5 mg OD PO up to 10 mg daily
- *Diltiazem*—standard release: initially 60 mg TDS PO, max 360 mg daily; modified release: 60–180 mg BD or 120–480 mg once-daily preparations
- *Verapamil*—immediate release: initially 40–120 mg TDS PO, modified release: 120–240 mg in 1–2 doses, max. 480 mg daily; for supraventricular arrhythmias can give 5–10 mg IV (over 2 min) and an additional 5 mg after 5 min if necessary

Calcium-channel blocker toxicity

Clinical features

- Nausea, vomiting, dizziness
- Slurred speech, confusion, convulsion
- Hypotension
- Hyperglycaemia, metabolic acidosis
- DHP group (e.g. nifedipine, amlodipine):
  - Sinus tachycardia
- Non-DHP group (e.g. diltiazem, verapamil):
  - Sinus bradycardia, AV block
  - Reduced myocardial contractility, pulmonary oedema

Investigations

ECG—as for β-blockers

Management

- Consider activated charcoal or gastric lavage
- Sustained release preparations may require further charcoal every 4 hours, plus a single dose of osmotic laxative (e.g. lactulose, $MgSO_4$)
- Monitor for at least 4 hours (at least 12 hours if sustained-release preparation)
- Calcium chloride

For severe clinical overdose

Dose: 0.2 mL/kg of 10% solution, up to 10 mL, IV over 5 min
Calcium gluconate is an alternative
Can be repeated every 10–20 min up to 4 doses
May reverse prolonged intracardiac conduction times

- Glucagon

For severe myocardial depression or hypotension

Dose: 10 mg IV every 3 min
Consider infusion (3–6 mg/hour) if good response

- Consider atropine, pacing, and inotropes as for β-blockers
- Prognosis is worsened in those taking concomitant β-blocker therapy

Diuretics

Main indications

- Congestive cardiac failure—loop diuretics primarily, or metolazone for refractory oedema
- Heart failure with reduced ejection fraction—aldosterone antagonists shown to reduce mortality
- Hypertension—thiazides
- Post-MI with EF < 40% —aldosterone antagonists, but primarily eplerenone

Mechanism of action by type

- Thiazides—e.g. bendroflumethiazide, metolazone; inhibit Na^+/Cl^- co-transporter at distal tubule yielding ↑ Na^+ and water excretion
- Loop diuretics—e.g. furosemide, bumetanide; inhibit Na^+–K^+–$2Cl^-$ symporter at the loop of Henle (medullary thick ascending limb)
- K^+ sparing diuretics—e.g. amiloride (inhibits epithelial Na^+ channels), spironolactone, eplerenone (aldosterone antagonists); inhibit Na^+/K^+ exchanger at cortical collecting ducts

Contraindications

- Hypersensitivity
- Gout
- For thiazides—caution in dyslipidaemia, erectile/sexual dysfunction, diabetes, prostatism, renal and hepatic impairment

Side effects

- *Cardiac*—hypotension, arrhythmias secondary to electrolyte imbalance
- *GI*—nausea/vomiting, constipation, anorexia, pancreatitis
- *CNS*—confusion, coma, seizures, depression, paralysis (all rare)
- *Other*—hypo/hyperkalaemia, cramps, hyponatraemia, hypercalcaemia, hyperglycaemia, hyperuricaemia (gout), dyslipidaemia, metabolic acidosis (amilorides) or alkalosis (thiazides, loop diuretics)

Dosing

- *Furosemide*—initially 20–80 mg OD PO or IV, max 600 mg/day
- *Bumetanide*—initially 0.5–2 mg OD PO, max. 10 mg/day (1 mg bumetanide ~40 mg furosemide)
- *Bendroflumethiazide*—2.5 mg OD PO
- *Metolazone*—initially 2.5 mg once only to gauge response, then 2.5–5 mg OD PO, max 20 mg/day
- *Amiloride*—initially 5 mg OD PO, max 20 mg/day
- *Spironolactone*—initially 25–100 mg PO in 1–2 doses, max 400 mg/day
- *Eplerenone*—initially 25 mg OD PO, increased within 4 weeks to 50 mg OD

SGLT-2 inhibitors

Main indications

- Management of diabetes
- Heart failure with reduced ejection fraction
- Heart failure with preserved ejection fraction

Mechanism of action

- Inhibition of sodium-glucose co-transporter 2 in the renal proximal convoluted tubule
- Results in glycosuria, lowering blood glucose
- A diuresis follows the glycosuria
- Other effects are debated but the drugs have been shown to improve outcomes

Contraindications/cautions

- Risk of diabetic ketoacidosis (DKA) in patients with intercurrent acute severe illness or undergoing surgery, or those with limited β-cell reserve. Use with caution in patients with previous DKA
- Hold SGLTi during acute severe illness or surgery
- Test for ketones in unwell patients on SGLT2i
- Contraindicated in diabetes mellitus type 1

Side effects

- Urinary tract infection, including urethritis, balanitis
- Rare/very rare: DKA, Fourniere's gangene

Dosing

- *Empagiflozin*—10 mg/day
- *Dapagiflozin*—10 mg/day

Renin–angiotensin system inhibitors

Main indications

- Hypertension
- Heart failure with reduced ejection fraction
- Asymptomatic LV dysfunction—improve prognosis
- Post-MI—reduce adverse remodelling
- Ischaemic heart disease—2° prevention

Types

- ACE inhibitors, e.g. ramipril, lisinopril. Reduce angiotensin II
- Angiotensin II AT1 receptor blockers, e.g. losartan, candesartan, valsartan. Useful when ACEi not tolerated, e.g. persistent cough

Mechanism of action

- Peripheral vasodilatation—arterial vasodilators
- Increase stroke volume and cardiac output
- Reduced TPR and renovascular resistance
- Increased natriuresis—inhibition of aldosterone release
- Inhibition of ADH release
- Prevent adverse ventricular remodelling

Contraindications/cautions

- Angio-oedema
- Renal artery stenosis
- Pregnancy—especially 2nd and 3rd trimesters
- Caution in renal impairment, severe/symptomatic LVOT obstruction, and concomitant use with other K^+-sparing drugs

Side effects

- *Cardiac*—hypotension *(particularly 1st dose)*
- *Respiratory*—cough *(ACEi)*, sinusitis, rhinitis
- *GI*—nausea/vomiting, diarrhoea, constipation, abdominal pain
- *CNS*—headache, dizziness, insomnia, paraesthesia
- *Other*—hyperkalaemia, hypoglycaemia, myalgia, arthralgia, rash, angio-oedema, renal impairment, deranged LFTs, blood disorders

Dosing

- *Ramipril*—initially 1.25–2.5 mg OD, max 10 mg/day
- *Lisinopril*—initially 2.5–5 mg OD, max 80 mg/day
- *Enalapril*—initially 2.5–5 mg OD, max 40 mg/day in 1–2 doses
- *Perindopril*—initially 2 mg OD, max 8 mg/day
- *Losartan*—initially 25–50 mg OD, max 100 mg/day in 1–2 doses
- *Irbesartan*—initially 75–150 mg OD, max 300 mg/day in 1–2 doses
- *Candesartan*—initially 4 mg OD, max 32 mg/day in 1–2 doses
- *Valsartan*—initially 20–40 mg BD, max 160 mg BD

ARB/neprilysin inhibitor

Main indications

- Heart failure with reduced ejection fraction

Types

- There is only one drug in class: Entresto ® 7, a combination of the ARB *valsartan* and the neprilysin inhibitor sacubitril

Mechanism of action

- Neprilysin breaks down BNP
- By increasing levels of BNP, this results in diuresis and vasodilation
- The combination with valsartan results in vasodilation and natriuresis as in the previous section

Side effects

- *Cardiac*—hypotension, particularly postural
- *Renal*—acute kidney injury, hyperkalaemia
- *Other*—angio-oedema, when combined with ACE inhibitor

Dosing

- 3 combination strengths: 24/26 mg, 49/51 mg, and 97/103 mg
- Start at 24/26 mg BD and uptitrate to max 97/103 mg BD
- Allow a 36 hour wash-out period after discontinuing an ACE inhibitor before starting neprilysin

Nitrates

Main indication

- Rapid relief of angina (short-acting sublingual or IV preparations)
- Prophylaxis of angina (slow-release oral or patch preparations)
- Acute management of congestive cardiac failure
- Blood pressure control in hypertensive emergency

Forms

- Glyceryl trinitrate (GTN)
- Isosorbide mononitrate
- Isosorbide dinitrate
- Chronic use requires sustained release preparations for effective dosing—usually BD or OD dosing

Mechanism of action

- Highly effective vasodilators (arterial and venous)
- Angina treatment a combination of coronary artery vasodilation and venodilation to reduce cardiac preload
- In heart failure, venodilation reduces preload to acutely decongest while arterial vasodilation reduces afterload and hence cardiac work

Side effects

- Headache, hypotension, dizziness, nausea, diarrhoea, dyspepsia

Contraindications

- Severe LVOT obstruction
- Caution with concomitant use with other vasodilators, antihypertensives, and phosphodiesterase inhibitors (e.g. sildenafil)

Dosing

- Oral forms for angina prophylaxis: isosorbide mononitrate 10 mg BD PO, increasing to 120 mg daily in divided doses, or OD if long-acting sustained-release preparation
- Sublingual GTN (acute angina)—1–2 sprays under the tongue PRN
- IV GTN for unstable angina, congestive cardiac failure or blood pressure control: 1–10 mg/hour, titrated against blood pressure (requires close monitoring)

Other vasodilators

Nicorandil

- Activates K^+ channels to cause vasodilatation (venous > arterial)
- Work in a very similar way to nitrates
- Used to treat angina
- Reduces preload and hence cardiac workload
- *Side effects*—headache, flushing, palpitations, nausea/vomiting, dizziness, weakness, mouth/intestinal ulcers
- *Contraindications*—hypotension, CCF (with low filling pressures), cardiogenic shock and concomitant use with phosphodiesterase inhibitors (e.g. sildenafil)
- *Dose*—10 mg BD PO increasing to 30 mg BD max

α-blockers

- Arterial vasodilators; block α_1-adrenergic receptors in vascular smooth muscle
- Used in treatment of severe/resistant hypertension
- Useful in patients with benign prostatic hypertrophy, and in phaeochromocytomas where combined β- and α-blockade is required
- *Side effects*—dizziness, headache, nausea, postural hypotension, fluid retention, sexual dysfunction, rash, agitation, depression
- *Contraindications*—caution in concomitant use with other antihypertensives and phosphodiesterase inhibitors
- *Dose*—doxazosin 1 mg OD PO, doubling every 1–2 weeks to usual max. 8 mg daily; can be up to 16 mg in selected cases

Hydralazine

- Arterial vasodilator—relaxes vascular smooth muscle (reduced Ca^{2+} release from sarcoplasmic reticulum)
- Used as adjunctive treatment for severe hypertension and 1st-line antihypertensive in pregnancy
- *Side effects*—reflex tachycardia, palpitation, hypotension, fluid retention, flushing, headache, nausea, diarrhoea, anorexia, drug-induced SLE
- *Contraindications*—coronary artery disease, MS
- *Caution in*—cerebrovascular disease and severe renal impairment
- *Dose*—25 mg BD PO, increasing to 50 mg BD

Antiarrhythmic drugs

Categorized historically by Vaughan–Williams classification as below. Note that this classification is now incomplete and excludes some drugs, e.g. digoxin, adenosine

Class I (membrane stabilizers)

- Na^+ channel blockers, restricting fast Na^+ current in phases 0 and 4 of cardiac action potential (AP)
- Reduced spontaneous automaticity, increased excitation threshold

Class Ia

- Lengthen AP
- Prolong duration of repolarization (phases 3 and 4) and refractory period (K^+-channel blockade)
- Delay conduction—prolong PR, QRS, QT
- For example quinidine, procainamide, disopyramide

Class Ib

- Shorten AP
- Shorten duration of repolarization
- Minimal effect on refractory period—no K^+-channel blockade
- Increase fibrillation threshold
- Reduce automaticity
- For example lidocaine, mexilitene, tocainide, phenytoin

Class Ic

- Prolong refractory period (blockade of outward rectifying K^+ channels)
- Reduce repolarization rate and contractility
- Delay conduction—prolong PR, QRS
- For example flecainide, propafenone

Class II (β-adrenergic receptor blockers)

- Decrease Ca^{2+} influx responsible for automaticity
- Reduce heart rate and conduction

Class III (K^+-channel blockers)

- Decrease K^+ efflux during repolarization
- Prolong repolarization and effective refractory period
- For example amiodarone, sotalol, bretylium, dofetilide

Class IV (Ca^{2+}-channel blockers)

- Reduce SA and AV node automaticity and AV conduction

Flecainide

Class Ic antiarrhythmic agent; effective for many types of life-threatening SVTs and VTs.

Main indications

- AF/atrial flutter—acute control and maintenance of sinus rhythm
- AVNRT (SVT)
- WPW syndrome
- VT—non-ischaemic
- RVOT tachycardia

Mechanism of action

- Rate-dependent block of cardiac Na^+ channels
- Prolongs cardiac AP
- Slows conduction through His–Purkinje system and ventricular myocardium (delays repolarization)
- Prolongs ventricular refractory period
- Decreased ventricular myocardial contractility
- Dose-related increase in PR, QRS, and intra-atrial conduction

Contraindications

- Bradycardia
- AV block or sinus node disease
- Structural (including valvular) heart disease
- Ischaemic heart disease
- LV dysfunction/heart failure
- Caution in renal or hepatic impairment, with pacemakers (increased capture thresholds) and concomitant use with other drugs (digoxin, alcohol, amiodarone, propafenone, procainamide, quinidine, cimetidine, paroxetine, β- and Ca^{2+}-channel blockers)

Side effects

- *Cardiac*—pro-arrhythmia, bradycardia, AV block, heart failure
- *Respiratory*—dyspnoea, pneumonitis
- *GI*—nausea/vomiting, dyspepsia, anorexia, diarrhoea, jaundice
- *CNS*—headache, blurred vision, dizziness, tremor, ataxia, paraesthesia, insomnia, amnesia, hallucinations, confusion, depression
- *Other*—reduced red/white blood cells or platelets, rash, ↑ANA, corneal deposits, photosensitivity

Dosing

- *Acute cardioversion of AF*—2 mg/kg (max 150 mg) over 15 min IV
- *Prevention of paroxysmal SVT/AF*—initially 50 mg BD PO; can increase by 50 mg BD every 3–5 days to max of 300 mg/day
- *Life-threatening ventricular arrhythmias*—initially 100 mg BD PO; increase by 50–100 mg/day to max of 400 mg/day

Amiodarone

Class III antiarrhythmic agent (with weak class Ia, II, and IV effects). It is highly lipid-soluble and oral loading is prolonged (2–3 months). A similar length of time is required for amiodarone to be removed from the system. IV infusions provide a high plasma level within 1–2 hours, but levels fall rapidly once the infusion is stopped.The potential for side effects is high, and amiodarone is reserved for when other drugs are unsuitable.

Main indications

- Control of acute atrial/ventricular arrhythmias where rapid return to sinus rhythm is required (caution—often drops BP when given IV)
- Recurrent arrhythmias difficult to control by other means
- Recurrent haemodynamically unstable VT—as adjunct to ICD
- Shock-refractory VF—IV 300 mg bolus

Mechanism of action

- Prolongs cardiac AP
- Reduced automaticity of SA and AV nodes
- Coronary and peripheral vasodilator
- May non-competitively block α- and β-receptors

Contraindications/cautions

- Hypersensitivity
- Bradycardia, sinoatrial, or AV block—it is a weak AV node blocker
- Thyroid dysfunction
- Caution in pregnancy, respiratory disease, hepatic impairment
- Caution in patients on digoxin, flecainide, procainamide, quinidine, warfarin, phenytoin, β- and Ca^{2+}-channel blockers

Side effects

- *Cardiac*—hypotension, bradycardia, AV block, heart failure
- *Respiratory*—lung fibrosis (esp. with large cumulative long-term dose), eosinophilic lung infiltration, cough
- *GI*—deranged LFTs, jaundice, hepatomegaly, hepatitis, cirrhosis
- • *Eyes/skin*—corneal microdeposits, papilloedema, optic neuropathy, slate-grey skin discolouration, photosensitivity (all patients should be warned to avoid sunshine)
- *Endocrine*—hyperthyroidism, hypothyroidism
- *CNS*—smell/taste disturbance, tremor, ataxia, peripheral neuropathy, weakness

Dosing and administration

- IV: 300 mg/1 hour then 900 mg/24 hours infusion. IV amiodarone should be administered through a central line wherever possible. If essential to give peripherally this should be via a newly sited, large-bore cannula in a large vein (e.g. antecubital fossa). Extravasation of amiodarone may result in severe tissue damage
- Oral loading—200 mg TDS for 1 week, then 200 mg BD for 1 week
- Maintenance dose—200 mg OD orally

Lidocaine

Class Ib agent used in emergencies for treatment of ventricular arrhythmia.

Main indication

- Stabilization of incessant ventricular tachycardia or fibrillation
- Especially useful for ventricular arrhythmias post-MI

Mechanism of action

- Blockage of voltage-dependent sodium channels
- Reduces automaticity by slowing rate of spontaneous depolarization
- Binds primarily to inactivated sodium channels, decreasing the AP duration and increasing the effective refractory period
- This can can interrupt re-entry and increases ventricular fibrillatory threshold, esp. in ischaemic myocardium

Side effects

- Myocardial depression and circulatory collapse
- AV block, arrhythmias
- Anxiety, nausea, dizziness/nystagmus, seizures

Contraindications/cautions

- Bradycardia, sinoatrial or AV block
- Congestive cardiac failure or severe LV dysfunction
- Post-cardiac surgery
- Acute porphyria

Dosing

- *Normal circulation*: 100 mg bolus over a few minutes followed by 4 mg/min for 30 minutes then 2 mg/min for 2 hours then 1 mg/min for up to 24 hours
- *Impaired circulation* (i.e. cardiogenic shock): 50 mg bolus over a few minutes followed by 4 mg/min for 30 minutes then 2 mg/min for 2 hours then 1 mg/min for up to 24 hours
- If continuous infusion is unavailable, the initial bolus can be repeated up to twice at intervals of minimum 10 minutes

Digoxin

Purified cardiac glycoside derived from foxglove plant (*Digitalis lanata*)

Main indications

- Ventricular rate control in AF/atrial flutter—primarily in older patients with a resting rate > 100 bpm
- Congestive cardiac failure (esp for patients with AF)—it has weak inotropic effects

Mechanism of action

- Binds and inhibits α-subunit of cardiac Na^+/K^+ ATPase pump
- Results in increased intracellular Na^+, slowing Ca^{2+} extrusion
- Lengthens AP
- Reduces AV node conduction and increases refractory period (thus reducing ventricular rate)

Contraindications

- 2° or complete heart block
- Accessory pathways, e.g. WPW syndrome
- VT/VF
- HCM
- Caution in hypokalaemia and metabolic acidosis (increase digoxin toxicity), sick sinus syndrome, thyroid disease, hepatic/renal impairment
- Caution with concomitant use of verapamil, amiodarone, erythromycin, warfarin—digoxin competes for binding to albumin and may displace/be displaced by other albumin-bound drugs, with potentiation of effect of either the digoxin or the other drugs

Side effects (mostly if toxic dose)

- *Cardiac*—arrhythmia (bigeminy, VT/VF, paroxysmal atrial tachycardia with variable AV block)
- *GI*—nausea/vomiting, anorexia, diarrhoea, abdominal pain
- *CNS*—headache, confusion, blurred vision, xanthopsia (yellow-green vision), drowsiness, dizziness, agitation, delirium, depression, psychosis

Dosing

- Oral loading with 0.75–1.5 mg in 2–3 divided doses over 24 hours
- IV loading (if essential): with 500 mcg slow infusion followed cautiously by 125–250 mcg every 6–8 hours until clinical effect evident
- Maintenance dose of 62.5–500 mcg OD PO depending on response

Digoxin toxicity

Chronic toxicity may occur as a result of interactions with other albumin-bound drugs (e.g. amiodarone) or from progressive renal failure. Digoxin has a long half-life (16–20 hours); the half-life of digitoxin (a related compound) is 6 days.

Toxicity is more common following acute overdose if the patient is already on digoxin, or cardiovascular disease is present (Boxes 19.2 and 19.3).

Clinical features

- Nausea and vomiting
- Dizziness, slurred speech, confusion, visual disturbances (blurring, alteration in colour perception), and hallucinations
- Hyperkalaemia
- Arrhythmias, hypotension, cardiac arrest
- Life-threatening toxicity rare in healthy hearts if < 5 mg ingested. Those with cardiac disease are much more susceptible

Investigations

- ECG—marked sinus bradycardia, PR and QRS prolongation, sinus arrest, supraventricular arrhythmias, AV block, ventricular ectopics, VT, VF. A classical arrhythmia in chronic toxicity is paroxysmal atrial tachycardia with AV block
- Blood:
  - Serum digoxin level—immediate if acute overdose and severe toxicity present (digoxin antibodies being considered). Otherwise wait > 6 hours post dose. Normal therapeutic range 0.8–2.0 mg/L
  - Serum electrolytes (esp. K^+)
  - Magnesium

Box 19.1 Predisposing factors for digoxin toxicity

- Acute hypoxia
- *Electrolyte disturbance, esp. hypercalcaemia,* hypokalaemia
- Respiratory alkalosis
- Myocardial ischaemia
- Old age
- Drug interactions
- Impaired renal/hepatic clearance

Box 19.2 Poor prognostic indicators

- Older patients
- Underlying cardiac disease
- Hyperkalaemia (> 5 mmol/L)
- High-grade AV block
- Serum digoxin level > 15 ng/mL
- VT

Management

- Consider activated charcoal if < 1 hour from ingestion
- Monitor for at least 6 hours
- Cardiac monitoring and frequent BP measurement
- Treat hyperkalaemia aggressively—but avoid calcium gluconate as it may precipitate VF
- Correct hypokalaemia with oral or IV K+ supplementation
- Atropine for symptomatic bradycardia and AV block (1–2 mg IV)
- Lidocaine, atenolol, or amiodarone for VT
- Pacing wire if severe bradycardia/sinus arrest
- Digoxin-specific Ab (Digibind®)—given in severe cases if $K^+ > 5.5$ mmol/L or a satisfactory cardiac output is not achieved in patients with sinus arrest, AV block, severe bradycardia, or tachyarrhythmias. Patients usually respond within 1 hour. Cardiac monitoring required for 24 hours; can cause hypokalaemia, so monitor K^+ frequently. See Box 19.4 for dose

Box 19.3 Digoxin-specific antibodies (Digibind®): dosing

Dosage for toxicity during chronic therapy

- In adult patients in whom the steady-state digoxin level is known:

$$\text{Number of vials} = \frac{\text{Serum digoxin conc. (ng/mL)} \times \text{weight (kg)}}{100}$$

- In adult patients in whom the steady-state digoxin level is unknown, 6 vials of Digibind® (228 mg) usually reverses toxicity

Dosage for acute poisoning

- Methods for calculating dose are usually by an estimate of the amount of digoxin ingested in milligrams (***not*** micrograms):

$$\text{Number of vials} = \frac{\text{Total dose ingested (mg)} \times 0.8}{0.5\ \text{(mg of digitalis bound per vial)}}$$

- 20 vials of Digibind® (760 mg) usually reverses acute toxicity if the amount ingested is unknown

Ivabradine

Rate-limiting drug.

Main indications

- Heart failure as a β-blocker adjunct
- Angina
- Against inappropriate atrial tachycardias/POTS
- Useful when β-blockers contraindicated or not tolerated

Mechanism of action

- Selectively inhibits I_f current—mixed Na^+/K^+ inward current regulating pacemaker activity in sinoatrial node
- Reduces rate at the sinoatrial node directly

Contraindications

- Bradycardias (sick sinus syndrome, AV block)
- Atrial fibrillation/flutter (ineffective as no sinoatrial node activity)
- Cardiogenic shock, severe heart failure
- Long QT syndrome
- Recent MI/stroke
- Concomitant use with CYP3A4 inhibitors (e.g. ketoconazole, erythromycin, nelfinavir)

Side effects

- Bradycardia, 1° AV block
- Headache, dizziness, blurred vision, luminous phenomena (sensation of brightness in visual fields),
- Nausea, constipation, diarrhoea,
- Eosinophilia

Dose

- Initially 2.5–5 mg BD PO then increase to 7.5 mg BD after 1 month

Statins

Hugely important cholesterol-lowering drugs.

Main indications

- Should be used routinely in all patients as 2° prevention for cardiovascular disease (including coronary artery disease, stroke/TIA, peripheral vascular disease, hypertension), unless contraindicated
- Significantly reduce cardiovascular events and mortality with a wealth of trial data supporting their use
- Also used in 1° prevention for those at increased risk of cardiovascular disease

Mechanism of action

- Inhibit HMG-CoA reductase (rate-limiting enzyme in cholesterol synthesis), leading to up-regulation of LDL receptors and increased LDL clearance
- Reduce LDL, increase HDL, reduce triglycerides
- Additional likely pleiotropic effects including improvement of endothelial function and plaque stabilization

Contraindications

- Significant liver disease
- Pregnancy
- Untreated hypothyroidism
- Caution: increased risk of rhabdomyolysis if used with other lipid-lowering agents

Side effects

- Myalgia, myositis; rarely: rhabdomyolysis—usually reversible
- Headache
- GI disturbance
- Rash
- Paraesthesia
- Deranged LFTs

Dosing

- Lifelong prescription once indicated
- For secondary prevention, start at high dose (e.g. atorvastatin 80 mg OD) unless high risk of adverse effects
- All statins given once daily, at night:
    - *Simvastatin*—20–40 mg PO initially, max 80 mg
    - *Pravastatin*—10 mg PO initially, max 40 mg
    - *Atorvastatin*—10–20 mg PO low dose, up to 80 mg PO high dose
    - *Rosuvastatin*—5–10 PO mg initially, max 40 mg

Other lipid-modifying drugs

Fibrates

- Activate PPAR-α receptors primarily in muscle and liver
- Mainly lower serum triglyceride levels and increase HDL
- Often used alongside statins—but increase risk of rhabdomyolysis
- Thought to improve insulin resistance and dyslipidaemia in T2DM
- *Side effects*—myalgia, GI disturbance, anorexia, erectile dysfunction, gallstones
- *Contraindications*—severe renal/hepatic impairment, 1° biliary cirrhosis, nephritic syndrome, increased risk of rhabdomyolysis when used with statins
- *Dose:*
  - *Bezafibrate*—200 mg TDS PO
  - *Fenofibrate*—200 mg OD PO
  - *Ciprofibrate*—100 mg OD PO
  - *Gemfibrozil*—600 mg BD PO

Ezetimibe

- Inhibits cholesterol absorption from small intestine and increases uptake of LDL cholesterol into cells
- Often given in combination with statin but licensed for monotherapy
- No mortality benefit yet demonstrated
- *Side effects*—headache, dizziness, diarrhoea, myalgia, deranged LFTs, gallstones, hepatitis, pancreatitis, URTI, rhabdomyolysis
- *Contraindications*—concomitant use with statin in liver disease
- *Dose*—10 mg OD PO

PCSK9 inhibitors

- Blockade of PCSK9 reduces LDL receptor degradation and increases LDL clearance
- Used as a second-line drug only when LDL is elevated above target despite maximal tolerated statin therapy
- *Evolocumab*—side effects: arthralgia, back pain, flu-like illness—dose 140 mg SC every 2 weeks
- *Alirocumab*—side effects: nasal complaints, oropharyngeal pain, vasculitis—dose 75 mg SC every 2 weeks, increased up to 150 mg SC every 2 weeks if necessary
- *Inclisiran*—long-acting small interfering RNA (siRNA) which inhibits hepatic PCSK9 synthesis. Side effects: injection site reactions, inflammation of nasal passages/throat. Dose: initially 284 mg SC for 1 dose, followed by 284 mg SC after 3 months for 1 dose, then 284 mg SC every 6 months

Antiplatelet agents

Aspirin (acetylsalicylic acid)

- 1° and 2° prevention of coronary disease
- Inhibits COX enzyme suppressing prostaglandin and thromboxane A_2 formation—responsible for platelet aggregation
- *Side effects*—GI ulcers, haemorrhage, tinnitus, bronchospasm, angio-oedema
- *Contraindications*—NSAID hypersensitivity, active ulcers, and caution in asthma, gout, hepatic/renal impairment and G6PD deficiency
- *Dose*—300 mg PO loading dose (ACS) then 75 mg daily

Clopidogrel

- Used alongside aspirin after PCI for reduction of stent thrombosis
- Reduces risk of non-fatal MI for up to 1 year post-NSTEMI
- Can substitute for aspirin in 1° or 2° prevention where aspirin intolerance exists, or augment aspirin where additional antiplatelet activity is required
- Blocks ADP receptor on platelet cell membranes to inhibit platelet aggregation
- *Side effects*—bleeding (GI, cerebral, mucosal), dyspepsia, nausea, diarrhoea, pruritus, depression, headache, confusion, myalgia, bronchospasm, renal/hepatic impairment, rash, TTP, neutropenia, erectile dysfunction
- *Contraindications*—hypersensitivity, acute bleeding/high bleeding risk (trauma, surgery) and caution in concomitant use with other antiplatelets/anticoagulants
- *Dose*—300 mg PO loading dose then 75 mg daily. 600 mg given PO before 1° PCI

Ticagrelor

- Alternative to clopidogrel with greater efficacy in event reduction but slightly worse bleeding profile
- Indicated in MI pre- and post-stent insertion
- *Side effects*—bleeding, GI upset, dyspnoea (idiosyncratic reaction), headache, gout, skin reactions
- *Contraindications*—acute bleeding/high bleeding risk
- *Dose*—180 mg loading dose then 90 mg BD. May be extended beyond first year at 60 mg BD in individuals at high risk of MI

Prasugrel

- Alternative to clopidogrel with lower MI/mortality rates but greater bleeding risk
- Indicated in patients undergoing angiography in the context of MI
- *Side effects*—bleeding, GI upset, skin reactions
- *Contraindications*—acute bleeding/high bleeding risk
- *Dose*—60 mg loading dose followed by 10 mg OD under 75 years old or 5 mg a day over 75 years old

Cangrelor

- Intravenous alternative to clopidogrel, prasugrel, or ticagrelor
- Useful in patients who cannot take an oral platelet inhibitor
- *Side effects*—dyspnoea, bleeding, skin reactions
- *Contraindications*—recent stroke/TIA, acute bleeding
- *Dose*—30 mcg/kg bolus followed by 4 mcg/kg/minute infusion for at least 2 hours, maximum 4 hours

Glycoprotein (GP) IIb/IIIa inhibitors

- Used in treatment of ACS, particularly when persistent symptoms or high thrombotic burden despite conventional treatment
- Given by IV infusion during and after PCI (with or without intracoronary stent placement)
- Block GP IIb/IIIa platelet surface receptors to inhibit platelet aggregation and thrombus formation
- *Side effects*—bleeding, thrombocytopenia, GI upset, headache, bradycardia
- *Contraindications*—hypersensitivity, coagulopathy, active bleeding, vasculitis, cerebral neoplasia, recent surgery, recent stroke, thrombocytopaenia and caution in concomitant use with other antiplatelets/anticoagulants
- For example abciximab, tirofiban, eptifibatide

Cardiotoxic drugs in overdose

Tricyclic antidepressants

Clinical features

- Dry mouth, blurred vision, urinary retention, dilated pupils
- Palpitation, supraventricular and ventricular arrhythmias
- Hyper-reflexia, extensor plantar responses
- Syncope, agitation/seizures, reduced level of consciousness

Investigations

- *ECG*—sinus tachycardia, prolonged PR interval, and QRS duration (> 100 msec, significant; > 160 msec, severe—risk of ventricular arrhythmias), supraventricular and ventricular arrhythmias
- *Blood*—arterial blood gas (metabolic acidosis), U&Es

Management

- Consider activated charcoal if ingestion < 1 hour previously
- Cardiac monitoring
- Supportive measures including IV fluids, vasopressors
- Sodium bicarbonate (reducing pH alters myocardial binding)

Dose: give 50 mmol (350 mL of 1.26% or 50 mL of 8.4% [through a central line]) over 20 min if any of: pH < 7.1; QRS duration > 160 msec (even in the absence of acidosis); arrhythmias; significant hypotension

- In general, antiarrhythmic drugs should be avoided and aggressive measures to correct the underlying metabolic and clinical state (hypoxia, hypotension, acidosis, hypokalaemia) should be prioritized
- IV diazepam for convulsions. Phenytoin is contraindicated

Theophylline

Clinical features

- Agitation, tremor, drowsiness, convulsions, status epilepticus
- Hypokalaemia, acidosis
- Sinus tachycardia, AF, hypotension, SVT, VT, VF

Investigations

- *ECG*—sinus tachycardia, SVT, VT, VF
- *Bloods*—U&E (esp. K^+), Mg, ABG, theophylline levels

Management

- Consider activated charcoal
- Cardiac monitoring
- Suuportive measures including IV fluids, vasopressors
- Check K^+ and blood gases regularly (1–2 hourly in severe cases)—initial K^+ may not reflect total K^+ depletion
- Benzodiazepines or phenytoin for convulsions
- β-blockers or verapamil for symptomatic or compromising SVT
- VT—synchronized DC cardioversion or $MgSO_4$
- Haemodialysis may be required in in very severe cases (life-threatening arrhythmia, seizure, levels > 100 mcg/ml)

Recreational drugs with cardiac effects

Cocaine

Clinical features

- Euphoria, agitation, paranoia
- Sweating, hyperthermia, convulsions
- Tachycardia, hypertension, chest pain, pulmonary oedema
- Coronary/carotid spasm—can be severe enough to cause MI/stroke
- Coronary artery dissection causing MI
- Intracerebral haemorrhage

Investigations

- *ECG*—ST segment elevation/depression if coronary ischaemia, supraventricular and ventricular arrhythmias
- *Bloods*—U&Es, CK, arterial blood gases

Management

- Cooling if core temperature > 41°C; aim for < 39°C
- IV diazepam to control agitation or convulsions
- Nitrates may relieve myocardial ischaemia and hypertension, e.g. GTN 1–10 mg/kg/hour IV infusion
- Adenosine 6–18 mg IV or verapamil 5 mg IV for sustained, haemodynamically tolerated SVTs
- Phentolamine for hypertension and coronary spasm (2–5 mg IV bolus)
- Primary PCI should be considered if persistent ST segment elevation
- Broad complex tachycardia can be treated with sodium bicarbonate (see Tricyclic antidepressants, p.311 for dose)
- β-blockers should be avoided—risk of unopposed α-receptor-mediated vasoconstriction leading to severe hypertension and coronary vasoconstriction

Amphetamine

Cardiac features and management of amphetamine overdose are comparable to those of cocaine overdose—see above

Ecstasy (MDMA)

Clinical features

- Nausea, muscle pain, hyperthermia, ataxia, rhabdomyolysis
- Euphoria, agitation
- Hyper/hypotension, tachyarrhythmias
- Hyponatraemia, hyperkalaemia, ARDS

Investigations

- Blood—U&Es (esp. Na^+), LFTs, ABGs
- ECG—sinus tachycardia or SVT

Management

- Cooling—to decrease core body temperature to < 39°C (e.g. tepid sponging, chilled IV fluids). Consider dantrolene (1 mg/kg IV over 15 min)
- β-blocker to treat SVT, e.g. metoprolol 5–10 mg IV
- Hypertension—IV nitrates or benzodiazepines

Drug-induced QT prolongation

Many factors influence acquired QT prolongation, including genetic susceptibility (separate from congenital long-QT syndromes), metabolic state (including hypokalaemia and hypomagnesaemia), other concomitant drugs, and heart rate. The concurrent use of agents that prolong QT interval and/or inhibit hepatic cytochrome P_{450} isoenzyme (e.g. fluoxetine) should also be avoided. Thus the emergence of QT prolongation relies not just on the drug ingested but on a combination of this and many predisposing factors. The occurrence with any particular drug is therefore unpredictable, but several drugs have been shown to be associated (Box 19.4):

The main risk is of polymorphic VT (torsade de pointes).

Box 19.4 Some causative drugs

- Class 1a antiarrhythmics—quinidine, procainamide, disopyramide
- Class 1c antiarrhythmics—flecainide
- Class III antiarrhythmics—sotalol, amiodarone, dofetilide
- Tricyclic antidepressants—amitryptiline, imipramine, clomipramine
- Psychotropic agents—lithium, chlorpromazine, haloperidol
- Antihistamines—terfenadine, loratadine
- Antimicrobials— erythromycin, clarithromycin, quinine, chloroquine, ketoconazole
- Immunosuppressants—tacrolimus
- Recreational drugs—cocaine

Clinical features

- Recurrent dizziness or syncope
- Palpitations
- Polymorphic VT/torsade de pointes

Investigations

- *ECG*—VT, torsade de pointes (Fig. 19.1)
- *Blood*—serum electrolytes (esp. K^+, Mg^{2+}, Ca^{2+})

Management

- Identify and withdrawing the offending drug(s)
- Avoid empirical antiarrhythmic therapy
- For torsade de pointes:
  - *$MgSO_4$*—8 mmol (2 g) over 15 min, then 20 mmol over 6–12h
  - *K^+*—keep at 4.5–5 mmol/L
  - *Pacing*—overdrive pacing for VT; prevention of VT in bradycardia with long QT (temporary/permanent pacing)

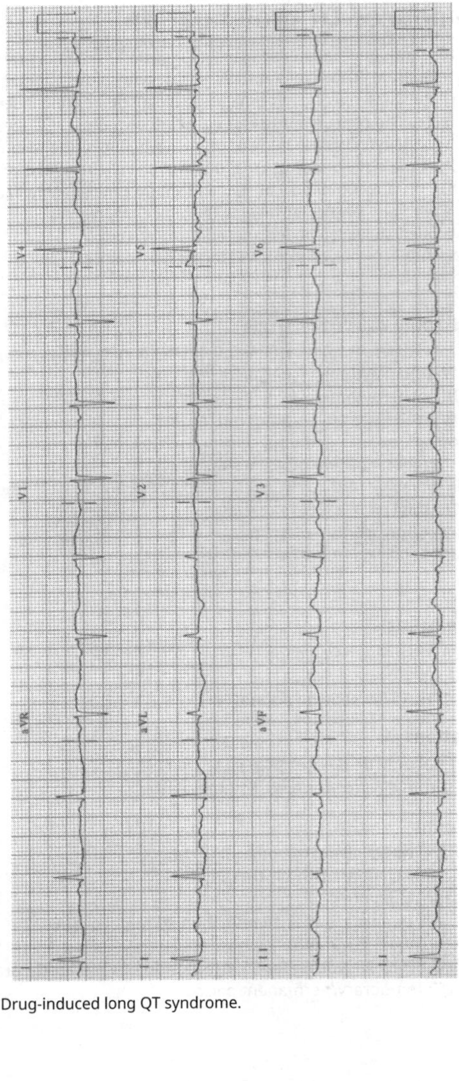

Fig. 19.1 Drug-induced long QT syndrome.

Drugs used in cancer

A number of oncological therapeutic agents are known to be cardiotoxic. In the majority, these effects are cumulative, but a number of medications have acute cardiac side effects:

Interleukin-2

- Causes a capillary leak syndrome (hypotension, oedema, effusions, arrhythmias)
- Stop infusion, administer steroids, antihistamines, and consider adrenaline

5- Fluorouracil

- May cause myocardial ischaemia and acute MI
- Stop 5- FU treatment and treat with conventional antianginal therapy

Anthracyclines (e.g. doxorubicin, daunorubicin)

- Chronic dose-related cardiomyopathy
- Arrhythmias

Herceptin

- Class III/IV heart failure
- Chronic dose-related cardiomyopathy
- Arrhythmias

Others

- Cisplatin —acute myocardial ischaemia
- Cyclophosphamide—heart failure, haemorrhagic pericarditis
- Mitomycin C—myocardial injury
- Vincristine—MI
- Vinblastine—MI
- Taxol—bradycardia

Cardiotoxic effects of cancer drugs

Specific effects

Cardiomyopathy

- Presenting with heart failure, may be acute or may be years after the chemotherapy regime
- Investigation: echocardiography, cardiac MRI
- NT-proBNP may be useful in monitoring

Myocarditis

- Variable presentation from mild symptoms and signs to fulminant myocarditis
- Patients may be symptomatic of typical chest pain, may develop pericardial effusion, or present with heart failure or cardiogenic shock
- Typically associated with immune checkpoint inhibitors
- Investigation: troponin, echocardiography, cardiac MRI, PET, ECG

Accelerated atherosclerosis

- Presentations with angina, MI
- Investigation: CT coronary angiogram, invasive angiography, functional testing

Arrhythmia

- Variable depending on drug, ranging from increased ectopy, atrial fibrillation to ventricular arrhythmias (paclitaxel, cisplatin, romidepsin, monoclonals, immune checkpoint inhbitors)
- Some drugs may cause bradycardias (capecitabine, paclitaxel, alemtuzumab, trastuzumab, pazopanib, alectinib, crizotinib, brigatinib, trametinib)

Pulmonary hypertension

- Either primary pulmonary hypertension or secondary from venous thromboembolism causing chronic thromboembolic pulmonary hypertension
- Patients present with breathlessness, chest pain, and right heart failure
- Investigations: echocardiography, right heart catheterization, CT pulmonary angiography

Pericardial disease

- Pericardial effusion, often related to myocarditis
- Patients may progress to tamponade, e.g. with cyclophosphamide
- Some therapies are associated with pericardial constriction, or following radiation beam therapy

Conventional chemotherapy drugs

Drug	*Cardiomyopathy*	*Arrhythmia*	*Vascular*	*Other*
Anthracyclines (doxorubicin, epirubicin, idarubicin)	+++	+++		
Cyclophosphamide	++	+	+	
Busulphan		+++	+++	Pericardial effusion)
5- Fluorouracil	++	++	+++	
Capecitabine	+	++	++	
Clofarabine	+	+++		
Gemcitabine			+	
Paclitaxel	+	++	++	
Docetaxel	+	+	+	
Vinca alkaloids (vincristine, vinblastine)			+	
Platinum based (cisplatin, oxaliplatin)	+	+	++	
Bleomycin			+	
Lenalidomide	+	++	++	
Thalidomide		+	+++	
Radiation beam therapy	++	+	++	Valvular disease, pericardial disease, restriction

Small molecule therapies

Drug	*Cardiomyopathy*	*Arrhythmia*	*Vascular*	*Other*
Proteasome inhibitors (bortezomib, carflizomib)	++	+	++	
HDAC inhibitors (panobinostat, romidepsin, vorinostat)		++	++	
Abemaciclib (CDK4/CDK6)			+	
Ribociclib (CDK4/CDK6)		++		
Everolimus (mTOR)	++	++	+++	Hypertension
Temsirolimus (mTOR)			+++	

Immune checkpoint inhibitors

- Antibody-based therapies
- Myocarditis is the principal complication
- Variable presentation, from asymptomatic with troponin elevation, mild symptoms, and echo abnormalities to decompensated heart failure
- Takotsubo and other cardiomyopathies have been reported

Drug	*Cardiomyopathy*	*Arrhythmia*	*Vascular*	*Other*
Ipilimumab (anti- CTLA4)	+	+	+	
Anti-PD1 (nivolumab, pembrolizumab)	+	+	+	
Anti-PLD1 (atezolizumab, avelumab, durvalumab)	+			

Monoclonal antibodies

Drug	Cardiomyopathy	Arrhythmia	Vascular	Other
Alemtuzumab (anti-CD52)	+	++	++	
Rituximab (anti-CD20)	+	+	++	Hypertension
Cetuximab (anti-EGFR)		+	++	
Necitumumab (anti-EGFR)			+++	
Panitumumab (anti-EGFR)			+	
Trastuzumab (anti-HER2)	+++	++		
Aflibercept (anti-VEGF)	+		++	Hypertension
Bevacizumab (anti-VEGF)	++		++	Oedema and hypotension
Ramucirumab (anti-VEGF)			++	
Erlotinib (EGFR)		++	+++	Pulmonary toxicity
Osimertinib (EGFR)	++	++		Pulmonary toxicity
Dacomitinib (EGFR)			++	Pulmonary toxicity
Lapatinib (HER2)	++	+		

Drug	Cardiomyopathy	Arrhythmia	Vascular	Other
Axitinib (VEGFR3)	+		++	Hypertension
Lenvatinib (VEGFR3)	++	++	++	Hypertension, oedema
Pazopanib (VEGFR3)	+++	+++	++	Hypertension, pulmonary toxicity
Sorafenib (VEGFR3)	++	+	++	Hypertension
Sunitinib (VEGFR3)	+++	+	+++	Hypertension
Vandetanib (VEGFR)	++	+++	++	Hypertensive crisis, pulmonary toxicity
Regorafenib (VEGFR2)			++	Hypertension
Bosutinib (BCR-ABL)		++	++	Pericardial effusion
Dasatinib (BCR-ABL)		++	++	Pulmonary hypertension
Imatinib (BCR-ABL)	+	++	++	Palpitations
Nilotinib (BCR-ABL)		++	+++	
Ponatinib (BCR-ABL)	++	+++	+++	Hypertensive crisis
Ibrutinib (BTK)		+++		Hypertension
ALK inhibitors (Alectinib, Brigatinib, Ceritinib, Crizotinib, Lorlatinib)		++ to +++		Pulmonary toxicity, Ceritinib pericardial effusion
Dabrafenib (BRAF)	++			Hypertension
Encorafenib (BRAF)		+		
Vemurafenib (BRAF)		+++		Hypertension
Gilteritinib (FLT3)	++	++		Pericardial effusion / pericarditis
Ruxolitinib (JAK)		+		
Cabozantinib (MET)		++	++	Hypertension
Binimetinib (MEK)	++		++	Hypertension
Cobimetinib (MEK)	+++			Hypertension
Trametinib (MEK)	+++	++		Hypertension

(+ = uncommon, < 1%, ++ = common, 1–10%, +++ = very common > 10%)

Tables adapted from Herrmann et al, *Nature Reviews Cardiology* 2020; 17(8): 474–502

CAR T-cell therapy

- Reprogramming of T-cells to target cancer antigens
- Associated with cytokine release syndrome (CRS), similar to SIRS, causing tachycardia, arrhythmias, and LV depression in severe cases
- Small numbers of reports of T-cell mediated severe acute myocarditis causing fulminant heart failure

Chapter 20

Hypertensive emergencies

Definition

The ESC/ESH guideline defines hypertension as a blood pressure reading of 140/90 mmHg and above with the goal of achieving a BP of 130 to < 140/ 70–79 mmHg for all and targeting to < 130/70–79 mmHg or lower in those at high cardiovascular risk defined as diabetes, post-stroke, and coronary artery disease (Fig 20.1).

Blood Pressure	Systolic—mmHg	Diastolic—mmHg
Normal	120 and below	80 and below
Prehypertension	121–139	81–89
Hypertension—Stage 1	140–159	90–99
Hypertension—Stage 2	160 and above	100 and above
Hypertensive crisis	180 and above	110 and above

Fig. 20.1 Normal blood pressure and stages of hypertension.

Hypertensive crisis

1–2% of the population will experience a hypertensive crisis, which includes urgent and emergency hypertensive crisis. The absolute value of the BP is not as important as the presence of end-organ damage, the systolic BP is usually > 180 mmHg and/or the diastolic BP is > 120 mmHg.

Classification

Urgent hypertensive crisis

Acute severe hypertension without any signs of target organ damage. Whilst these patients require BP reduction, they do not usually require admission to hospital, and BP reduction is best achieved with oral medication with urgent outpatient follow-up to ensure effective treatment.

Emergency hypertensive crisis

These are clinical situations in which severe hypertension (grade 3) is associated with acute hypertension-mediated organ damage, which can be life-threatening and requires immediate intervention.

Presentation

The clinical presentation will depend on the organs affected, but can include headache, visual disturbances, chest pain, dyspnoea, and dizziness.

Hypertensive encephalopathy can present with somnolence, tonic clonic seizures, cortical blindness, and loss of consciousness.

Focal neurological features should raise the suspicion of stroke due to intracranial haemorrhage. Nausea, vomiting, altered consciousness, seizures (hypertensive encephalopathy).

Angina, shortness of breath (left ventricular failure, acute myocardial infarction),

Sudden onset, severe interscapular pain (aortic dissection).

Haematuria (acute renal failure).

During pregnancy (eclampsia, pre-eclampsia).

Catecholamine excess (phaeochromocytoma, recreational drug overdose).

Causes of hypertensive crisis (malignant hypertension)

- Essential hypertension—non-compliance with anti-hypertensive medication, poor BP control (most common)
- Cardiac emergencies—acute pulmonary oedema/acute left ventricular failure, coronary ischaemia/infarction
- Vascular emergencies—aortic dissection, recent vascular surgery
- Renal emergencies—acute deterioration in renal function
- Neurological emergencies—hypertensive encephalopathy; acute head injury—trauma; cerebral embolism—thrombotic stroke; acute ischaemic stroke; acute intracranial haemorrhage; subarachnoid haemorrhage
- Pregnancy-related emergencies—pre-eclampsia/eclampsia
- Epistaxis—unresponsive to conservative treatment (packing)
- Catecholamine excess state—pheochromocytoma, phenylcyclidine, cocaine, sympathomimetic drugs

- Tyramine containing foods in a patient on monoamine oxidase inhibitors
- Withdrawal of centrally acting α2 agonists—clonidine, methyldopa
- Perioperative hypertension
- Hypertension after organ transplantation
- Hypertension related to burns

Management

Key steps

1. Establish which organs are involved
2. Determine whether there is an identifiable cause
3. Select a pharmacological approach to BP reduction (agent, extent of reduction, time frame)
4. Patients with hypertension emergencies are usually admitted to hospital for bed rest, haemodynamic monitoring, and IV BP treatments.

The initial goal of therapy

Reduce mean arterial BP by no more than 25% (within 30 minutes to 1 hour). Then to 160 mmHg systolic and 100–110 mmHg diastolic within the next 2–6 hours.

Excessive falls in blood pressure may precipitate renal, cerebral, or coronary ischaemia and hence should be avoided. Exceptions to this general rule are patients with aortic dissection, phaeochromocytoma crisis, and severe pre-eclampsia or eclampsia. Selected patients with spontaneous intracerebral haemorrhage may also require acute blood pressure lowering; careful titration in these patients is required to ensure continuous smooth and sustained control of BP.

Medications

IV blood pressure control using short half-life agent has the advantage of rapidity of control and the ability to titrate dose to response.

Intravenous—labetalol, nitrates, nitroprusside infusion.

A combination of β-blockers, calcium-channel blockers, ACE inhibitors, oral β-blocker (atenolol), or long-acting calcium antagonist (amlodipine), and other antihypertensive agents are often necessary to normalize blood pressure.

Management in specific conditions

- Aortic dissection—labetalol injection of 50 mg over 1 minute followed by a continuous infusion of 1–2 mg/minute) or vasodilator sodium nitroprusside infusion are the first-line therapies of choice. A rapid reduction in BP is necessary to lower systolic blood pressure to less than 120 mmHg
- Subarachnoid haemorrhage—nimodipine infusion 0.5–2 mg/hour via central line or oral therapy of 60 mg every 4 hours
- Phaeochromocytoma—initial therapy with α-blocker phentolamine 2–5 mg intravenously followed by β-blocker therapy if necessary
- Pregnancy—expert advice is a must. First-line therapy with methyldopa 250 mg TDS orally and or hydralazine 5–10 mg IV, repeated after 30 minutes in severe hypertension. Calcium antagonists and β-blockers are second-line agents. Avoid nitroprusside because of foetal toxicity. Obtain emergency obstetric support. Consider delivery
- Cocaine abuse—IV benzodiazepines (diazepam 5–10 mg IV) and IV nitrates recommended
- Monoamine oxidase inhibitors—IV benzodiazepines (diazepam 5–10 mg IV) and a short-acting anti-hypertensive sodium nitroprusside infusion (0.5–1.5 mcg /kg/minute increasing in steps of 0.5 mcg/kg/minute every 5 minutes)

Table 20.1 Management in specific conditions

Clinical presentation	Timeline and target for BP reduction	First-line treatment
Malignant hypertension with or without acute renal failure	Several hours Reduce MAP by 20–25%	Labetalol Nicardipine
Hypertensive encephalopathy	Immediately reduce MAP by 20–25%	Labetalol, nicardipine
Acute coronary event	Immediately reduce SBP to <140 mmHg	glyceryl trinitrate (GTN) labetalol
Acute cardiogenic pulmonary oedema	Immediately reduce SBP to <140 mmHg	Nitroprusside or glyceryl trinitrate (GTN) (with loop diuretic)
Acute aortic dissection	Immediately reduce SBP to <120 mmHg AND heart rate to <60 bpm	Esmolol and nitroprusside or glyceryl trinitrate (GTN) or nicardipine
Eclampsia and severe pre-eclampsia/HELLP	Immediately reduce SBP to <160 mmHg AND DBP to <105 mmHg	Labetalol or nicardipine and magnesium sulfate

Adapted from 2018 ESC guidelines (OUP)

Further reading

2018 ESC/ESH Guidelines for the management of arterial hypertension. The Task Force for the management of arterial hypertension of the European Society of Cardiology (ESC) and the European Society of Hypertension (ESH). *European Heart Journal* 2018; 39: 3021–104.

Advanced heart failure and transplant emergencies

Definition and classification

The deteriorating patient in need of advanced therapies

One of the greatest challenges with advanced heart failure patients is recognizing that they are decompensating and could benefit from specialist therapies or referral.

Consider the following criteria:

I-NEED-HELP

Patients with advanced HF may be identified by the following:

- I – Intravenous inotropes
- N – NYHA IIIB to IV/ NT-proBNP persistently elevated
- E – End organ dysfunction
- E – EF < 35%
- D – Defibrillator shocks
- H – Hospitalizations (more than 1)
- E – (O)Edema (despite diuretic escalations)
- L – low systolic blood pressure (≤ 90), high heart rate
- P – prognostic medications: intolerance or down-titration of goal directed medical therapy

European Society of Cardiology definition of advanced HF

All 4 of:

- Severe and persistent NYHA III/IV
- Severe cardiac dysfunction: 1 of
    - EF ≤ 30%
    - Non-operable severe valve abnormality
    - Non-operable severe congenital abnormality
    - Isolated RV failure
    - Persistently high/increasing BNP/NT-proBNP and severe LV diastolic dysfunction/structural abnormality
- > 1 unplanned heart failure hospitalization in the last 12 months
- Severe impairment of exercise capacity

Classifying advanced heart failure and cardiogenic shock

INTERMACS Class

This can be used to determine how rapidly intervention should take place. Prognosis with LVAD support correlates with INTERMACS class, with 1-year survival 53% for class 1, but 93% for class 5

1. Critical cardiogenic shock: 'Crash and burn'
   Patients with life-threatening hypotension despite escalating inotropic support, critical organ hypoperfusion, worsening acidosis and/or lactate levels
2. Progressive decline despite inotropes: 'Sliding on inotropes'
   Worsening renal function, nutritional depletion, inability to restore volume balance, or an inability to tolerate inotropes
3. Stable but inotrope dependent: 'Dependent stability'
   Stable blood pressure, organ function, nutrition and symptoms on inotropes (or mechanical support) but an inability to wean from them

4. Resting symptoms:
   Daily symptoms of congestion at rest or during activities of daily living. High diuretic doses
5. Exertion intolerant: 'Housebound'
   Comfortable at rest and with activities of daily living but may have refractory elevated volume status, often with renal dysfunction
6. Exertion limited: 'Walking wounded'
   No evidence of fluid overload, comfortable at rest and with minor exertion but is easily fatigued
7. Advanced NYHA III Living comfortably with limited meaningful activity.

Modifiers:

- TCS: Temporary circulatory support
- A: Arrhythmia

Eligibility for advanced heart failure therapies

In the UK, durable LVAD or supporting with temporary MCS in a heart without the prospect of recovery is only licensed as a bridge to heart transplant. Hence any patient referred for advanced HF therapies must be free of contraindications to transplantation.

- Age is not an absolute contraindication but patients over the age of 60 are selected on an individual basis
- Active infection (patients with chronic viral infection e.g. hepatitis B/C or HIV may be considered if viral load is undetectable with treatment and no evidence of organ damage)
- Symptomatic cerebral/peripheral vascular disease
- Diabetes mellitus with end-organ damage. Poor control (HBA1c persistently > 58 mmol/mol) is a relative contraindication
- Current/recent neoplasm (an oncology opinion may be required)
- Severe lung disease (FEV1 and FVC < 50% predicted)
- Irreversible renal dysfunction (eGFR < 30 mL/min/m2)
- Irreversible liver dysfunction (cirrhosis)
- Recent (within 3 months) pulmonary embolism
- Recent stroke
- Pulmonary hypertension (PA systolic pressure > 60mmHg, transpulmonary gradient > 15mmHg, PVR > 5 Wood units). This is an absolute contraindication if irreversible with pharmacologic manipulation or mechanical LV unloading
- Psychosocial factors (history of non-compliance with medication, inadequate support, substance misuse, current smoker)
- Obesity (BMI 35 kg/m^2 / weight > 140% ideal body weight)
- Other multisystem disease with poor long-term survival

Temporary mechanical circulatory support

Intra-aortic balloon counterpulsation

IABP is the most widespread and oldest form of MCS. Studies to date would suggest it does not alter mortality in cardiogenic shock, but its relative simplicity and low cost of use means that its use is still advocated in some centres.

Mechanism

- The intra-aortic balloon inflates in diastole and deflates during ventricular systole, reducing afterload and LV end-diastolic pressure
- Balloon inflation during diastole also improves coronary perfusion and myocardial oxygenation

Contraindications

- Peripheral vascular disease preventing access
- Aortic dissection preventing placement of the balloon
- Aortic regurgitation (> mild) as the balloon's inflation in diastole will exacerbate this, further loading the LV

Management

- The patient should remain supine while the IABP is in place
- If there are concerns about positioning, a CXR should be obtained: the marker on the tip should be at the proximal descending aorta, just below the aortic knuckle and the origin of the left subclavian. If the IABP is positioned too low, it can occlude the splanchnic arteries
- Most centres (not all) will anticoagulate patients with IABP. If the balloon is left deflated without anticoagulation, clots can form around it and embolize, hence it should be removed promptly if not in use

Settings

- The degree of balloon inflation ('augmentation') can be varied (0–100%) and the ratio of augmented beats can be set (i.e. 1:1 meaning every beat is augmented; at 1:8 only every 8th beat is augmented). Setting 1:2 or 1:3 may improve augmentation in tachycardic patients
- As the patient recovers, the balloon may be weaned down: this can either be done by slowly reducing augmentation or increasing ratio
- Where LV function is poor, the augmented pressure will be higher than the native systolic pressure. As the LV recovers, native systolic pressure becomes higher

Complications

- Ischaemic—embolism or direct blockage of vessels by the balloon
- Bleeding—from concurrent anticoagulation
- Access site—bleeding, dissection, or pseudoaneurysm

Impella

Impella is a continuous flow microaxial pump positioned across the aortic valve, with the power provided by a driveline to an external power source.

Devices

A variety of models with different maximum flow rates are available:

- Impella 2.5: 13 Fr introducer, 2.5 L maximal flow, percutaneous femoral/axillary implant, max support 4 days
- Impella CP: 14 Fr introducer, 3.7 L maximal flow, percutaneous femoral/axillary implant, max support 4 days
- Impella 5.0: 23 Fr introducer, 5 L maximal flow, femoral/axillary cut-down, max support 14 days
- Impella 5.5: 23 Fr introducer, 5.5 L maximal flow, axillary cut-down/aortic implant, max support 30 days
- Impella RP: right heart support up to 4.4 L, 23 Fr introducer, percutaneous femoral vein implant, max support 14 days (note can be used with a left-sided Impella)

Contraindications

- Peripheral vascular disease preventing access
- Aortic stenosis
- Mechanical aortic valve replacement
- Left ventricular thrombus
- Ventricular septal defect

Management

- The Impella system will display the flow through the device, device power, the native cardiac output, cardiac and arterial BP, and the cardiac power output (a metric calculated as CO × MAP/451)
- The device is set at a power output of P1 to P9, a linear scale of increasing flow
- Systemic anticoagulation is required to prevent thrombus formation
- Monitor cardiac power output, MAP, indices of organ function (e.g. urine output) and indices of tissue perfusion (e.g. lactate)
- In general, increase Impella support until MAP is above 60, lactate is low, and central venous oxygen saturation is > 50%
- If there is good ventricular contractility (pulsatile flow from the LV exceeding pressure generated by the Impella) and/or cardiac power index is > 0.6 W with MAP above 60 and indices of organ perfusion are good, Impella support can be weaned

Complications

- Access site complications depending on point of insertion
- Haemolysis (typically when mispositioned, and at higher flow rates): measure haptoglobin, LDH, and plasma-free haemoglobin daily. Reposition the device under echo guidance, and/or reduce flow rate
- Thombosis (typically at lower flow rates)
- Damage to cardiac structures: upon removal of devices which have been present for more prolonged periods and have tangled in chordae or become adherent to the ventricular cavity

Temporary VAD and ECMO

Temporary ventricular assist devices (VAD) and extra-corporeal membrane oxygenation (ECMO) are managed in specialist centres and their use is outside the scope of this chapter. An understanding of these devices is important, however, to guide referral for advanced support in selected patients.

Temporary VAD

- These are percutaneously placed devices where the pump is extracorporeal and connects via tubing to the patient
- Tubing placement may be peripheral (into femoral/axillary/jugular vessels) or central (directly into great vessels via a sternotomy and tunnelled out via the upper abdominal wall)
- VAD support may be for both ventricles (BiVAD), left only (LVAD), or right only (RVAD)
- Central VAD—more invasive but once the sternotomy has healed, patients may be mobilized to prevent muscle atrophy while awaiting transplant
- Peripheral VAD—less invasive but the LVAD outflow competes with LV outflow and may cause clot formation within the LV and on the aortic valve, preventing recovery

Extra corporeal membrane oxygenation (ECMO)

- ECMO may be veno-venous (VV), where deoxygenated blood is pumped out of a large vein, oxygenated and then returned to the venous circulation, or veno-arterial (V-A), where venous blood is pumped out, oxygenated, and then returned to the arterial circulation at arterial pressure
- Any VAD system which has an oxygenator added to it is, technically speaking, ECMO. Like temporary VAD, ECMO can be central or peripheral
- Peripheral V-A ECMO may be rapidly placed by cannulating large peripheral vessels. Like peripheral VAD, this carries the drawback of LVAD outflow competing with LV outflow, and some centres advocate the use of 'ECMELLA' where an Impella is added to offload the LV

Durable LVAD emergencies

A durable left ventricular assist device (LVAD) is an internally implanted pump which draws blood from the left ventricle and pumps it into the aorta and connects to external batteries to allow a patient to be ambulant with the device. There are several generations of LVAD available, the most recent being HeartMate 3, however older devices such as HeartWare HVAD or HeartMate 2 are still in use. Most of these patients will have an emergency contact at their transplant centre who should be first port of call.

Monitoring LVAD patients

- Patients have continuous rather than pulsatile blood flow. Their pulse will often be impalpable and a standard BP cuff may not work
- BP should be measured with a cuff and a Doppler probe, to give a single mean arterial pressure value. Target MAP is 70–80 mmHg
- The patient will have a driveline, typically emerging from an incision in the abdominal wall and attached to a controller. The driveline should be monitored for cleanliness and signs of infection
- The controller will in turn be attached to 2 battery packs or to a mains adaptor. The control device attached to the LVAD will produce a wealth of data; the patient may attend emergency services owing to an alarm from a high or low parameter (Table 21.1)
- Patients with LVAD should be anticoagulated with warfarin, with an INR range of 2–3 to reduce the risk of pump thrombosis. They may be bridged with heparin if required for surgery but any interruption should be minimized as much as possible
- The pump power, rotor speed, flow, and pulsatility index may be cycled through on the control device display or displayed by connecting to a mains adaptor
- Pump speed is set, and the control device will read out the power in watts needed to maintain that speed. Flow is calculated in litres per

Table 21.1 Device alerts

Alert	Meaning
High pump power	Mechanical drag on pump rotor, usually due to thrombus
High flow	Decreased peripheral resistance from increased vasodilation (sepsis or vasodilator drugs)
Low flow	Decreased preload (hypovolaemia or arrhythmia)
High pulsatility index	Decrease in pump speed Myocardial recovery
Low pulsatility index	Increase in pump speed Poor ventricular contraction (arrhythmia / progression of disease) Low preload
Low battery	

minute. Pulsatility index is calculated over 15 seconds and gives an idea of how much blood the ventricle is pumping

Low flow alarms

Hypovolaemia

- These are commonly caused by inadequate preload due to hypovolaemia
- Attempt a straight leg raise
- Give cautious fluid boluses as needed (e.g. 4 mL/kg), targeting a MAP > 60 mmHg
- Be aware that LVAD patients are at higher risk of bleeding owing to anticoagulation, and be sure to rule out GI bleeding

Arrhythmia

- Ventricular tachycardia compromising RV function or AF compromising atrial function
- Restoring sinus rhythm should be the goal, either with chemical cardioversion (patients may tolerate VT with relative stability given the support from the LVAD) or DC cardioversion (contemporary LVADs are not susceptible to damage from a shock). Most patients have ICDs and ATP or shocks can be used
- Atrial arrhythmia may be due to inadequate LVAD flow causing raised atrial pressures, and ventricular arrhythmia may be due to flow which is too high causing 'suck down' so the patient may require changes to their LVAD settings

RV failure

- This will result in reduced flow through to the left heart. Echocardiography is helpful

Tamponade

- Echocardiography should be performed to rule out tamponade
- LVAD patients may develop elevating filling pressures but maintain systemic pressures owing to the device

Outflow obstruction

- Blockage of the LVAD outflow tubing by kinking or thrombosis will increase resistance and reduce flow
- A contrast CT study is the best way to examine the outflow but may require specialist radiographers or interpretation

High flow alarms

Sepsis

- This causes peripheral vasodilation and as the LVAD works against less resistance, its flow will increase
- Patients should be worked up in the normal fashion for sepsis, with specific attention to a driveline infection (see below)

Vasodilator

- Vasodilator drugs can cause similar changes. Review the patient's medication history for recent alteration

High power alarm

As the LVAD will be set at a specific pump speed, resistance due to drag on the rotor will cause the power consumption of the motor to rise. This may occur over time as thrombus gradually accumulates and patients may have heart failure symptoms or haemolysis in addition. CT angiography may show the cause and echocardiogram may show biventricular dilation. Thrombolysis has had poor results and should only be used by experts. Treatment often involves device explant but sometimes may be managed by an intensification of anticoagulation.

Suction event

If the LVAD is pumping blood faster than the LV is filling, the inflow cannula will intermittently 'suck down' onto the wall of the ventricle. This can sometimes result in ventricular arrhythmia from irritating the ventricle. The LVAD will detect suction events as a large fall in the pulsatility index and will ramp down to a low speed to allow the ventricle to refill before slowly ramping back up to the original speed. Anything reducing LV inflow can cause suction events: hypovolaemia, excessive diuresis, right heart failure, PE, tamponade. A mispositioned inflow cannula can also cause this.

Anaemia

GI bleeding

- Owing to anticoagulation and/or acquired von Willebrand disease

Haemolysis

- Due to shearing of red blood cells within the VAD, sometimes in the context of pump thrombus. This was defined as plasma-free haemoglobin > 40 mg/dl and LDH > 1000 mg/dl in the Heartmate II trial. Reducing pump speed may help

Infection

Infections in LVAD patients may be divided into three categories:

- LVAD specific: involving the pump, the cannula, the pocket it sits in or the driveline
- LVAD related: infective endocarditis, mediastinitis, bloodstream infections
- Non-LVAD related

Driveline infection

- Ultrasound or CT may be needed to see deeper seated pockets of infection along the course of the driveline. Depending on severity, this may need increased dressing changes, oral or IV antibiotics, or surgical revision of the device

Device infection

- These are difficult to eradicate and may require lifelong antibiotics. Infection which cannot be eradicated or is progressive may be an indication for urgent transplant listing

Stroke

LVAD patients are at risk of ischaemic and haemorrhagic stroke, with ischaemic being slightly more common. There is a high risk of haemorrhagic transformation of ischaemic strokes so careful anticoagulant monitoring is needed.

Cardiac arrest in the LVAD patient

- Remember that you will not be able to feel a pulse in these patients: look for signs of circulation with a normal capillary refill, no signs of cyanosis or pallor, a mean BP (recorded with BP cuff and Doppler probe) above 60 mmHg and end tidal CO_2 if available
- As early as possible, discuss with the patient's VAD centre. Patients may have tailored plans in the event of arrest
- If the LVAD display is available, check parameters are normal (flow should be > 3 L/min). The Heartmate III's default state is a blank screen and it will wake after pressing any buttons. If the screen is persistently blank, either the controller has failed or the power source is completely depleted
- Fully expose the whole LVAD system to see the whole driveline and power/control system
- Check for LVAD function: if there is a loud alarm from the external controller or there is no audible hum from the device when auscultating with a stethoscope, assume LVAD failure. Restoring LVAD function is the most effective resuscitation tool available

LVAD failure

- In the event of LVAD failure, first expose all connections and ensure they are firmly attached
- Check battery power by pressing the charge indicator button. Replace batteries (one at a time) or connect to mains if available
- If the controller has failed, attach a spare battery to a backup controller and quickly change the driveline to the backup controller
- If none of the above cause the LVAD to restart, consider a cable fracture and try gently manipulating the driveline to see if this restores function
- If LVAD function cannot be restored, follow conventional ALS guidelines including CPR (there is a theoretical risk of dislodging the cannula, however this is rare while withholding CPR; where a VAD has failed in a pulseless patient this will of course be fatal). It is recommended to delay CPR by no more than 2 minutes while attempting to restore LVAD function
- In persisting inadequate circulation, immediate escalation to temporary mechanical support (e.g. Impella or VA ECMO) should be considered and initiated within 60 minutes. A mechanical CPR device should only be considered to facilitate these

If the LVAD is functioning

- Look for causes of low-flow, high-power, or suction events as above. Consider a straight leg raise in a low flow alarm and IV fluid bolus for hypovolaemia
- If the patient is in VT or VF, only shock if the patient is unstable: use 3 stacked shocks if required. If the patient is stable, discuss with local VAD center regarding DC cardioversion under GA or chemical cardioversion

Post-transplant care and complications

Transplant patients are at a higher risk of other medical issues than healthy patients of equivalent age. In particular, they are at risk of rejection and opportunistic infection owing to immunosuppression.

General principles

- Liaise with the patient's transplant centre: they will want to know that the patient has been admitted to hospital and will be able to fine-tune management or arrange transfer if required
- Do not discontinue or alter doses of immunosupressive medications without discussion with the transplant centre: it may be tempting to reduce immunosuppression in the context of infection but you could inadvertently induce rejection
- Take trough (pre-dose) levels of immunosuppressants to help guide treatment
- Caution when prescribing drugs which interact with liver enzymes (see below)

Drugs post transplant

Standard therapy after transplantation

- Maintenance immunosuppression: usually consists of steroid (methylprednisolone), calcineurin inhibitor (tacrolimus— Adoport or Modigraf, ciclosporin, or alternatively sirolimus) and proliferation inhibitor (mycophenolate mofetil— Myfenax, mycophenolic acid, or azathioprine)
- Infection prophylaxis (for the first 6 months after transplant): co-trimoxazole against pneumocystis jirovecii, valganciclovir against cytomegalovirus, and nystatin against oral candida

Drug interactions

Multiple drugs can interact with immunosuppressants, especially drugs affecting CYP450 enzymes. Common drugs interacting with ciclosporin, tacrolimus, and sirolimus are shown below. Caution—this list is not definitive and where possible, discussion with your local transplant centre and/or pharmacist is recommended.

- *Increase* immunosupressant plasma level: amiodarone, clarithromycin, triazole antifungals (fluconazole, itraconazole, etc.)
- *Decrease* immunosuppressant plasma level: carbamazepine, phenytoin, rifampicin
- Increase risk of nephrotoxicity: aminoglycosides, AmBisome (liposomal amphotericin), foscarnet, NSAIDs
- Increase risk of hyperkalaemia: ACE inhibitors, mineralocorticoid receptor antagonists

Renal failure

- Calcineurin inhibitors are strongly associated with nephrotoxicity. Chronic renal failure is common, although acute renal failure can be associated with CNI toxicity
- Part of the work-up should include drug-level monitoring

Rejection

Patients with rejection may present with heart failure symptoms, atrial or ventricular arrhythmias, an asymptomatic decline in systolic function, or no symptoms at all (detection via biopsy screening). Therapy is largely based on consensus and varies from centre to centre, the figures quoted below are intended as representative examples.

Acute cellular rejection (ACR)

- This T-cell-mediated process is most common in the first 3 months post transplant and becomes less frequent after 6 months
- All centres will take regular surveillance biopsies in the first 6 months post transplant and usually beyond this
- Any transplant patient presenting with clinical evidence of heart failure or a suspicion of rejection should undergo biopsy
- Rejection is managed differently depending upon the presence or absence of haemodynamic compromise, which is defined as a fall in ejection fraction of more than a quarter, a cardiac index less than 2.0 L/min/m^2, or the need for inotropic or mechanical cardiac support

ACR with haemodynamic compromise

- Typically treated with IV corticosteroids and/or anti-thymocyte globulin (ATG)/alemtuzumab
- Methylprednisolone is used at a dose of 10 mg/kg/day for three days before switching to oral corticosteroids
- Heart failure medications, inotropes, or MCS may be required in addition

ACR without haemodynamic compromise

- Typically treated with a short (i.e. 3 day) course of high-dose oral steroid
- Prednisolone is used at a dose of 1 mg/kg/day, then tapered at 5 mg intervals back to baseline dose
- Any patient receiving high-dose steroids should also be prescribed antimicrobial prophylaxis (nystatin, co-trimoxazole, valganciclovir)

Antibody-mediated rejection (AMR)

- AMR typically occurs in the few months after transplant but may occur late. Again, it is diagnosed on biopsy but elevated levels of donor specific antibodies will provide useful information
- Therapy consists of corticosteroids, therapeutic plasma exchange, and intravenous immunoglobulin. The number of cycles of plasma exchange will depend on the patient, with IVIg being administered after completion of plasma exchange

Infection

Immunosuppression predisposes to infection. The types of infection which are most common vary with the time from transplant, with nosocomial infection predominating early.

< 1 month: Nosocomial/Technical

- Antimicrobial resistant species (MRSA, VRE, *Candida*)
- Aspiration

- Catheter infection
- *Clostridium difficile*
- Donor-derived infection (rare)
- Recipient derived infection (colonization): *Aspergillus*, pseudomonas

1–6 months: Activation of latent infection

- With PJP and antiviral prophylaxis: polyomavirus BK, *C. difficile* colitis, HCV, adenovirus, *Cryptococcus neoformans*, *Mycobacterium* tuberculosis
- Without prophylaxis: pneumocystis, herpesviruses (HSV, VZV, CMV, EBV), HBV, listeria, nocardia, toxoplasma, strongyloides, leishmania, T cruzi

> 6 months: Community acquired

- Community acquired pneumonias, urinary tract infection
- Aspergillus, atypical moulds
- Nocardia, rhodococcus
- Late viral infections (CMV colitis/retinitis), hepatitis (HBV, HCV), HSV encephalitis, JC polyomavirus
- Skin cancers/lymphomas (post-transplant lymphoproliferative disease)

Specific infections after heart transplantation

- ***Clostridium difficile***: similar presentation to normal hosts but the disease may be more severe. Oral vancomycin is the preferred therapy
- ***Mycobacterium tuberculosis:*** reactivation occurs in up to 2% of patients. Presentation is similar to that in immunocompetent individuals but is more likely to be disseminated. Caution using rifampicin as it will interact with immunosuppressants
- ***Cytomegalovirus*** (CMV): classically presents with fever, malaise, myalgias, and bone marrow suppression but may cause end organ disease in GI tract, lungs, heart, liver, or brain. CMV PCR should be undertaken to quantify viral load for detection. Treatment is with IV ganciclovir and/or oral valganciclovir until there is resolution of symptoms and negative CMV PCR. Foscarnet or cidofovir may be used in resistant cases
- ***Epstein Barr virus*** (EBV): This causes a mononucleosis type syndrome with fever, malaise, fatigue, and pancytopaenia but is also related to post-transplant lymphoproliferative syndrome (see later). There are no specific antiviral agents
- ***Candidiasis***: commonly involves the oesophagus; treated with fluconazole
- ***Aspergillus***: causes pneumonia; usually treated with voriconazole
- ***Cryptococcus***: usually begins with pulmonary disease and disseminates, with a propensity to meningitis, osteomyelitis, and cellulitis. Diagnosis is by detecting cryptococcal antigen in serum and/or CSF. Amphotericin and fluconazole are standard treatments
- ***Pneumocystis jirovecii pneumonia*** (PJP): previously known as PCP, this is less common due to widespread use of prophylaxis. It usually presents with dry cough, shortness of breath, and hypoxia. It is diagnosed on sputum/bronchoalveolar lavage. It is treated with high dose co-trimoxazole

Cardiac allograft vasculopathy

- CAV affects the coronary arteries diffusely, typically causing a narrowing throughout the entire arteries (unlike discrete stenoses commonly seen in atherosclerotic disease)
- As the transplant heart is denervated, ischaemia does not tend to cause pain and events are silent
- Patients may present with worsening shortness of breath representing atypical angina, a sudden deterioration in function representing an infarct, or with dysrhythmias Patients typically undergo screening angiography (invasive or via CT), although typical ischaemia patterns on echo, ECG, or stress testing may be helpful
- Angiography should be performed in patients with new dyspnoea and arrhythmia which is not due to rejection. IVUS may be useful in measuring luminal area. PCI can be effective against more discrete stenoses but restenosis rate tends to be higher. CABG is challenging due to the diffuse nature of the disease
- Statins reduce incidence and severity of CAV. Immunosupressive therapies have not been shown to be helpful

Malignancy

- The risk of malignancy in the transplant population is substantially higher, and tends to follow a more aggressive course
- Transplant patients are also at risk of post-transplant lymphoproliferative disorder (PTLD), usually caused by EBV

Inherited cardiac conditions

Cardiomyopathies

Cardiomyopathies are primary disorders of heart muscle and are the commonest forms of Mendelian inherited heart disease, affecting around 1 in 500 of the adult population.

They are generally classified by morphological features (summarized in Fig. 22.1). Congenital forms of cardiomyopathy are rare and often severe; most commonly the condition develops in late childhood/adolescence or in adult life.

Cardiomyopathies can cause a variety of emergency presentations, including:

- Atrial arrhythmia including atrial fibrillation (AF) ➲ p.151
- Syncope ➲ p.37
- Ventricular arrhythmia and sudden cardiac death (SCD) ➲ p.167
- Acute heart failure and cardiogenic shock ➲ p.11
- Stroke and systemic embolism is also substantially more common in patients with cardiomyopathy ➲ p.217

Inheritance can be monogenic (usually dominantly inherited, but recessive, X-linked, and mitochondrial inheritance can be seen) but there is increasing evidence of polygenic or oligogenic inheritance in other cases, and there is an important interaction with environmental factors (e.g. blood pressure, obesity, toxins such as alcohol or chemotherapy). The main long-term management decision in cardiomyopathies is usually whether and when to implant an ICD. This decision is often complex and depends on disease type and patient factors.

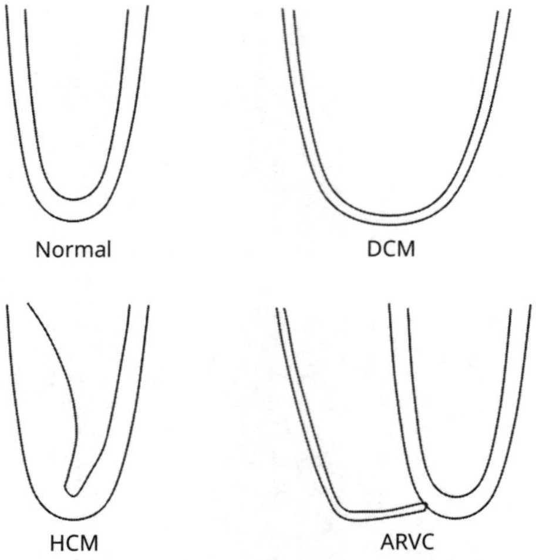

Fig. 22.1 Schematic representation of the ventricular morphology in more common forms of cardiomyopathy. DCM—dilated cardiomyopathy, HCM—hypertrophic cardiomyopathy, ARVC—arrhythmogenic right ventricular cardiomyopathy (a form of arrhythmogenic cardiomyopathy).

Hypertrophic cardiomyopathy

Hypertrophic cardiomyopathy (HCM) is characterized by increased wall thickness in any left ventricular (LV) myocardial segment (15 mm or greater in an adult), unexplained by loading conditions (e.g. hypertension, obesity, aortic stenosis). Dynamic LV outflow tract obstruction is common—present in 30% at rest, and 60% on exercise or Valsalva. This is due to a combination of hypertrophy and mitral valve (MV) abnormalities, leading to MV systolic anterior motion (SAM). Risk stratification can be assisted using a calculator (HCM Risk-SCD). HCM affects around 1 in 500 of the population, though only a proportion have the more severe 'sarcomeric' form of the disease.

Inheritance

Approximately 50% of patients have a monogenic ('sarcomeric') form of HCM. This tends to present at a younger age and carries a higher risk of AF, heart failure, stroke, and SCD. It is dominantly inherited with incomplete penetrance. The remainder have the polygenic ('non-sarcomeric') form of the disease, wherein a combination of common polymorphisms (in combination with environmental factors—especially hypertension and obesity) leads to disease. This form presents later in life and carries a lower risk of complications and of familial transmission (approximately 5% will have affected first degree relatives). The two forms can be distinguished by clinical context, imaging features, and genetic testing.

Presentation

- Commonly found incidentally due to abnormal ECG or echocardiography
- May present with chest pain, shortness of breath, or palpitation
- May present with unheralded cardiac arrest, particularly during exertion

Signs

- Predominantly relate to obstruction so may be absent in 30%
- Ejection systolic murmur, left sternal edge, augments with Valsalva
- Jerky carotid pulse

Investigations

- *ECG*—large voltages, pathological Q waves, axis deviation, ST depression, non-ischaemic type T wave inversion (may be widespread, especially in apical forms)
- *Echocardiography*—asymmetric septal hypertrophy ± outflow tract obstruction, apical (usually non-sarcomeric), concentric, or spiral hypertrophy, LV systolic impairment is more common in sarcomeric disease
- *CMR*hypertrophy as above plus patchy/hazy fibrosis, most commonly in the hypertrophied segments

Management

- Acute management of heart failure, AF, or ventricular arrhythmia is as standard ➲ p.73
- Volume depletion (e.g. due to diuretic overdose or diarrhoea) can cause intractable outflow tract obstruction and even cardiogenic shock. Treatment is based on IV fluids to improve filling and β-blockade. Severe cases may require invasive management including surgery

Dilated cardiomyopathy

Dilated cardiomyopathy (DCM) is characterized by LV dilatation and systolic dysfunction. Increasingly, other forms of the disease are recognized and patients may have dilatation alone or LV systolic dysfunction with a normal sized ventricle (sometimes termed 'hypokinetic non-dilated cardiomyopathy'). It can lead to progressive heart failure, atrial or ventricular arrhythmia, stroke, and SCD. Prevalence is difficult to estimate due to differences in diagnostic criteria, but primarily genetic DCM is uncommon, affecting less than 1 in 1000 of the adult population.

Inheritance

DCM can be sporadic or familial. Even in clear familial disease, monogenic inheritance occurs only in a minority (30–40% of cases). The most common cause of monogenic DCM is truncation of TTN; though these variants can also be seen at relatively high frequency in the normal population (~1–2%). Other genotypes show additional or extra-cardiac features (*LMNA* variants show early heart block, *SCN5A* variants can overlap with early conduction disease and Brugada syndrome, *DMD* variants can cause variable degrees of muscular dystrophy). Certain genotypes carry an elevated risk of sudden cardiac death, even with relatively preserved systolic function (e.g. *LMNA*, *RBM20*, *PLN*, *FLNC*) and the presence of such variants would influence risk stratification and ICD implantation. The presence or absence of fibrosis on CMR appears to be a particularly important risk marker in this group.

Presentation

- Commonly found incidentally due to abnormal ECG or echocardiography
- May present with shortness of breath, ankle swelling, or palpitation
- May present with unheralded cardiac arrest, particularly during exertion

Signs

- Fluid overload (ankle swelling, raised venous pressure, third heart sound)
- Usually no signs when euvolaemic

Investigations

- *ECG*—very variable and can be normal. LBBB is more common in DCM and is a marker for more severe disease. AF may be present as a cause or consequence of DCM. Certain genotypes may have a distinctive ECG (e.g. *PLN*-related disease with very low voltages)
- *Echocardiography*—LV dilatation and systolic dysfunction, raised pulmonary pressures
- *CMR*—mid-wall fibrosis, commonly in interventricular septum

Management

- Acute management of heart failure, AF, or ventricular arrhythmia is as standard ➲ p.73
- Cardiogenic shock is managed with inotropes ± mechanical support
- DCM is the most common condition leading to heart transplantation in the UK

Arrhythmogenic cardiomyopathy

Arrhythmogenic cardiomyopathy (ACM) encompasses disease of the right ventricle (ARVC), biventricular and left-dominant ACM. Some authorities include high-risk DCM genotypes in this classification. ACM is characterized by a progressive replacement of ventricular myocardium (either RV or LV or both) by fat and fibrous tissue. This leads to ventricular arrhythmia, which can be frequent and sustained, and can occur early in the course of disease. Progressive heart failure can occur later in disease. Stroke is also common and prophylactic anticoagulation should be considered carefully. Sudden cardiac death can occur with minimal ventricular dysfunction and risk calculators are available to assist in decisions over ICD implantation (e.g. at ARVCrisk.com). ACM is uncommon, affecting approximately 1 in 1200 of the adult population.

Inheritance

ACM is caused by monogenic variants in around 70% of cases. Environmental factors are also very important and, in particular, endurance exercise is a risk factor for severe disease. Genetic variants are in desmosomal genes (e.g. *PKP2*, *DSP*, *DSC*) and inheritance is usually autosomal dominant. Homozygotes and compound heterozygotes usually show substantially more severe disease with extra-cardiac features.

Presentation

- Commonly presents with sustained ventricular arrhythmia causing palpitations or syncope
- May present with unheralded cardiac arrest, particularly during exertion
- May present with stroke in association with AF

Signs

- Irregular heart rhythm due to frequent ectopy
- Fluid overload (ankle swelling, raised venous pressure, third heart sound)

Investigations

- *ECG*—ARVC: anterior T wave inversion (to V3/V4) with epsilon waves (low amplitude, short duration deflections in the terminal QRS). Left dominant disease: lateral T wave inversion. *DSP*-related disease may show low voltages in the limb leads
- *Holter*—frequent ventricular ectopics, non-sustained VT
- *Echocardiography*—ARVC: RV dilatation and systolic dysfunction, with regional wall motion abnormalities. Left-dominant ACM: LV systolic impairment ± dilatation. Patients frequently have biventricular involvement
- *CMR*—features as above plus fibrofatty replacement of RV, fibrosis in LV (particularly ring-like or epicardial)
- *Endomyocardial biopsy*—rarely used in most centres but can show fibrofatty replacement and inflammation

Management

- Acute management of heart failure or AF is as standard ➲ p.73

- Arrhythmia storm should be treated with maximal β-blockade, additional anti-arrhythmic medications and may require sedation and intubation to achieve control ➲ p.175
- Useful anti-arrhythmic medications include amiodarone, sotalol, and sodium-channel blockers such as mexiletine or flecainide
- Combination sotalol and sodium-channel blocker can give safe and effective long-term control
- Monomorphic ventricular tachycardia is often amenable to ablation (usually requiring an endocardial plus epicardial approach)
- Heart transplantation may be required due to progressive heart failure or intractable arrhythmia

Other cardiomyopathies

Restrictive cardiomyopathy

Restrictive cardiomyopathy is characterized by restrictive LV filling in the absence of severe hypertrophy or pericardial constriction. It can be genetic in a minority of cases (commonly associated with sarcomeric gene variants) or caused by infiltrative diseases such as amyloidosis. Atrial arrhythmia, especially AF, is common and may precipitate decompensation. Patients are often exquisitely sensitive to filling status, with pulmonary oedema in response to overfilling, and circulatory collapse with dehydration. It is often challenging to manage and the prognosis in highly symptomatic disease is poor.

Excessive trabeculation

Cardiomyopathy with excessive trabeculation (formerly known as LV non-compaction) is an unclassified cardiomyopathy. Excessive trabeculation is an imaging finding that may be seen in normal individuals (particularly athletes), in association with other cardiac diseases (e.g. congenital heart disease) or, rarely, with cardiomyopathy. In these cases, the most common causative gene changes are in sarcomeric genes. It is not clear whether the finding of trabeculation confers any additional risk of SCD or stroke over and above the underlying cardiomyopathy itself. It was previously believed to be due to a failure of compaction of ventricular myocardium during foetal life, though latest evidence suggests that the condition is usually not present at birth and, indeed, that this specific developmental process does not in fact occur.

Channelopathies

Channelopathies are inherited primary disorders of heart rhythm. They are rare, affecting < 1 in 2000 of the UK population. However, clinically unaffected carriers of gene changes causing long QT syndrome are more common than this. Channelopathies generally cause fast ventricular arrhythmia leading to syncope (if self-terminating) or sudden cardiac death. Shorter or slower bouts of arrhythmia may present with palpitations.

Long QT syndrome

Long QT syndrome (LQTS) is caused by alterations in (primarily) cardiac potassium and sodium channels. Changes in channel function cause prolongation of repolarization and increase the 'vulnerable window'. Gene carriers may have overt QT prolongation or a normal ECG at rest. Certain medications can exacerbate QT prolongation and may be very dangerous, even in previously asymptomatic individuals. New medications should be checked against a list of known QT-prolonging drugs (various lists available online, e.g. crediblemeds.org). So-called acquired LQTS is characterized by variable QT prolongation at rest and a high sensitivity to QT-prolonging medications; there is likely to be a strong polygenic tendency to low repolarization reserve in such individuals though this is not well understood.

Inheritance

The majority of LQTS is dominantly inherited. LQT1 is caused by variants in *KCNQ1*, LQT2 by variants in *KCNH2*, and LQT3 by variants in *SCN5A*; together these represent > 95% of genetically proven LQTS. Homozygotes for LQT1 usually have a severe phenotype and congenital deafness (the Jervell and Lange-Nielsen syndrome—JLN).

Presentation

- May present with syncope or palpitation
- Sudden cardiac death may be first presentation
- May be identified in clinical screening or cascade genetic screening due to family history of SCD or LQTS
- Variants in *KCNQ1*, *KCNE1*, and *KCNE2* are commonly found incidentally during genetic testing for congenital deafness
- Schwartz score is used to assess likelihood of a diagnosis

Signs

- Diagnosis is suggested by prolongation of QTc on resting ECG (> 450 ms in a man, > 460 ms in a woman) in the absence of structural heart disease, ischaemia, electrolyte abnormalities, or QT-prolonging drugs (Fig. 22.2)

Investigations

- *ECG*—very variable and can be normal in asymptomatic gene carriers
- *ETT*—failure of QTc shortening in early exercise (LQT1), sudden lengthening of QTc in recovery (LQT2)
- *Ambulatory ECG*—QTc is variable through the day and may aid diagnosis, ectopy can be a marker of risk (particularly in LQT2)
- Echocardiography/CMR/angiography—should be normal

Management

- Lifestyle measures: avoid intense exercise or swimming (particularly LQT1), loud noises, or intense emotion (particularly LQT2); arrhythmia classically occurs at rest or asleep in LQT3
- Avoid QT-prolonging drugs

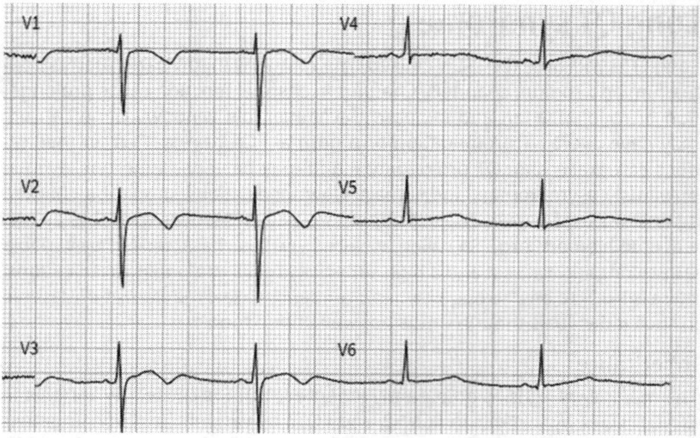

Fig. 22.2 ECG of a 13-year-old female with long QT syndrome type 2. There are biphasic anterior T waves (normal for age) with flat and slurred T waves in the lateral vectors. The QT interval is 500 ms (corrected to 480 ms by Bazzett's).

- Non-selective β-blockers (e.g. nadolol, propranolol, carvedilol) are most effective
- Mexiletine may be useful in LQT3
- Cervical sympathectomy can be useful (particularly in LQT1)
- ICD is generally reserved for secondary prevention or rare very high-risk individuals (e.g. JLN, LQT3 with QTc > 550 ms)
- Risk stratification depends on QTc, genotype, gender, and age

J wave syndromes (Brugada and early repolarization syndrome)

Brugada syndrome (BrS) is a rare channelopathy caused by disturbance in sodium-channel function. It is more common in East Asia (especially northern Thailand, where it can affect up to 1 in 200 young men) than in Europe and Africa. In a minority of patients (~20%), BrS is part of a wider spectrum of sodium channel disease and can associate with early conduction disease and DCM.

Early repolarization syndrome (ERS) is diagnosed in survivors of VF arrest with J waves and ST changes, particularly in the inferior leads, on the resting ECG. It is important to recognize that the ECG finding of early repolarization in healthy individuals is common and does not seem to confer any particular risk.

Inheritance

A disease-causing gene change in *SCN5A* is found in ~20% of individuals with BrS. The remainder of cases are likely to be caused by a combination of common variants in other genes and potentially by phenocopies (other conditions causing a similar ECG). Certain specific *SCN5A* genotypes cause an overlap of BrS and LQT3. ERS is usually sporadic and it is unusual to find affected family members. Genetic testing typically does not reveal convincing pathogenic variants in ERS and its aetiology is incompletely understood.

Presentation

- May present with syncope or palpitation
- Sudden cardiac death may be first presentation
- May be identified in clinical screening or cascade genetic screening due to family history of SCD or BrS
- Shanghai score is used to assess likelihood of a diagnosis

Signs

- Diagnosis of BrS is suggested by the presence of a type 1 ECG (coved ST elevation > 2 mm terminating in a negative T wave in any of V1–V3, Fig. 22.3A) at rest or provoked by drug challenge or fever. Further supporting evidence for a diagnosis (syncope, family history, genetics) is required in the latter cases
- ERS is diagnosed in a survivor of unexplained cardiac arrest with features of early repolarization (Fig. 22.3B) on the ECG, particularly in inferior vectors

Investigations

- *ECG*—type 1 Brugada ECG at rest or on provocation. ECG should include high RV leads (e.g. V5 and V6 leads moved to 1 intercostal space above V1 and V2). Type 2 ECG may warrant further investigation but is not diagnostic
- *12-lead ambulatory ECG*—may reveal a spontaneous type 1 ECG in an individual with a normal ECG at rest
- *Echocardiography/CMR*—should be normal. Some individuals have evidence of epicardial fibrosis in the RVOT (BrS) and inferior LV wall (ERS)

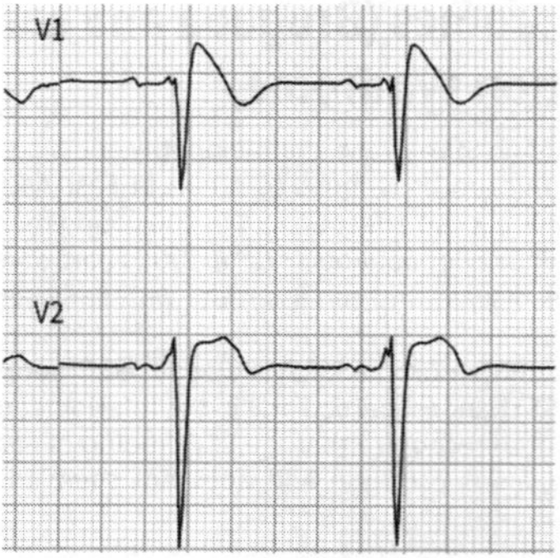

Fig. 22.3 ECG showing type 1 Brugada pattern (coved ST elevation) in lead V1 and type 2 pattern (saddleback ST elevation) in V2 in a 52-year-old male.

Management

- Lifestyle measures: aggressive management of fever, avoid binge drinking alcohol or very heavy meals
- Avoid high-risk medications (brugadadrugs.org)
- ICD is indicated for secondary prevention or high-risk individuals
- Quinidine/hydroquinidine appears to be effective in BrS and ERS
- Ablation of RVOT substrate may be useful in BrS with recurrent VF
- Risk stratification is based on features such as spontaneous type 1 ECG, FH, syncope
- There is increasing evidence that *SCN5A* gene positive individuals carry more risk

Ryanodinopathies (CPVT and CRDS)

Catecholaminergic polymorphic ventricular tachycardia (CPVT) and its counterpart, calcium-release deficiency syndrome (CRDS), are caused by disturbances in the function of the sarcoplasmic reticulum. They are thought to be very rare, affecting < 1 in 10,000 of the population, but the true prevalence is unknown.

Inheritance

CPVT and CRDS are most commonly caused by variants in *RYR2*, which encodes the cardiac ryanodine receptor (a calcium channel). Gain of protein function causes CPVT, loss of function causes CRDS. Recessive inheritance can be seen in a small minority of cases of CPVT.

Presentation

- CPVT usually presents with recurrent syncope provoked by exertion or emotional stress. It often presents in childhood. SCD may be the first presentation
- CRDS usually presents with SCD or aborted SCD, prior symptoms are uncommon
- May be identified in clinical screening or cascade genetic screening due to family history of SCD or CPVT

Signs

- CPVT is suggested by frequent/complex ectopy, non-sustained monomorphic or polymorphic VT (classically, bidirectional VT) on an exercise test
- CRDS patients typically have normal standard tests (ECG/Holter/ETT) though there may be subtle features

Investigations

- *ECG*—the resting 12-lead ECG is usually normal in both CPVT and CRDS
- *12-lead ambulatory ECG*—may reveal ectopy or NSVT (frequent in CPVT, uncommon in CRDS)
- *ETT*—frequent or complex ectopy, NSVT, bidirectional or polymorphic VT at peak exercise in CPVT (Fig. 22.4); ectopy NSVT may be seen in early exercise/recovery in CRDS
- *Echocardiography/CMR*—should be normal
- *Programmed ventricular stimulation*—may be useful in diagnosis and management of CRDS, no known value in CPVT

Management

- Lifestyle measures: avoid known triggers (stress/exercise) in CPVT; arrhythmia typically occurs at rest or while asleep in CRDS
- Non-selective β-blockers (e.g. nadolol, propranolol, carvedilol) are most effective for CPVT, possibly harmful in CRDS
- Flecainide and quinidine may be effective in CRDS

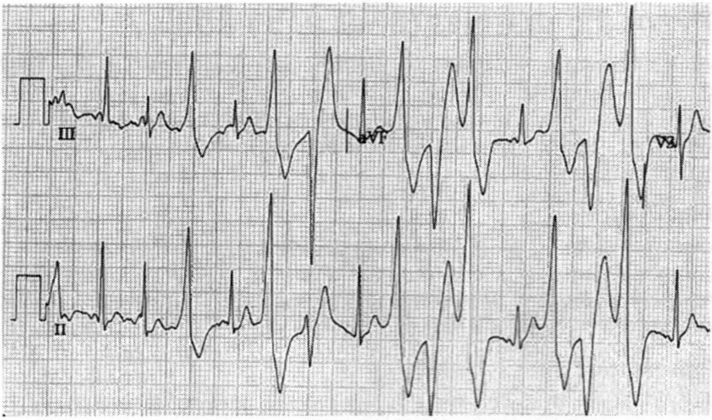

Fig. 22.4 ECG showing multifocal ectopy at high exercise workload in a 17-year-old male with CPVT.

- Cervical sympathectomy can be useful in CPVT
- ICD therapy is controversial in CPVT as shocks can cause recurrent arrhythmia, some authorities recommend avoiding as much as possible; indications for ICD therapy in CRDS (apart from secondary prevention) are unknown

Part 3

Procedural

Practical procedures

General considerations

There is always time to think

There are very few emergencies that require an *immediate* response. A focused period of reflection and planning, supported when required by the opinion and contribution of others, is an essential prelude to the successful performance of a practical procedure—especially in the demanding setting of an acute clinical problem.

Is the proposed procedure indicated?

This may seem an odd first question but it is the correct starting point. Many a practical procedure is abandoned after prolonged, fruitless (and often painful and dangerous) attempts with an observation to the patient that 'We can do without it'. Consider the indications for the proposed procedure and any special factors that may affect the likelihood of success or the risk. Review all alternative approaches to the problem. Commit to a procedure only if the intervention is considered essential or has much to offer, at a risk judged acceptable to your patient, ideally with informed consent though this may not always be possible or appropriate.

Do you have the skills to perform the procedure?

To thine own self be true.

It is your professional duty to act within your established competence. Never hesitate to ask for help or guidance or to refer to an appropriate specialist. This text aims to serve as a practical aide-memoire and is not a substitute for formal training and practical experience.

Even if experienced and confident in a procedure, never underestimate the role and importance of assistants or other professionals that will be involved (e.g. radiographers in temporary pacemaker insertion). The full range of skills will be required.

Do you have the setting and equipment for the procedure?

Remember the rule of the 12 Ps:

> Proper Prior Preparation and Planning and Perfect Patient Positioning, Prevents Poor Performance of Practical Procedures,

- If appropriate, inform your senior cover of your intentions
- Secure time, free of likely interruption—who will hold your bleep? Are there any competing urgent clinical concerns?
- Rearrange the room and furniture to secure optimum access. Adjust patient position, bed height, lighting, and remove obstructions
- Prepare and check all items of equipment that will be required
- For complex or unfamiliar procedures, perform a mental rehearsal—establish the sequence of your planned action; checklist all planned equipment requirements
- Ensure compatibility of items—will the pacing wire fit through the venous access line? Will the pacing wire fit to the pacing box?
- Prepare in advance items that do not demand sterile handling, e.g. infusions for central venous lines, transducers and monitors for pressure lines

Central venous lines

Choice of approach

The 3 main approaches to central venous cannulation are:

- Internal jugular vein
- Subclavian vein
- Femoral vein

You should aim to become familiar with at least 2 of these routes.

General points—applicable to all approaches

- *Ultrasound guidance has emerged as the standard of care in central venous access (to locate the target vein and identify related structures). You should seek training in the use of these imaging devices and use them when they are available*
- Pay attention to sterility. Prepare the skin and drape the area with sterile dressings. Wear sterile gloves and gown
- Positioned the patient with head-down tilt. This fills the central veins, increasing their available size for cannulation and minimizes the risk of cerebral air embolization during the procedure

Internal jugular approach

This has emerged as the most common route for central venous access. When compared to subclavian access, it has a lower risk of pneumothorax and allows compression haemostasis for patients with a disordered co-agulation or following thrombolysis. It is also ideal for the application of ultrasound guidance methods. The line position may, however, be more uncomfortable for patients, and there may be a tendency for displacement of temporary pacing wires. The right internal jugular is preferred to the left, as it is a straighter course to the SVC and avoids the thoracic duct.

Internal jugular cannulation with ultrasound guidance

Ultrasound-guided internal jugular (IJ) line insertion is a highly effective technique (and safer than non-image-guided approaches for central venous access, reducing complications such as arterial puncture and hematoma formation.

The procedure begins with the patient in a supine position, with their head turned slightly to the opposite side to expose the neck.

First, identify the internal jugular vein and common carotid artery using ultrasound. The internal jugular is typically located lateral and slightly posterior to the carotid artery. The ultrasound probe is placed transversely on the neck, just above the clavicle, and adjusted to visualize both structures.

- Infiltrate the skin and SC tissue with 5–10 mL lidocaine 1%
- Mount the needle on a syringe containing a few mL of normal saline
- Position the guidewire on the sterile field but within easy reach
- Make a small incision ('nick') the skin with a small (e.g. number 11) scalpel blade to facilitate advancement of the sheath/cannula
- Advance the needle, maintaining negative pressure by aspiration
- The needle is inserted at a 30–45° angle to the skin, directed toward the internal jugular vein
- Under real-time ultrasound guidance, the needle tip is visualized as it approaches the vein

- Once the needle tip is confirmed inside the vein, the guidewire is threaded through the needle, and the needle is removed
- After placing the guidewire, dilate the tissue using a dilator to accommodate the catheter. The catheter is then threaded over the guidewire, and the line is secured with sutures

Internal jugular cannulation without ultrasound guidance

N.B. Ultrasound guidance is recommended whenever possible

The approach

(See Box 23.1 and Fig 23.1 for details of technique.)

- Identify the apex of the muscle-free triangle between the clavicular and manubrial heads of the sternocleidomastoid muscle
- Palpate the line of the carotid artery and insert the needle lateral to this line at an angle of 45° to the skin, aiming for the right nipple area (or anterior superior iliac spine)
- The vein is superficial and cannulation should be achieved at a depth of a few centimetres. Do not advance beyond this, as the apex of the lung could be injured

Subclavian approach

The subclavian approach allows access to the patient if the area around the patient's head is unavailable (e.g. during a cardiac arrest). A line inserted by this route lies on the anterior chest, is comfortable for the patient, and easy to manage. The main limitations of the approach are a risk of pneumothorax and an inability to apply pressure to the target vessels in the event of multiple venous or inadvertent arterial puncture.

► It is unwise to attempt immediate subclavian puncture on the contralateral side after an initial unsuccessful attempt as this may result in bilateral pneumothoraces.

The approach

(See Box 23.1 and Fig 23.2 for details of technique.)

- Identify the junction between the medial 1/3 and lateral 2/3 of the clavicle. This is usually at the apex of a convex angulation as the clavicle sweeps laterally and cranially
- The skin incision point is 2 cm inferior and lateral to this point
- Infiltrate the skin and SC tissue at this point and up to the edge of the clavicle. Keeping the needle horizontal, move the needle tip gently down and behind the clavicle, infiltrating local anaesthetic
- Prepare the cannulation needle and follow the same initial track as the anaesthetic needle
- When the needle lies just below the clavicle, aim the needle at the nadir of the suprasternal notch
- Keeping the needle horizontal and parallel to the bed (avoiding lifting the hands off the body and angling the needle tip down) minimizes the risk of pneumothorax

Box 23.1 Technique for central venous line insertion

- Whenever possible use the Seldinger technique (needle over guidewire). Catheter over needle devices (similar to peripheral IV cannulae) are more difficult to place
- Infiltrate the skin and SC tissue with 5–10 mL lidocaine 1%
- Mount the needle on a syringe containing a few mL of normal saline
- Position the guidewire on the sterile field but within easy reach
- Make a small incision ('nick') the skin with a small (e.g. number 11) scalpel blade to facilitate advancement of the sheath/cannula
- Advance the needle, maintaining negative pressure by aspiration
- If the vein is not entered, withdraw the needle slowly maintaining syringe aspiration. Sometimes the needle transfixes the vein and cannulation is only evident on slow withdrawal
- After an unsuccessful pass:
  - Flush the needle to remove debris that may clog its lumen
  - Reassess the anatomical landmarks and identify a modified line for the next attempt. Be systematic in exploring the target region
- When the needle enters the vein and blood is aspirated, be prepared to make minor adjustments (advance or retract) to ensure free flow of blood
- Fix the needle with one hand and carefully remove the syringe
- Pass the flexible end of the guidewire (usually with 'J' tip) down the needle—the wire should pass with minimal resistance. Passage can sometimes be facilitated with minor rotation of the wire or needle (to change the angle of the bevel)
- If resistance persists, remove the wire and check the needle position by aspiration with a syringe before retrying
- When half of the wire is in the vein, remove the needle and place the sheath and its dilator over the wire
- Do not advance the sheath into the body until a short length of wire is visible protruding from the rear end of the dilator and is secured with a firm grasp
- If there is resistance to insertion of the sheath, consider enlargement of the skin incision. If there is resistance in the deeper layers (e.g. clavipectoral fascia for subclavian lines) it may be necessary to first advance a dilator of smaller calibre (without its sheath) to open the track
- Once the line is in place remove the dilator and secure the cannula with suture and a transparent occlusive dressing
- Radiographic examination (penetrated films) can be used to check the line position but this investigation should not preclude emergency use of a line following uncomplicated insertion

Femoral vein approach

The femoral approach allows easy cannulation of a great vein and is valuable in an emergency setting. The area can be compressed in the event of bleeding and temporary pacing can be achieved by this route. The main limitations relate to subsequent patient immobility and a probable ↑risk of line infection.

The approach

(See Box 23.1 and Fig 23.3 for details of technique.)

- The patient should be lying flat with the leg slightly adducted and externally rotated
- Shave the groin, prepare the skin, and drape
- Palpate the femoral artery below the inguinal ligament, over or slightly above the natural skin crease at the top of the leg
- The femoral vein lies medial to the femoral artery
- Infiltrate local anaesthetic at the skin surface and deeper layers
- Advance the cannulation needle at 30–45° to the skin surface, parallel to the direction of the femoral artery
- The vein usually lies ~4 cm from the skin surface

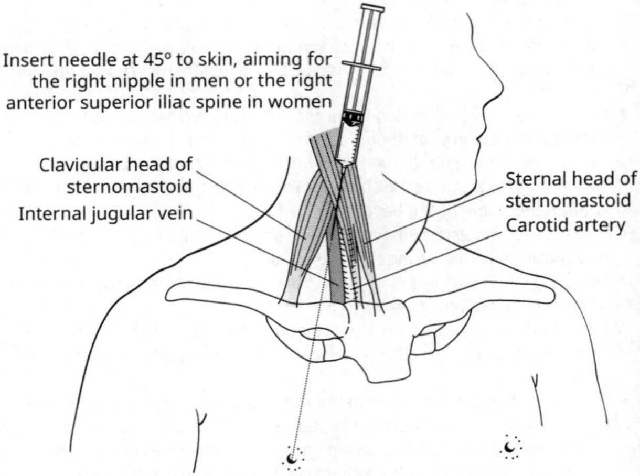

Fig. 23.1 Internal jugular central insertion.

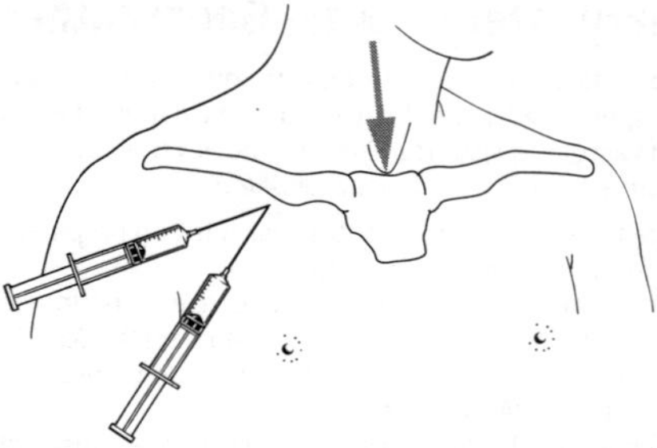

Fig. 23.2 Right subclavian vein central line insertion.

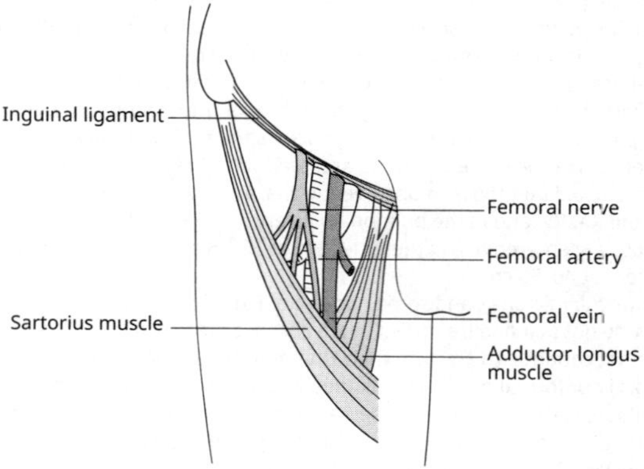

Fig. 23.3 Right femoral vein anatomy.

Pulmonary artery (Swan–Ganz) catheters

The main purpose of this intervention is to monitor intracardiac pressures. Other, more specialized catheters allow the calculation of indices of cardiac function and vascular resistance. They are, however, used less frequently in modern practice as their usefulness is debated.

- Ensure that the correct equipment is available and prepared including the pressure transducers and monitors
- Connect the patient to ECG monitoring and insert a peripheral IV cannula
- Secure central venous access via internal jugular (➲ p.358–9) or subclavian routes (➲ p.358–9) using a special sheath designed to allow the introduction of PA catheters
- Prepare the catheter by flushing its internal lumens—usually labelled distal, mid, and proximal, describing the exit lumen in the catheter. Most catheters include a soft balloon, inflated with air and designed to encourage floatation of the catheter tip (with blood flow), through the right heart and into the pulmonary vasculature. Test this balloon with inflation/deflation
- Attach real-time pressure monitoring to the distal channel of the catheter and insert into the great veins to a depth of 8–10 cm
- Inflate the balloon to encourage flow through the right heart. Deep inspiration can encourage passage across the tricuspid valve
- Progress of the catheter can be assessed with X-ray screening but the more usual method is to observe the characteristic waveforms recorded in the RA, RV, and in the pulmonary artery (Fig. 23.4). The right ventricle is usually entered at a catheter length of 25–35 cm and the pulmonary artery at 40–50 cm
- Ventricular ectopics and some non-sustained VT can occur during passage but do not demand treatment in the absence of circulatory collapse
- Do not continue to advance the catheter if there is no progress. This risks knot formation with the catheter coiling in a chamber. Deflate the balloon, withdraw to the RA, and attempt another passage. In patients with low cardiac output or established right heart pathology specialist help with X-ray imaging may be required
- When in the pulmonary circulation, advance the catheter tip to a position where the wedge pressure can be measured when the balloon is inflated. Deflation of the balloon between readings minimizes the risk of trauma or rupture of a pulmonary vessel
- A good wedge tracing exhibits a classic LA pattern with 'a' and 'v' wave morphology (if the patient is in sinus rhythm)—see Fig. 23.4 and Box 23.2. It is lower or equal to the PA diastolic pressure and has no dichrotic notch, seen in most PA tracings. The wedge pressure usually fluctuates with respiration. If the pressure tracing is damped and tends to increase in a ramp fashion this implies 'overwedging' and partial balloon deflation or catheter withdrawal may be required

Box 23.2 Normal ranges

- RA 0–8 mmHg
- RV systolic 20–25 mmHg; diastolic 6–12 mmHg
- PA systolic 20–25 mmHg; diastolic 4–8 mmHg
- PCWP 6–12 mmHg

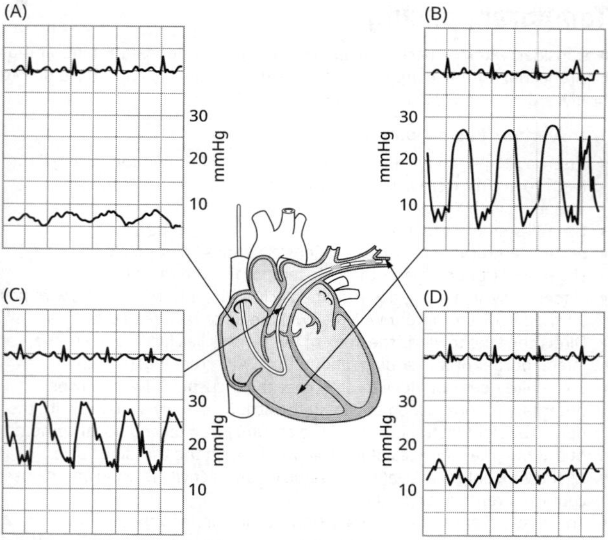

Fig. 23.4 Right heart catheterization. In each panel, the ECG is shown at the top with the corresponding pressure trace from the distal port of a PA catheter at the bottom. The characteristic pressure traces indicate the position of the catheter as it traverses the right heart. Record the pressures obtained from each location and the systemic arterial BP.

(A) (Top left) RA pressure trace in sinus rhythm. Atrial pressure is clearly lower than that of RV or PA. The 'a' wave coincides with atrial contraction while the 'v' wave reflects atrial filling against the tricuspid valve (closed during RV systole). The 'a' wave will be absent in AF. Large 'v' waves are indicative of tricuspid incompetence.

(B) (Top right) The RV pressure trace is characterized by large swings in pressure that correspond to RV contraction and relaxation.

(C) (Bottom left) In the PA, the systolic should be equal to RV systolic (in the absence of RVOTO or pulmonary stenosis). Note the dicrotic notch corresponding to closure of the pulmonary valve.

(D) (Bottom right) PCWP. With the PA catheter balloon inflated, the distal port is insulated from the right heart and it is effectively exposed to LA pressure. In the absence of PE or pre-capillary pulmonary hypertension then PA diastolic pressure should approximate closely to PCWP.

Temporary pacing

▶ Consider external pacing or pharmacological support (atropine and/or isoprenaline) if immediate support for haemodynamic compromise due to bradycardia is required.

Transvenous pacing wire insertion

- Insert a peripheral IV cannula and connect an ECG monitor—using limb leads to avoid external wires over the chest that will be visible when screening with X-rays
- Use full sterile precautions
- Secure central venous access (➲ Central venous lines, p.358–9) with a sheath of larger diameter than the temporary wire to be used
- Under X-ray screening, advance the pacing wire into the RA. The wire has a J-shaped distal contour which allows the tip to be directed by rotation
- Direct the wire towards the apex of the RV (this lies just medial to the lateral border of the cardiac silhouette on AP screening) (Fig. 23.5)
- If the wire does not move directly over the tricuspid valve it may be necessary to form a loop of wire in the atrium, usually achieved with the tip on the right lateral border of the atrium. Rotation and advancement of the wire may then result in prolapse through the tricuspid valve
- As the wire enters the ventricle, some ectopic activity is usual and helps confirm a ventricular position
- The wire can enter the coronary sinus (which drains venous blood from the myocardium to the RA), the orifice of which lies just above the tricuspid valve. A wire in the coronary sinus appears more cranial on AP screening and on a lateral view moves posteriorly) rather than the desired anterior direction of an RV position)
- Manipulate the wire so that the tip curves downwards to the apex of the ventricle (Fig. 23.5). In its final position the line of the wire should resemble the heel of a sock in the RA, with the toe in the apex of the RV
- Connect the lead to the pacing box (Box 23.3, Fig. 23.6) and test the threshold for capture
- Test the stability of the lead position by observing lead motion and the ability to pace the heart during patient manoeuvres of deep inspiration, coughing, and sniffing

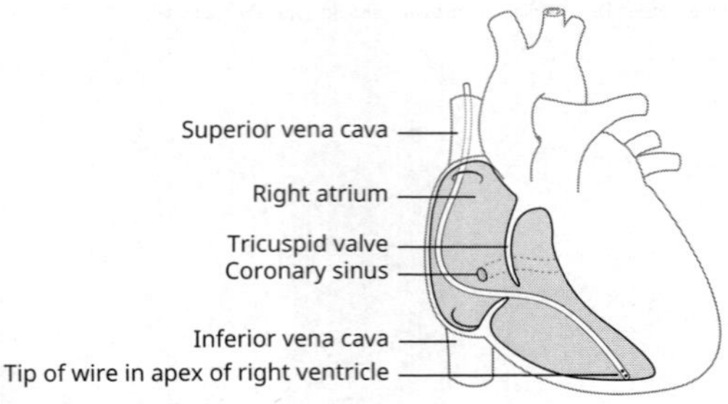

Fig. 23.5 Temporary pacing wire position.

Box 23.3 Configuring the pacemaker settings

- Set to **Demand** at a **rate** of 60–80 bpm
- The pacemaker will, on a beat-to-beat basis, **pace** when it does not detect ventricular activity above that rate
- The red **pace** light will illuminate on each occasion
- When the spontaneous ventricular rate is above the pacemaker rate, the box will inhibit and the red **sense** light will illuminate
- An **output** voltage set to at least 3 × pacemaker threshold will ensure that each impulse 'captures' the ventricle
- The **SENSITIVITY** should be adjusted to ensure that each intrinsic beat is detected but that skeletal muscle interference does not lead to pacemaker inhibition—the lower the setting, the more sensitive the pacemaker

- Suture the lead to the skin close to the entry point and apply transparent occlusive dressings
- Secure the external portion of the lead with tape or other fixatives

❶ Ensure that the pacemaker is set to DEMAND. Asynchronous pacing risks inducing ventricular arrhythmias.

❶ Note that instigating pacing may lead to pacemaker dependence.

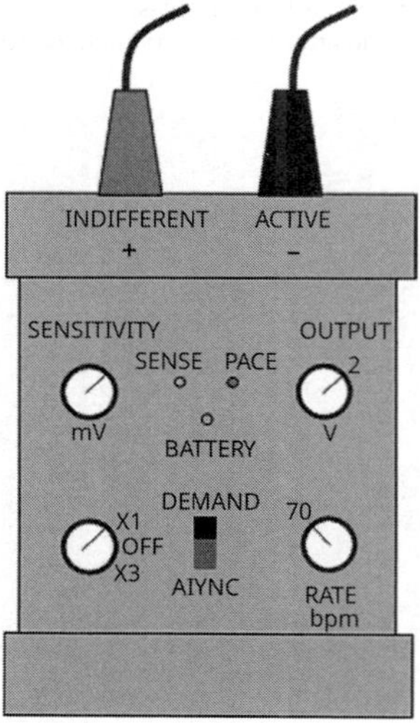

Fig. 23.6 Diagram of a typical temporary pacing box.

Inserting an arterial line

Although the femoral and brachial arteries can be used, the best approach is via the radial artery. This is a superficial vessel, easily palpated at the wrist medial to the radial styloid. In the vast majority of people, a dual blood supply to the hand (via the ulnar artery and palmar arch) ensures adequate distal limb perfusion even if the radial artery is occupied by a catheter or closes by subsequent thrombosis.

Procedure

- Position the patient's hand palm upwards. Place a support (bandage roll or 500 mL fluid bag) to support the lower forearm and allow the wrist to rest in passive extension
- Prepare (sterile field) and drape the wrist
- Infiltrate local anaesthetic at the skin surface and superficial SC layer
- Use a special radial artery catheter pack with small calibre needle, guide wire and cannula (Seldinger technique)
- Palpate the radial pulse
- Aim to cannulate proximal to the flexor skin creases to avoid the tough flexor retinaculum
- Advance the needle at 45° to the skin. As the artery is entered blood flow is observed in the needle hub
- Insert guidewire and cannula following the pattern of central venous line insertion (➲ Central venous lines, p.358–9)
- Secure the cannula and attach a pressure monitoring line, transducer, and flush facility

Pericardial drainage (pericardiocentesis)

Emergency drainage of the pericardial space is usually performed for the management of cardiac tamponade. When known or suspected tamponade has created a cardiac arrest situation, the procedure can and should be performed as an immediate and potentially life-saving measure (Box 23.4). In other, less critical cases, echocardiography should be performed first. This allows confirmation of the diagnosis and provides important information about the wisdom of and approach to pericardial aspiration.

Box 23.4 Emergency situations

Insertion of a pericardial drain requires specialized equipment (see Box 23.5). In a critical situation, however, symptoms and haemodynamic compromise will improve (at least in the short term) with simple drainage, sometimes of modest volumes of fluid. This can be achieved with simple aspiration using a syringe and a standard 'white' venepuncture needle or IV cannula, inserted at the position of the apex beat and directed towards the heart. This 'apical' approach' can also be used for inserting a drain, with appropriate echocardiographic guidance.

Box 23.5 Key equipment

A variety of manufacturers now supply composite pericardial drainage packs but the key items of equipment include:

- Long needle (15 cm) of at least 18G calibre; a short bevel is an advantage to avoid potential cardiac laceration
- 'J' tip guidewire—0.035″ (0.89 mm) diameter
- Dilator (5–7 Fr)
- Pigtail or other drainage catheter with multiple side-holes on the distal shaft
- Large calibre syringe for initial aspiration
- Drainage bag and connecting tubing

Aspiration should only be attempted if there is a substantial fluid collection between the pericardial layers at the access point of intended drainage (> 2 cm echocardiographic separation). Following cardiac surgery or with certain chronic and infective aetiologies, there can be localized tamponade of a cardiac chamber, not amenable to percutaneous drainage, and expert cardiac surgical advice should be sought for this.

Location and imaging

Both emergency and elective procedures can be performed without imaging but most authorities now recommend some form of guidance. A cardiac catheterization laboratory is the ideal environment with radiographic screening and pressure monitoring, though this is not essential, and echocardiographic imaging is commonly used. Some older texts refer to the use of ECG monitoring connected to the aspiration needle, though this is difficult to achieve with modern ECG recording equipment.

The subxiphisternal approach

- Position the patient at 45° to encourage pooling of the effusion at the inferior surface of the heart
- Prepare the skin and drape the patient in sterile fashion
- Conscious sedation may be required
- Infiltrate local anaesthetic along the drainage track
- The skin incision point lies just below the xiphisternum. Use a scalpel blade to make a small incision to reduce skin friction for the passage of the drainage catheter
- Advance the needle just under the costal margin, advancing behind the sternum, and aiming towards the tip of the left scapula
- Maintain negative pressure on an attached syringe and observe for the aspiration of fluid
- Remove the syringe and advance the guidewire through the needle so that it loops in the cardiac shadow on X-ray screening or is visible in the pericardial space with echo (bubble contrast may help to confirm position)
- Advance a dilator over the wire
- Advance the drainage catheter over the wire and into the pericardial space
- Initially fluid can be aspirated with a syringe—including samples for biochemical, immunological and microbiological analysis. Following this, the drainage bag is connected
- The drain is secured with sutures at the skin entry point and dressed with transparent occlusive dressings

Intra-aortic balloon counterpulsation

►The insertion, setup, and maintenance of an IABP is a specialist skill beyond the scope of this text. This device can however be valuable, sometimes life saving, and those involved in the management of acute conditions should be aware of its potential. The following points may be of value in managing patients under your care, and it may be possible to make some initial preparation to assist a cardiac team en route to your patient.

Practical considerations

- Most patients receive systemic anticoagulation with IV heparin
- IABP therapy is less effective in patients with tachycardia, especially if the rhythm is irregular. These patients may need specialist review with inflation/deflation cycles being triggered by changes in aortic pressure rather than the surface ECG
- In the event of IABP failure (balloon rupture, exhausted helium supply, ECG trigger failure) pumping must be resumed in 20–30 min or the balloon catheter removed. A static IABP is a potential source of clot formation and distal arterial embolization
- Some patients require weaning from IABP support. The usual method is to reduce the balloon inflation frequency to every second, and later to every 3rd cardiac cycle
- Though it is possible to draw arterial blood samples from the pressure monitoring line of an IABP, this should be avoided as the calibre of the line is narrow and prone to blockage if contaminated with blood

Preparation for IABP insertion

- An IABP can be inserted in a general ward area but many centres prefer insertion to take place in a facility with radiographic screening and improved sterility. Ask if you should secure the use of a cardiac catheterization laboratory or other clinical area
- Shave and clean both groins and the anterior aspects of both thighs
- Position extra ECG monitor electrodes for use by the IABP system
- Check and document the peripheral pulses in the lower limbs
- Check clotting status

Box 23.6 lists the indications for IABP insertion and Box 23.7 gives a brief description of how IABPs work.

IABP removal

If the device ceases to function and regular balloon inflation and deflation cycles cannot be restored, the intra-vascular balloon should be removed within 20–30 min, as it creates a significant risk of clot formation in the descending aorta.

► The puncture hole in the artery is large however (at least 7.5 Fr in size; diameter ~2.7 mm) and there is a risk of bleeding, bruising, or other vascular compromise on removal. ***Do not remove an IABP unless you are competent in the manual compression of arteries following the removal of large bore catheters.***

Box 23.6 IABP insertion (see also p.83)

Indications
- Cardiogenic shock
- Severe pulmonary oedema
- Acute LV dysfunction, e.g. MI, with severe cardiac failure
- Acute severe MR with cardiac failure, e.g. post-MI
- VSD with severe cardiac failure, esp. post-MI
- Intractable myocardial ischaemia
- Support during CABG and coronary angioplasty

Contraindications
- Significant AR
- Significant AS
- Hypertrophic obstructive cardiomyopathy with significant gradient
- Thoracic aortic pathology, e.g. dissection, aneurysm, clot
- Significant peripheral vascular disease—relative contraindication

Cautions
- May sometimes worsen renal blood flow
- Peripheral vascular compromise can occur, usually affecting the leg on the side of insertion, though ischaemia of the contralateral limb can also occur. A cold, pale, and painful limb with reduced pulses demands immediate specialist attention.

Box 23.7 How IABPs work
- A long (34 or 40 cm) balloon is placed in the proximal descending aorta, nearly always via an entry site in the proximal femoral artery (as for an angiogram). Rapid expansion of the balloon in diastole displaces blood and promotes flow distally to the mesenteric, renal, and lower limb vessels
- Augmented flow also occurs proximal to the balloon, to the head and neck vessels, and coronary arteries
- Flow in coronary vessels mainly occurs in diastole and use of an IABP is associated with a substantial improvement in coronary perfusion
- Abrupt balloon deflation at the start of systole decreases the afterload resistance to LV contraction, improving performance, and decreasing cardiac work
- The balloon is inflated and deflated with helium via a pressurized line, fed from a reservoir cylinder
- Inflation and deflation cycles are timed from the surface ECG and adjusted so that the balloon inflates immediately after aortic valve closure and deflates at the end of diastole

Procedure

- Stop IV (unfractionated) heparin and aim for ACT < 200, as a guide
- Remove the dressings over the balloon pump insertion site and any further dressings along the line of the balloon shaft down the thigh
- Identify and cut any sutures, placed to secure the device
- Inject 10 Ml of 1% lidocaine into the SC tissues around the puncture site
- Consider pre-medication with an opiate
- Have ready and available 600 mcg of atropine and a unit of IV fluids as vagal reactions with bradycardia and hypotension are common following the removal of large-bore arterial lines
- Switch off balloon inflation
- Prepare a receiver surface for the balloon pump (e.g. incontinence pad) as the IABP is very long and will be covered with blood
- IABP catheters can be inserted directly or via a sheath into the femoral artery. At the time of removal, the used balloon will not however retract through the sheath. If a sheath is present, the IABP catheter should be withdrawn slowly until the balloon reaches the sheath. At this point resistance will be encountered
- Place 2 or 3 fingers of 1 hand over the presumed arterial puncture site (2–5 mm cranial to the skin puncture site)
- The sheath ± balloon catheter are pulled out together as a single unit
- Maintain firm pressure to secure haemostasis over a 10–15-min period, until haemostasis occurs
- Insist on continued flat bed rest for at least 2 hours following sheath removal

Exercise stress testing

The exercise ECG is a widely available, well-established, inexpensive test designed for investigating exercise tolerance and potential IHD (Box 23.9 and 23.10). The predictive value is affected by the pretest probability of IHD based on symptoms and risk factors. Patients with a low pretest probability will have a high rate of false positive tests.

- Overall sensitivity 68% and specificity 77% for the diagnosis of IHD
- Specificity is reduced in females and in patients with diabetes

Performing the exercise test

- Prior examination and ECG are important to assess contraindications and conditions making interpretation unreliable (see Box 23.8)
- Full resuscitation equipment must be available
- Continuous ECG monitoring, BP, and workload are recorded

Box 23.8 Indications, contraindications, and complications for exercise stress testing

Common indications

- Assessment of patients with suspected IHD
- Risk stratification following ACSs
- Prognosis and management in patients with medically treated stable angina, or those with known IHD who develop worsening symptoms
- Other indications include:
  - Preoperative evaluation
  - The assessment and response to treatment of selected patients with arrhythmias

Contraindications

Absolute

- Symptomatic severe AS
- Uncontrolled symptomatic heart failure
- Acute MI—within 2 days
- Unstable angina
- Acute myocarditis or pericarditis
- Acute PE
- Acute aortic dissection

Relative

- Left main coronary stenosis
- Severe hypertension—systolic ^{3} 200 mmHg /or ^{3} 110 mmHg
- Tachyarrhythmias with uncontrolled ventricular rate, e.g. AF
- Mental or physical impairment leading to inability to cooperate
- High degree AV block

Complications

- Although rare, exercise testing can be associated with serious complications
- For every 10,000 tests there are approximately 3.5 MIs, 4.8 serious arrhythmias, and 0.5 deaths

Box 23.9 Interpreting exercise tests

- If a patient completes 12 min of the Bruce protocol without symptoms or ECG changes, it represents a negative test for cardiac ischaemia and puts the patient in a low-risk group for cardiovascular events
- Tests terminated prematurely for any of the reasons highlighted in ➲ Test end-points, p.378 have to be interpreted carefully to manage the patient appropriately
- Be careful about signal-averaged ECGs (often labelled 'linked medians' or have a '*' on them)—these can include artefact and under- or over-report ST segment change. Computer-generated reports often don't recognize these artefacts—always examine the raw data alongside computer-averaged traces

Indicators of a 'positive' test

- Significant anginal symptoms, esp. if accompanied by ECG changes
- Significant planar or downsloping ST segment depression (^{3} 1.5–2 mm in lateral leads at 80 msec beyond 'J' point) (Fig. 23.7)
- ST elevation
- New bundle branch block
- Ventricular tachyarrhythmias
- Exertional hypotension—systolic BP lower than pretest standing BP

► Exercise time is important—a low distance covered indicates poor functional reserve and in itself can be an indicator of poor prognosis, even without other changes (esp. < 3 min. of a Bruce protocol).

Box 23.10 Duke scoring

The Duke University treadmill score is the most popular validated scoring system that risk stratifies patients based on three exercise parameters:

Score = **exercise time** (minutes based on the Bruce protocol)
minus (5 × maximum **ST segment deviation** in mm)
minus (4 × **exercise angina** [0= none, 1= non-limiting, 2= limiting])

Score 5-year survival	Score	5-year survival
Low risk ^{3}+5 97%	≥+5	97%
Moderate -10 to +4 90%	-10 to +4	90%
High risk £-11 65%	≤-11	65%

- The exercise treadmill is the most common modality used, often with the Bruce protocol which has been extensively validated. It involves a series of 3-min stages of increasing incline and speed
- The modified Bruce protocol is often used for risk stratification of patients 5–7 days after an ACS and in those with reduced mobility. It adds 2 low-workload stages at the beginning of the standard Bruce protocol

Test endpoints

Generally there is little clinical reason to continue a Bruce protocol beyond 12 min as any additional information gained is unlikely to be of diagnostic or prognostic significance. There are a number of reasons to terminate an exercise tolerance test:

Patient determined

- Patient wants to stop or is unable to maintain exercise
- Significant chest discomfort
- Marked fatigue or severe dyspnoea
- Other limiting symptoms

Operator determined

- Patient looks unwell
- Exertional hypotension (systolic BP lower than pre-test standing BP)*
- Systolic BP > 250 mmHg or diastolic BP > 120 mmHg

ECG endpoints

- Planar or downsloping ST segment depression (usually ^{3} 1.5 mm)*
- ST elevation*
- New bundle branch block* or AV block
- Ventricular tachyarrhythmias*
- Supraventricular tachyarrhythmias

Protocol-determined endpoints

Achieving ^{3} 85% of the maximal predicted heart rate for age (or 70% if post ACS).

*Also suggests a positive test

Conditions making ECG interpretation unreliable

Not suitable for exercise tolerance testing if ECG changes are important for assessment, but exercise tolerance may be reliably assessed.

- Pre-excitation—WPW syndrome
- Paced ventricular rhythm
- More than 1 mm of ST depression at rest
- Complete LBBB
- RBBB—makes interpreting ECG changes in leads V1–V3 unreliable
- Patients taking digoxin
- ECG criteria for LV hypertrophy
- Electrolyte abnormalities, esp. hypokalaemia

Further management

- Patients with significantly positive tests or high-risk Duke scores will generally be considered for coronary angiography
- The management of patients with intermediate scores or inconclusive tests will be based on the clinical picture. This may involve further non-invasive testing or coronary angiography

Other (imaging) modalities of stress testing

Indications

- Patients unable to perform an exercise test
- Resting ECG abnormalities making interpretation unreliable
- As further assessment of equivocal exercise ECG tests

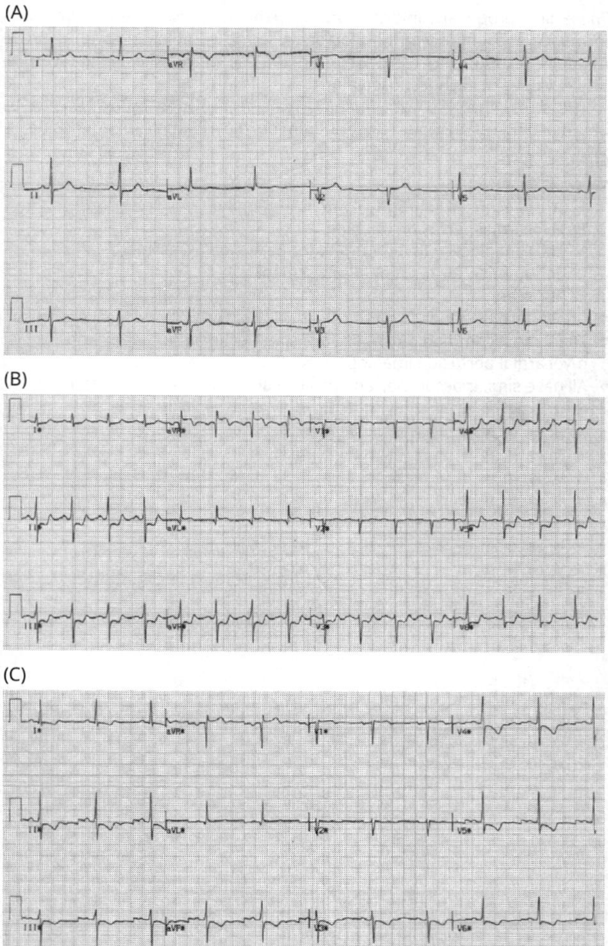

Fig. 23.7 Exercise ECG recordings at rest (A), peak exercise (B), and recovery (C) of a patient presenting with exertional chest pain. Note the significant downsloping ST depression in multiple lead groups during exercise that persists into recovery suggestive of significant coronary disease.

These give prognostic information independent of exercise treadmill performance and underlying risk factors. Used in combination with exercise treadmill testing, they can vastly improve the positive and negative predictive values of each test used alone.

The stress involved with imaging may be provided by exercise or by pharmacological methods (e.g. dobutamine, dipyridamole, or adenosine).

Choice of test

- Available tests:
  - Stress echocardiography—with dobutamine
  - Myocardial perfusion imaging
  - CMR imaging—with adenosine for perfusion assessment, or dobutamine for functional assessment
  - PET scanning
- Choice largely depends on the availability of the test and local expertise
- The 2 most common modalities are stress echocardiography and myocardial perfusion imaging
- All have similar accuracies and positive and negative predictive values

ECG recognition

Physiology of the ECG

Electrical conduction

- Electrical spread is facilitated either by direct cell-to-cell depolarization (e.g. in the atria), or, as in the ventricles, via the specialized conduction system, termed the *His–Purkinje system*
- Cell-to-cell depolarization is relatively slow, producing more slurred, widened patterns of tracing, e.g. P waves, delta waves
- His–Purkinje conduction is rapid, giving rise to the sharp deflections as normally seen in the QRS complex
- In the presence of a bundle branch block (p.387), conduction through the ventricles is initially via the His–Purkinje system, and so begins as a sharp deflection in the QRS complex, followed by cell-to-cell depolarization which leads to QRS prolongation
- In pre-excitation (p.413) the ventricles are starting to depolarize via an anomalous ('accessory') pathway before the His–Purkinje system, thus the complex begins slurred before becoming sharper (depending upon the balance of activation between the accessory pathway and His–Purkinje system)

The origin of the waves of the ECG

- A single cardiac myocyte produces an electrical signal when it 'fires' (depolarizes), followed by another signal when it 'recovers' (repolarizes)
- The P wave represents atrial depolarization. It occurs from cell-to-cell, and thus is relatively slow in onset and duration giving a typical broad 'dome' shape
- The QRS wave is produced from depolarization via the His–Purkinje system. It is normally fast, and the whole of the RV and LV myocardium is depolarized in under 120 msec—hence the normal QRS duration of ≤ 120 ms
- The T wave represents ventricular repolarization ('resetting'). Thus measuring the onset of the QRS until the end of the T wave gives a measure of the time taken for ventricular myocytes to depolarize and repolarize ('fire and reset'). This is termed the QT interval

Interpreting the ECG

The art of ECG recognition

ECG interpretation is a fundamental art of medicine. Basic principles are learnt and applied to each and every ECG encountered. Time and experience makes 'pattern recognition' possible. Combining both pattern recognition and fundamental principals is the cornerstone to the 'art of ECG recognition'. The following points will hopefully aid with the understanding of some aspects that are traditionally not well explained. The ECG recordings included hereafter will have salient features pointed out, and serve as an aid for pattern recognition.

ECG fundamentals

- An electrogram can be recorded from any site upon the body surface; however, convention dictates a 10 different electrode configuration to produce what we know as *the routine 12-lead ECG*
- Other electrode configurations may be of use clinically (RV electrodes, and posterior electrodes)

Assessment of rate

- Check that the ECG is recorded using standard settings (25 mm/s)
- In regular rhythms, dividing 300 by the number of large squares between consecutive QRS complexes will give the rate in bpm (e.g. 3 large squares between complexes = 100 bpm)
- In irregular rhythms, it may be easier to count the number of complexes across the rhythm strip and multiply by 6 (e.g. 12 complexes = 72 bpm)

Determining the rhythm

- Is the rhythm regular?
- Is the QRS complex narrow?
- Is each QRS complex preceded by a p wave, and is each p wave followed by a QRS complex?
- If the answer to each of these questions is yes, then the rhythm is likely to be normal sinus rhythm
- If the ECG rhythm is abnormal, the following are rules of thumb:
  - If the rhythm is irregularly irregular and there are no visible p waves, it is likely to be atrial fibrillation
  - If there are more p waves than QRS complexes, there is likely to be some form of heart block
  - If there is a tachycardia, the width of the QRS complexes is critical to the likely aetiology (narrow complex tachycardia—likely supraventricular; wide complex tachycardia—likely ventricular)

Cardiac axis

Leads and direction of electrical activity

Each ECG lead 'looks at' a mean voltage of the entire electrical activity in the heart from a particular 'point of view' (Fig. 24.1, Table 24.1)

- An electrical wavefront moving towards an electrode appears as a positive deflection above the isoelectric line
- An electrical wavefront moving away from an electrode appears as a negative deflection below the isoelectric line

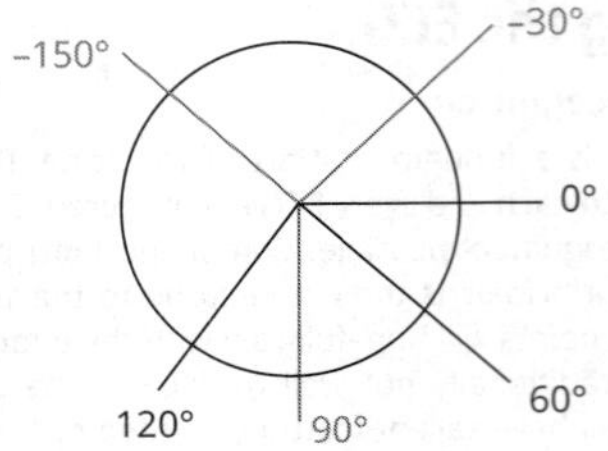

Fig. 24.1 ECG lead vectors.
The augmented leads (aVR, aVL, and aVF) are spaced at 120°. The standard leads (I, II, and III) are spaced at 60°

Table 24.1 Areas related to each ECG lead

ECG lead	Area that lead 'looks at'
Leads I and aVL	Lateral aspect of the whole myocardium
Leads II, III, aVF	The inferior (caudal) aspect of the whole myocardium
Lead aVR	Right lateral heart
V1 and V2	Atria (with the RA moving towards these electrodes and the LA moving away) and the base of the ventricles
V3 and V4	The septum and mid LV
V5 and V6	LV lateral wall and apex

Table 24.2 ECG normal values

	Milliseconds	Small squares*
PR interval	0.12–0.2	3–5
QRS duration	≤ 0.12	Not > 3
Axis	–30° to +90°	
QT interval	0.35–0.43†	9–11
P-wave duration	< 0.11	< 3

*assuming paper speed of 25 mm/sec; †must be corrected for heart rate

- Hence, V1 which 'looks at' the base of the heart towards the RV has predominantly a negative QRS, as the major vector of myocardial depolarization is away from that lead, towards the apex of the LV
- V6, which 'looks at' the LV apex, is correspondingly predominantly a strongly positive complex

Determining the cardiac axis

- The normal cardiac axis is, by convention, between –30° and +90°
- Hence, if the largest QRS deflection is 'positive' in lead I and lead II, the axis is normal (see Fig 24.1 and Table 24.2)

- If lead I is 'positive' and lead II is 'negative', there is left axis deviation
- If lead I is 'negative' and lead II is 'positive', there is right axis deviation
- If both lead I and lead II are 'negative', the most likely causes are, depending on the clinical scenario, a technical error in ECG acquisition (limb lead transposition) or ventricular tachycardia
- Much has been made of the ECG axis, although in reality there are only a few important patterns to recognize:
  - RBBB and left or right axis deviation in bifascicular block
  - Left anterior hemiblock
  - 'Upward' or 'northward' axis (e.g. in fascicular VT, see Fig. 24.36)
  - Right axis deviation in RV strain/overload, e.g. chest disease, including acute PE

ECG changes with myocardial injury

- A myocyte damaged by any cause cannot regulate normal ionic transport. The earliest process to be affected is repolarization and thus the earliest changes seen on the ECG are usually in the ST segment of the ECG—i.e. the period at the very end of depolarization to repolarization
- An injured myocyte produces an action potential which has a 'lower' (i.e. *more negative*) baseline. Taken as a group of cells, this gives the appearance of ST segment *elevation* when viewed from an electrode position directly adjacent to the damaged area
- In cardiac ischaemia, the endomyocardium becomes ischaemic first, as it is relatively less well perfused. The ST elevation is directed in an inward vector manifesting as ST segment depression when observed on surface electrodes
- In acute MI the full thickness of myocardium is in jeopardy and so ST elevation is seen in those leads which 'look at' the affected territory (Table 24.1) (ECG: pp.392–395)
- In temporary (and permanent) pacing, endomyocardial electrode contact is confirmed by a local signal of ST elevation obtained from the pacing-electrode tip. Conversely ST depression suggests penetration of the electrode through the ventricular wall into the pericardium

Box 24.1 'High take-off'

- This is a term which refers to fixed physiological ST elevation
- It is more often seen in the anterior leads (V1, V2, V3) where the ST segment often lies 1 mm or so above the isoelectric line
- It is less commonly seen in inferior leads and occasionally it is affected by posture, e.g. moving from lying to standing
- In either case, clinical assessment is critical before making any conclusions about coronary ischaemia or MI
- In the presence of LBBB, V1 and V2 almost always show some degree of ST elevation
- In RBBB, V1 and V2 again often show ST elevation—but be aware that you are not missing Brugada syndrome (p.351, ECG p.419)

Some patterns of ST segment abnormalities

See Figs 24.2–24.4.

True posterior myocardial infarction

- Differentiating between true posterior MI and ischaemic ST depression may be difficult
- The key is to look at the 'shape' of the ST elevation from a posterior point of view using either true posterior leads or holding the ECG up to the light and looking at V1–V3 reversed (i.e. from behind, upside down)
- Fig. 24.6 shows (A) V1–V3 in standard fashion, with (B) the leads reversed, such that V3 is uppermost
- The pattern in reversed V1 (lowermost complex, B) looks like typical ST elevation

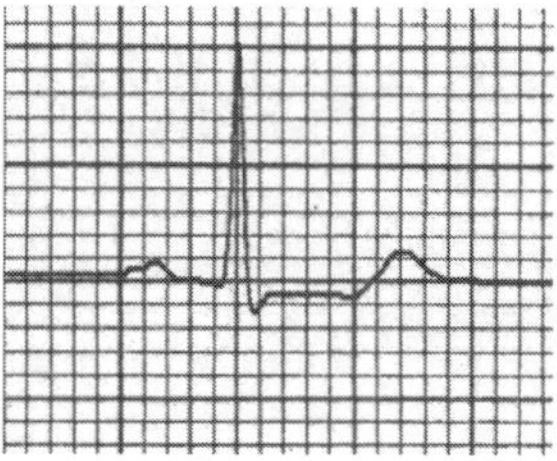

Fig. 24.2 Typical, planar ST depression.

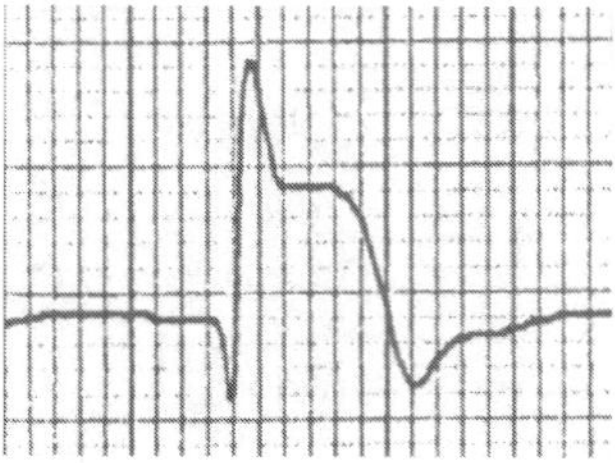

Fig. 24.3 ST elevation due to MI.

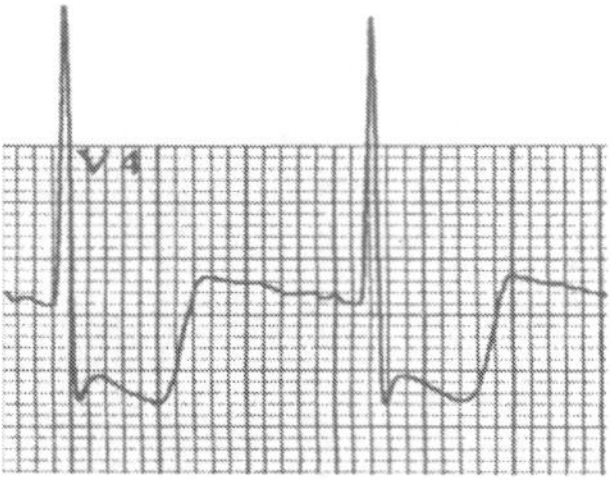

Fig. 24.4 ST depression. This exaggerated response is often found in LV hypertrophy and ischaemia—particularly during exercise tests. 'Strain' pattern can sometimes be this severe, especially in severe AS and HCM.

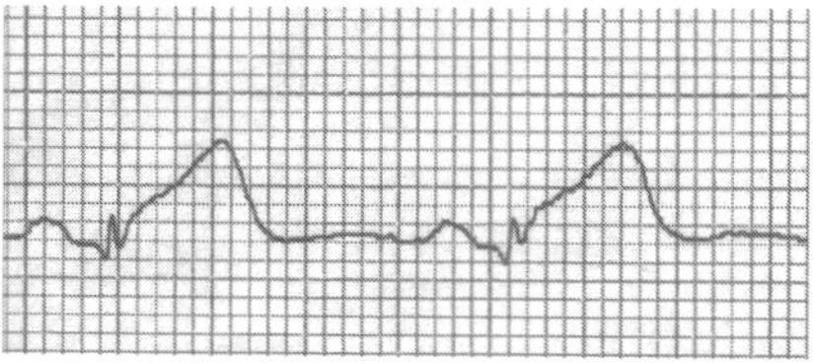

Fig. 24.5 'Hyper-acute' ST changes. Often this is the first sign of ST shift in acute MI. It may also be seen in hyperadrenergic states, including subarachnoid haemorrhage and post-arrest (especially after adrenaline has been given) where it does not necessarily represent infarction.

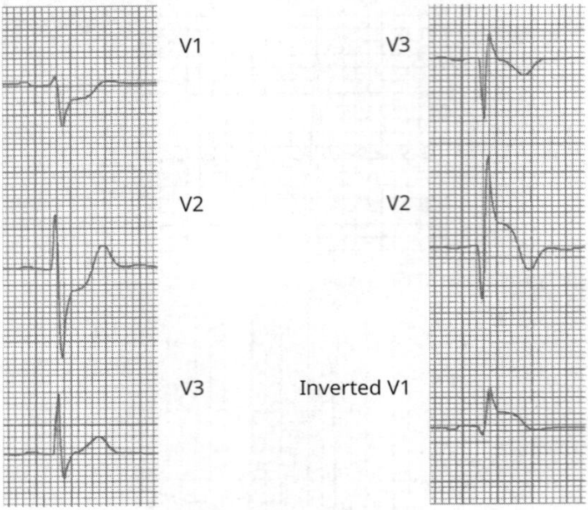

Fig. 24.6 ECG of posterior myocardial infarction.

Helpful tips

Left ventricular hypertrophy

This is difficult to diagnose on the ECG as most criteria are only up to 50% sensitive, making them clinically unhelpful. QRS size may also be influenced by body size and shape, as well as lead positioning.

- Quick measurements consistent with LV hypertrophy are:
  1. (S in V1 or V2) + (R in V5 or V6) > 35 mm (over age 35)
  2. R in AVL > 12 mm
- LV hypertrophy with strain pattern is the presence of:
  - LV hypertrophy with T-wave inversion, *and*
  - ST depression (usually in V5–V6, I, and aVL)
- The ST depression in LVH is thought to represent chronic ischaemia within the endomyocardium. Myocytes produce a current of injury which is interpreted by the external leads as ST depression

Dominant R wave in V1

A useful tip for ECG interpretation is that a dominant R wave in lead V1 is usually associated with one of the following:

- RBBB
- Left-sided accessory pathway
- Posterior MI
- RV hypertrophy
- Dextrocardia
- Infancy

Localization of accessory pathways

The acute management of patients with pre-excitation does not require accurate localization of the pathway. Localization is important to guide the electrophysiology approach to ablation, however. There are some simple rules of thumb:

- Dominant R wave in V1 suggests left-sided accessory pathways— i.e. looks more like RBBB because left heart is being stimulated prematurely via the accessory pathway
- LBBB-like pattern suggests right-sided accessory pathway
- The negative delta wave 'points' to the accessory pathway's position e.g. left free wall accessory pathways usually have negative delta wave in aVL, posteroseptal pathways (actually, inferiorly situated in true anatomy) have negative delta waves in II, III, and aVF
- As septal pathways move from posteroseptal, to mid-septal and anteroseptal, the delta wave tends to become more positive in the inferior leads in sequence—i.e. II, then aVF, and then III

Thus, in basic terms, localization may be simplified as follows:

- Dominant R wave in V1?
  - Yes—left sided
  - No—right sided
- Negative delta wave in inferior leads?
  - Yes—posteroseptal likely
  - No—free-wall likely

Electrolytes and the ECG

- As a rule of thumb hyPO PrOlongs the QT interval
- With hypokalaemia, the T wave flattens, the ST segments depress, and U waves can develop (Fig. 24.7):

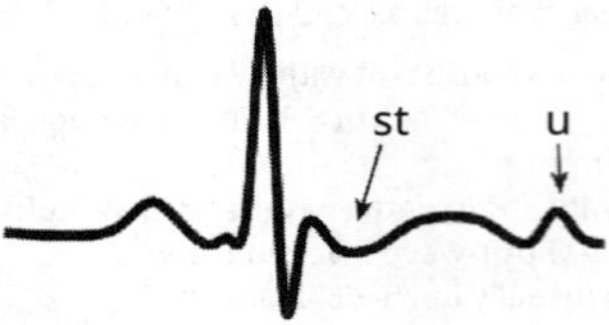

Fig. 24.7 Hypokalaemia.

- HYPERkalaemia is an important and classic ECG which typically shows a broad QRS, flattened P waves with high peaked T waves (Fig. 24.8):

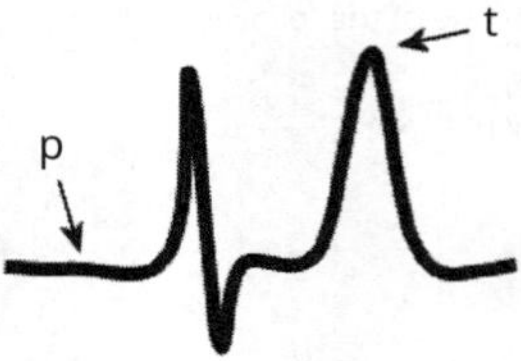

Fig. 24.8 Hyperkalaemia.

- As the potassium concentration increases the ECG may simply show a sine wave appearance—this is a medical emergency

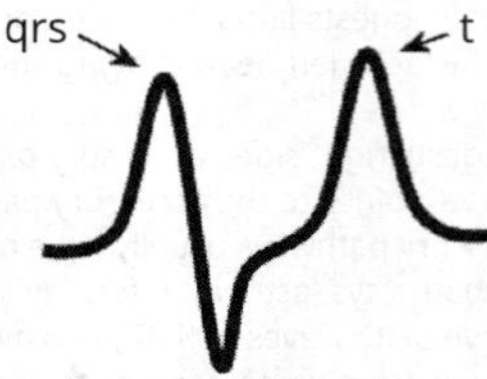

Fig. 24.9 Severe hyperkalaemia with QRS prolongation and 'sine wave'.

- ECG changes of hypomagnesaemia resemble that of hypokalaemia
- ECG changes of hypermagnesaemia resemble that of hyperkalaemia
- Hypercalcaemia *shortens* the QT interval; hypocalcaemia *prolongs* it

Further reading

El Hamriti M. *et al.* EASY-WPW: a novel ECG-algorithm for easy and reliable localization of manifest accessory pathways in children and adults. *EP Europace* 2023; 25(2): 600–09.

Bundle branch block

The bundle of His exits the AV node within the interventricular septum and bifurcates into the left and right bundle branches. The left bundle subdivides further into the left posterior and anterior fascicles. The bundles can develop conduction block from a variety of sources, both transient and permanent. Characteristic changes may then be observed on the ECG.

Left bundle branch block

(Also see ECG, p.400.)

- Activation proceeds through the bundle of His and into the right bundle as normal, activating the RV early. This is rapid, and hence there is a sharp deflection initially
- Septal and left ventricular activation is delayed, hence the QRS configuration similar to normal activation but 'wider'
- As septal depolarization is reversed (now occurring from right-to-left) there is an initial Q wave in V1 and an R-S-R' pattern in V6—i.e. V1 is W shaped and V6 is M shaped
- In true LBBB there can be no initial Q wave in 'left-looking' leads, V5, V6, and I, no matter how small the deflection

Clinical significance of LBBB

- Almost always associated with organic heart disease, e.g. ischaemia, cardiomyopathy, conduction tissue disease, hypertensive heart disease, infiltration
- ST elevation is very difficult to interpret and thus cannot be relied upon to diagnose acute MI
- New-onset LBBB with ischaemic sounding chest pain is supportive of acute MI and thus is considered an indication for primary PCI activation

Right bundle branch block

(Also see ECG, p.401.)

- RV activation occurs via the left bundle branch and thus is delayed
- The interventricular septum is depolarized in the normal fashion (left-to-right)
- Because the RV is activated just after the LV it typically produces an R-S-R' pattern in V1 (M shape)
- In V6 it may produce a deep S wave, giving a modified W type pattern, although often this is not apparent. The changes in V1 are much more constant

Clinical significance of RBBB

- May be normal, especially in the young and the fit
- May be a sign of right heart strain, e.g. acute PE, RV overload due to shunts
- Often seen in ASDs, with right axis deviation in atrial septal type ('secundum') defects and left/upright axis in AV canal defects ('primum')

'William and Marrow'

- William and Marrow are often used aide memoirs to recognize and differentiate LBBB and RBBB

- The first letter of each word refers to the appearance of the QRS complex in V1 and the last letter in V6
- The double letters in the middle give the type of BBB. In practice, 'WiLLiaM' for LBBB tends to work quite well as a rule of thumb, but as mentioned earlier, 'MaRRoW' tends to fall down because V6 often does not look like an M shape (see Figs 24.10 and 24.11)

Alternating LBBB/RBBB

- A sign of advanced conduction tissue disease, and high risk of complete heart block
- Permanent pacemaker implantation should be considered

Bifascicular and 'trifascicular' block

- Conduction delay, usually due to widespread fibrotic disease, is present within the AV node, His bundle, and bundle branches
- Left anterior hemiblock usually results in left axis deviation
- Left posterior hemiblock usually results in right axis deviation
- 'Trifascicular' block is a misnomer, as it really represents conduction delay. Logically, if all 3 fascicles were actually blocked there would be complete heart block
- Bifascicular block is most commonly seen with RBBB and left anterior hemiblock. Hence there is RBBB and left axis deviation
- In trifascicular block, the classic ECG shows 1° heart block, RBBB and left axis deviation (p.402)
- In an asymptomatic patient with trifascicular block, permanent pacing is not indicated. In the presence of unexplained syncope however, a bradycardic cause is likely and permanent pacemaker implantation should be considered

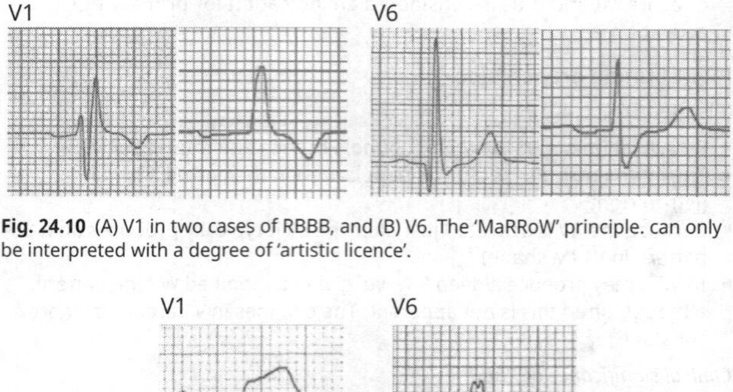

Fig. 24.10 (A) V1 in two cases of RBBB, and (B) V6. The 'MaRRoW' principle. can only be interpreted with a degree of 'artistic licence'.

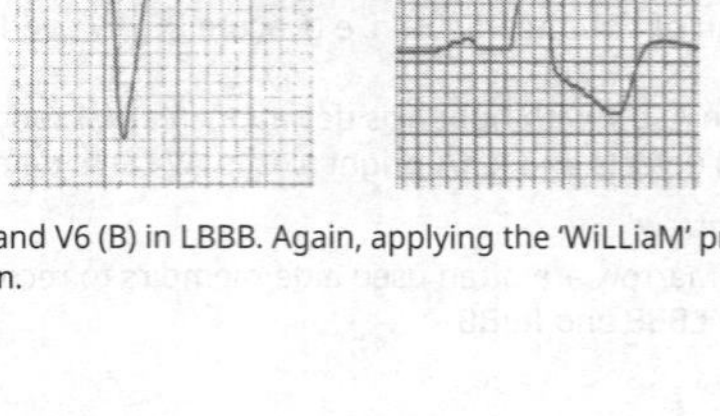

Fig. 24.11 V1 (A) and V6 (B) in LBBB. Again, applying the 'WiLLiaM' principle requires a little imagination.

- Risk of complete heart block (may be transient) is 2–6% per annum, with asymptomatic patients forming the lower percentage, and those with unexplained syncope the higher

Bundle branch block and cardiac catheterization

- Direct trauma to a bundle may produce BBB (so-called mechanical bundle block); this may last for several hours or even days
- In pre-existing BBB, catheter-based procedures on the contralateral side may produce complete heart block, with acute compromise. This occurs most typically during right heart procedures with pre-existing LBBB (e.g. Swan–Ganz lines, pacing, etc.)

Paced complexes and VT morphology

- Pacing from the RV apex causes the septum and LV to be activated right-to-left, rather like LBBB. Thus paced complexes have the LBBB 'WiLLiaM' type morphology. In LV pacing (as part of cardiac resynchronization therapy) the pure LV paced complex has RBBB morphology (fig. 24.12)
- For similar reasons, VT with LBBB type morphology may be exiting within the right heart, and RBBB morphologies may be exiting within the left heart
- Conduction system pacing (left bundle area pacing or His bundle pacing) aims to activate the conduction system below any area of block and should result in a narrow paced QRS complex

Box 24.2 Bundle branch block and SVT rate

When a BBB develops during SVT it is often labelled a 'rate-related' BBB. However, careful attention should be paid to the tachycardia rate. If the rate or cycle-length actually slows, then an accessory pathway ipsilateral to the block is implicated—i.e. LBBB with slowing implicates a left free-wall accessory pathway, and RBBB suggests a right-sided accessory pathway. The mechanism is due to the extra time the head of the re-entrant wave takes to cross the septum after it leaves the AV node and spreads through the His–Purkinje system.

Example: *In AVRT with a left-sided free-wall accessory pathway, the circuit travels down the AV node, through both LV and RV, before climbing the accessory pathway back into the LA, and so on. If LBBB develops, the wavefront must travel down the right bundle, across the septum, and into the LV using cell-to-cell spread. This adds about 40–60 msec to its journey and results in an increase in tachycardia cycle length by the same amount.*

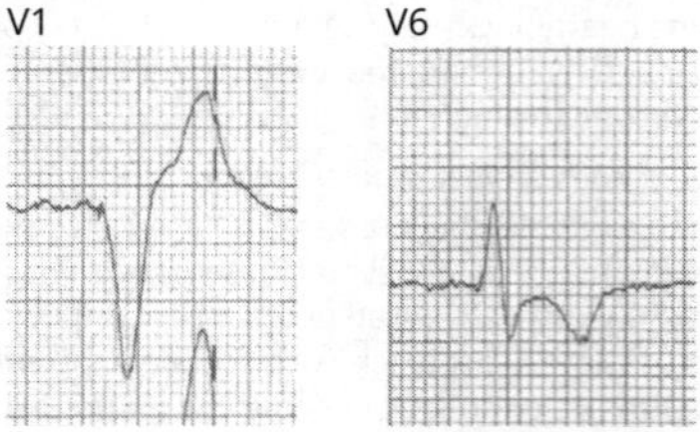

Fig. 24.12 Paced rhythm from RV apex, with V1 (A) and V6 (B) shown. Depolarization initiating from the RV apex 'mimics' to a certain degree, LBBB, as reflected in the tracings. RBBB-paced patterns are due to inadvertent LV capture via an ASD/PFO, VSD, or coronary sinus branch. With a biventricular pacemaker it may represent a LV lead or programming problems.

ECG library

The following collection of ECGs is presented to act as a reminder of the 12-lead ECG patterns of common (and a few uncommon) cardiac conditions.

Anterior myocardial infarction

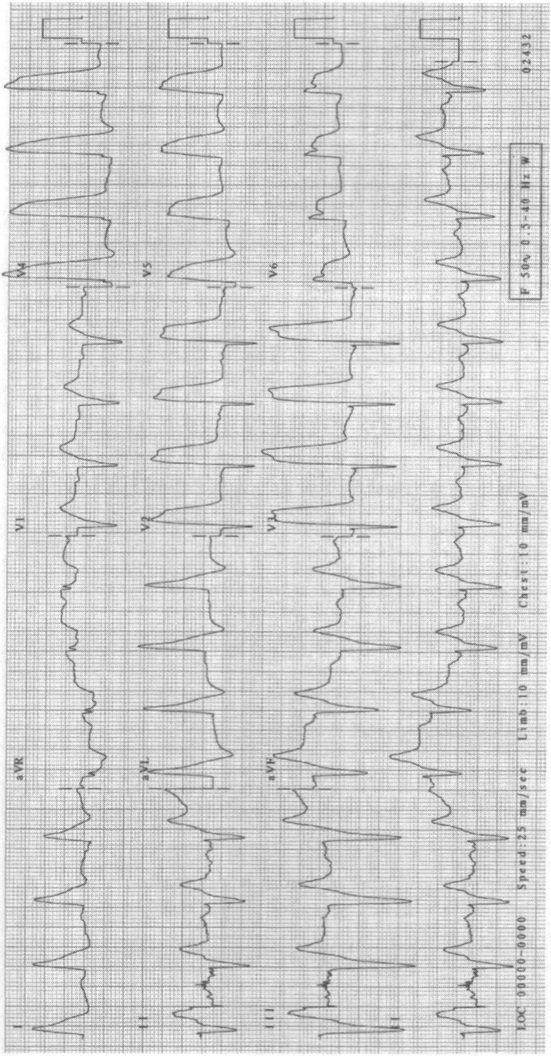

Fig. 24.13 There is ST elevation of > 30 mm in anterior leads (V2–V4). For management see p.53.

Anterolateral myocardial infarction

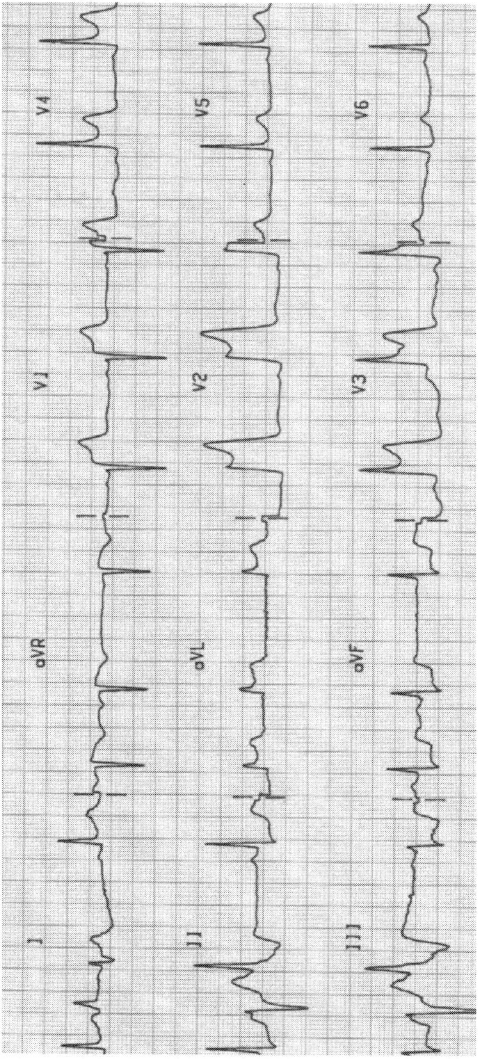

Fig. 24.14 There is marked ST segment elevation in leads V1–V4 and aVL. Reciprocal ST segment depression is present in leads II, III, and aVF. For management see p.53.

Inferior myocardial infarction

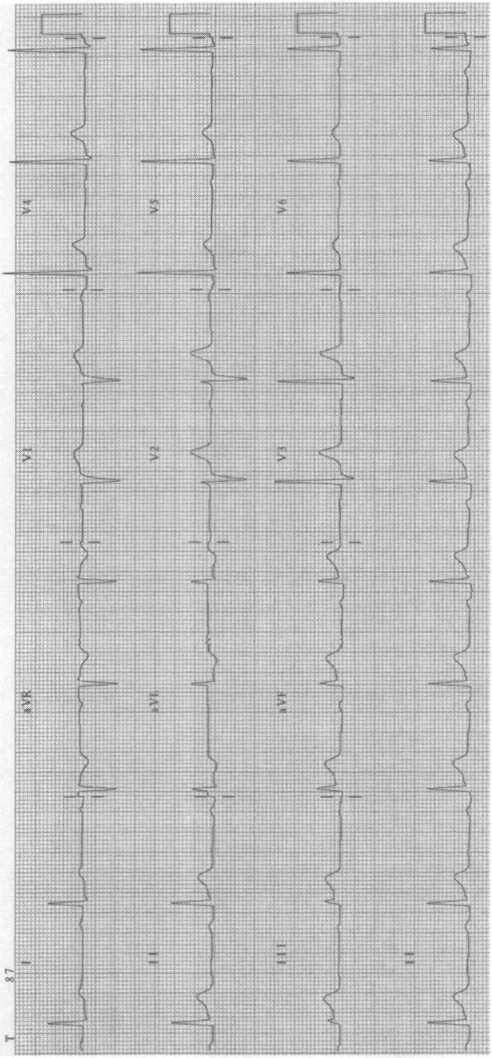

Fig. 24.15 There is ST elevation of > 1 mm in the inferior leads (II, III, and aVF). There is also 1° AV block (PR interval >200 msec). For management see p.53.

Anterolateral myocardial infarction

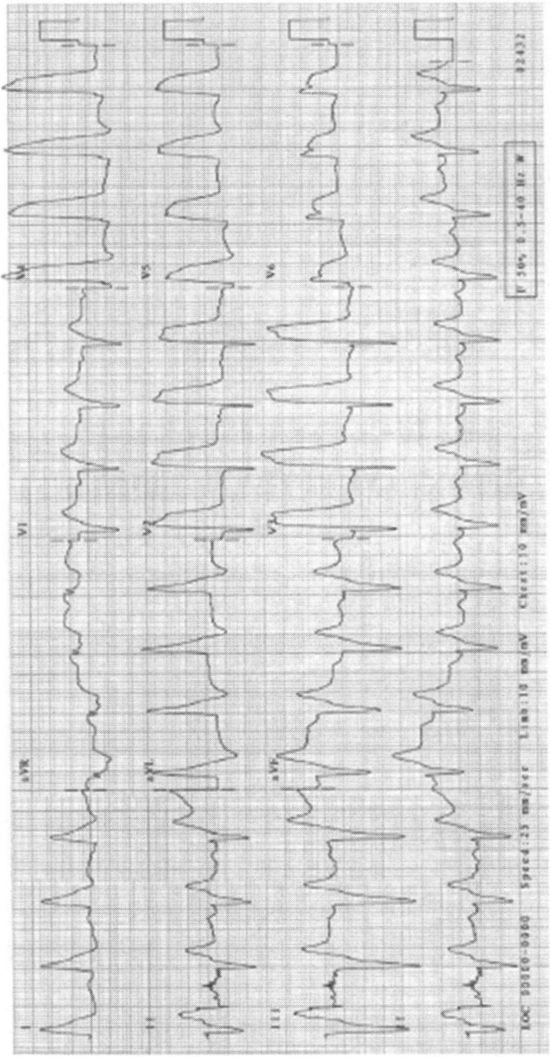

Fig. 24.16 There is ST elevation of >1mm in the anterior leads (V2-V4) and lateral leads (I, aVL, V5-6). For management see p.53.

Myocardial ischaemia

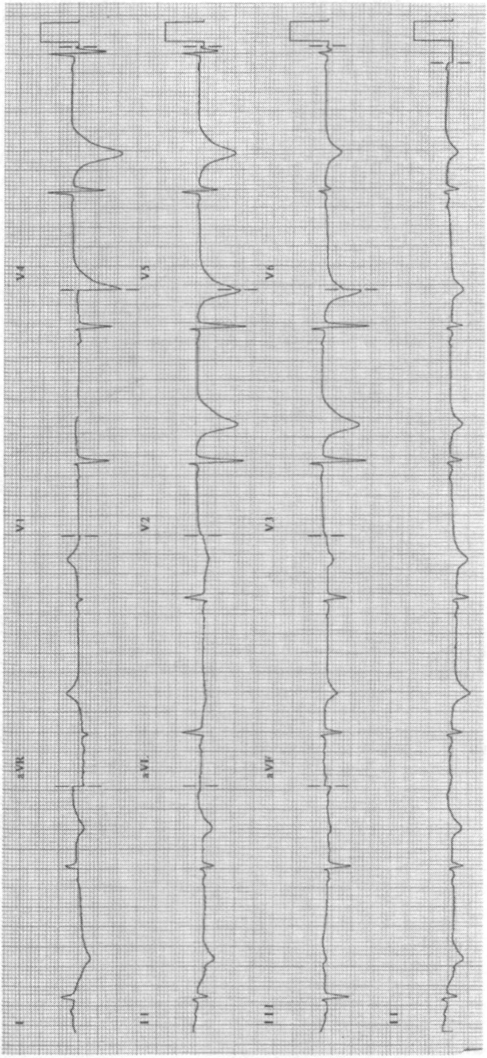

Fig. 24.17 Deep T-wave inversion across the anterior leads. A stenosis of the proximal left anterior descending coronary artery lesion is commonly the culprit. For management see p.68.

Pericarditis

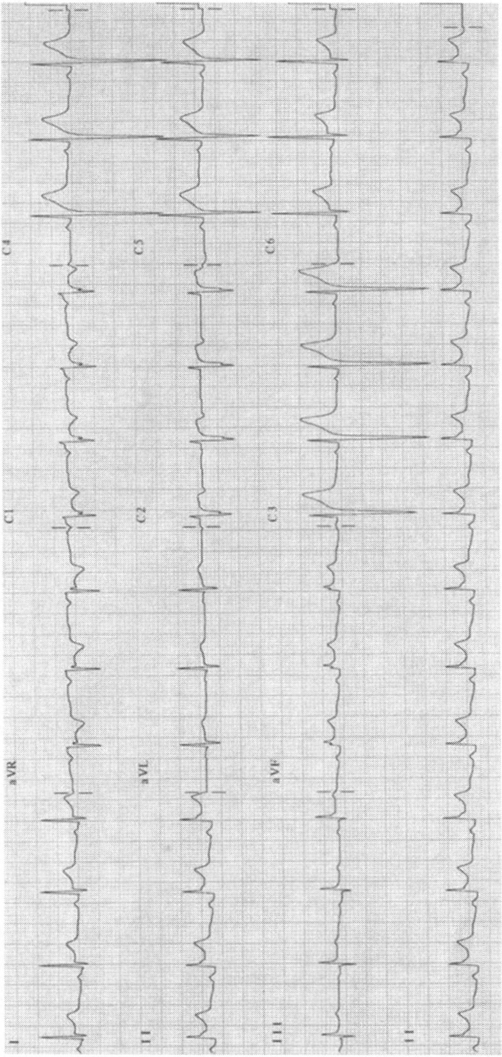

Fig. 24.18 Saddle-shaped ST elevation across several, non-contiguous leads. There is PR segment depression (particularly in leads II and aVF). For management see p.198.

Pulmonary embolism

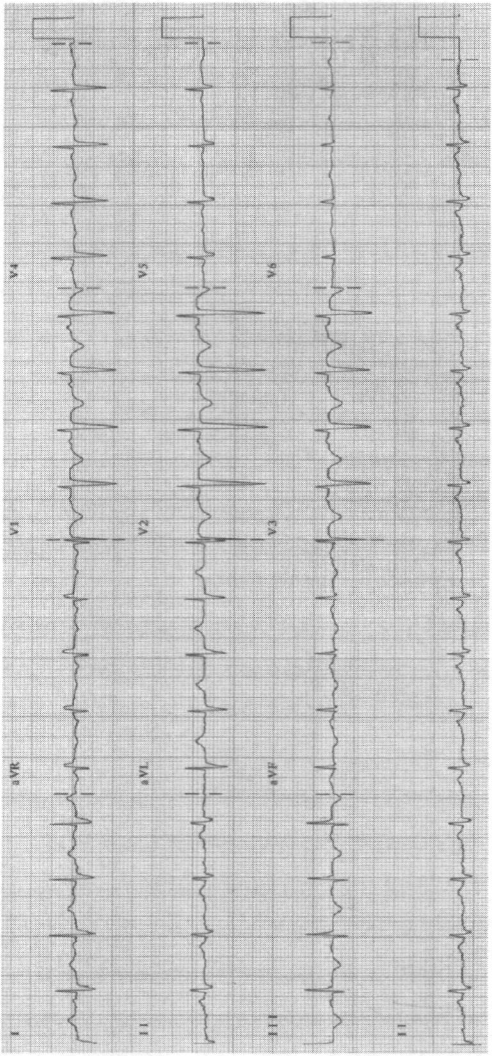

Fig. 24.19 Sinus tachycardia with widespread T-wave inversion. There is a large S wave in I with a Q wave and T inversion in lead III. NB this is rare—the most common ECG finding in PE is sinus tachycardia.

Pulmonary hypertension

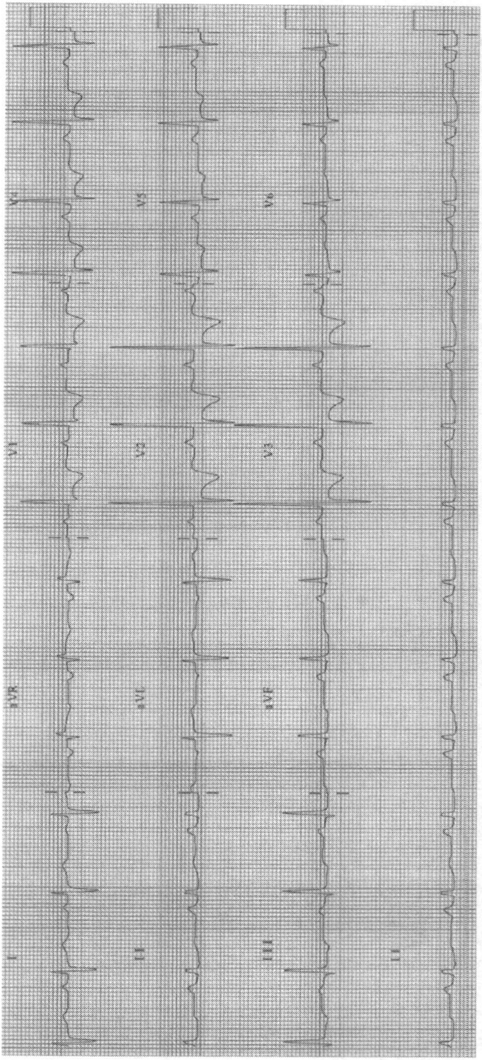

Fig. 24.20 RV hypertrophy is demonstrated by right axis deviation, large R waves with T-wave inversion in leads V1–V3 and a prominent p wave (p pulmonale).

Left bundle branch block

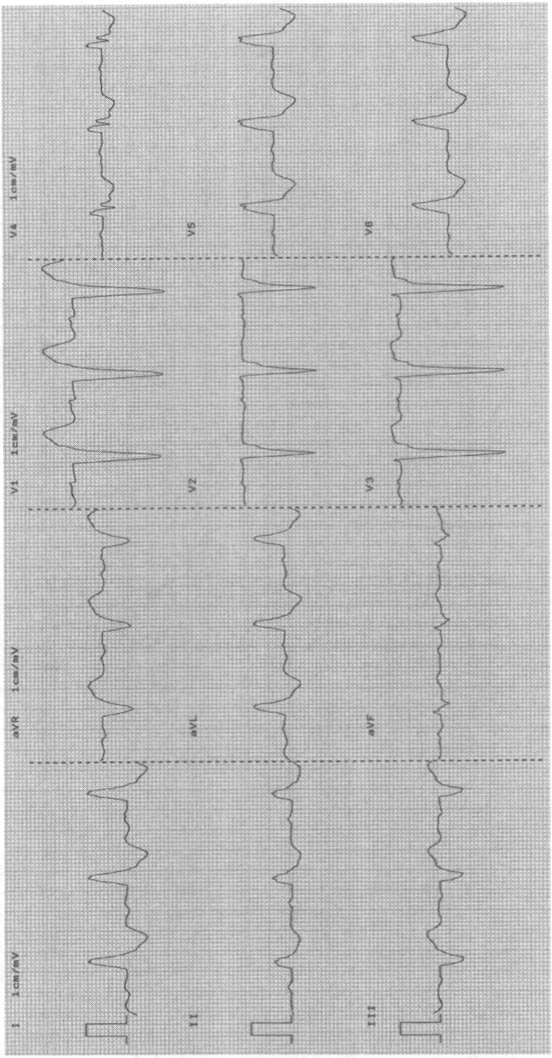

Fig. 24.21 LBBB. Broad QRS complex with a Q wave in V1 ('W') and RSR pattern in V6 ('M'). See p.387.

Right bundle branch block

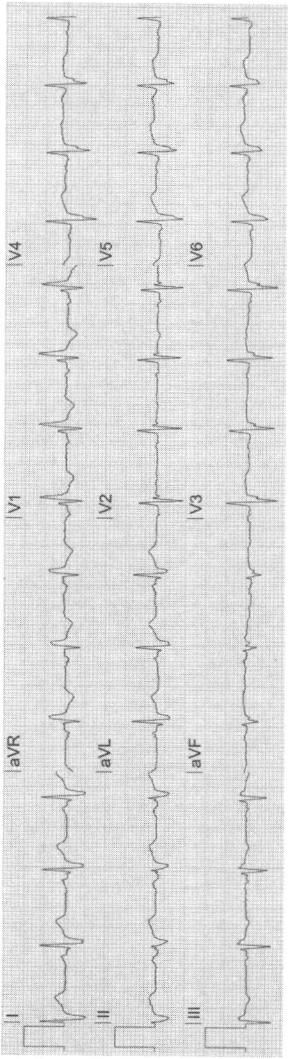

Fig. 24.22 RBBB. Broad QRS complex with an RSR pattern in V1 (M shape) and an S wave in V6 (W shape). There is also 1° AV block. See p.387.

Trifascicular block

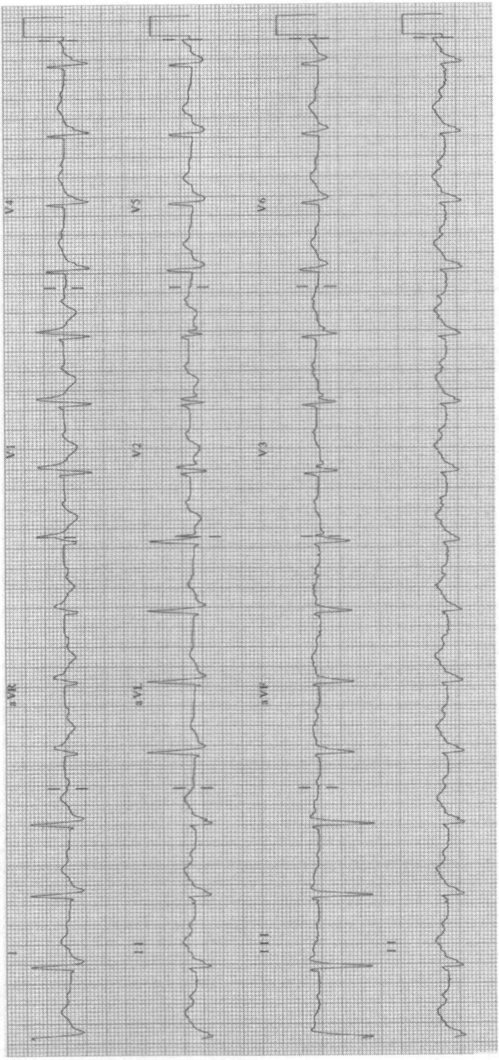

Fig. 24.23 There is RBBB, 1° degree AV block, and left anterior hemiblock (left axis deviation). See p.387.

Junctional rhythm

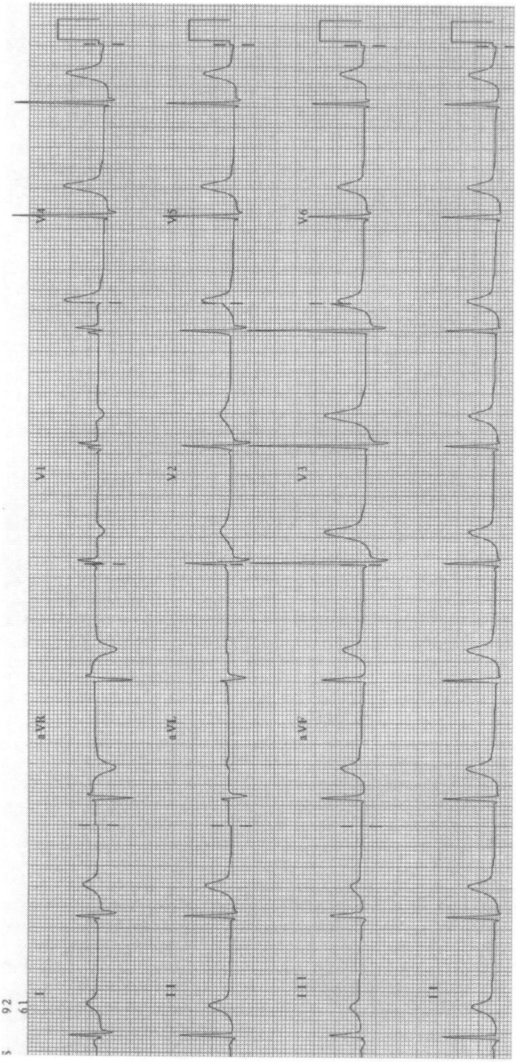

Fig. 24.24 P waves are seen before the first complex but then are buried within the QRS complex. See p.137.

First degree heart block

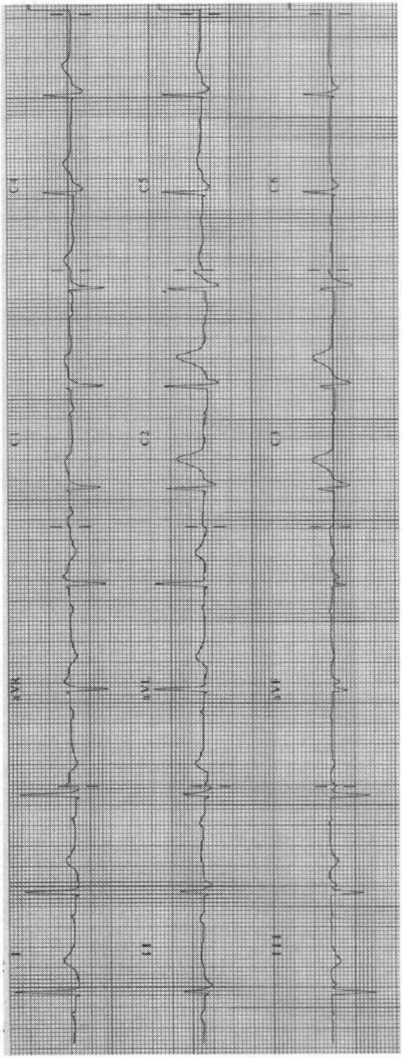

Fig. 24.25 P waves are seen before each QRS complex. The PR interval is prolonged (289 ms). See p.139.

Second degree heart block (Mobitz I)

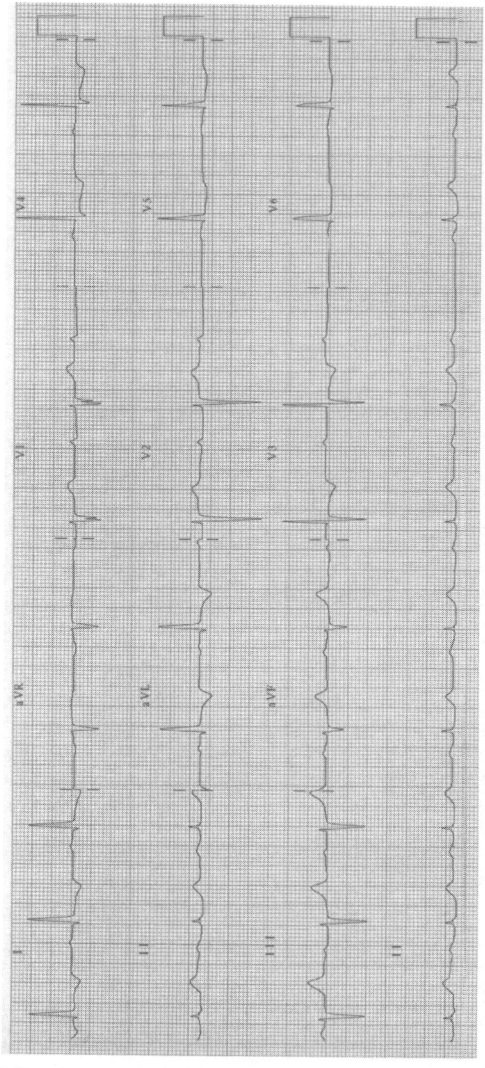

Fig. 24.26 There is progressive lengthening of the PR interval until a P wave is nonconducted and a QRS is dropped (Wenckebach). The PR interval after the dropped beat is the shortest. See p.139.

Complete heart block

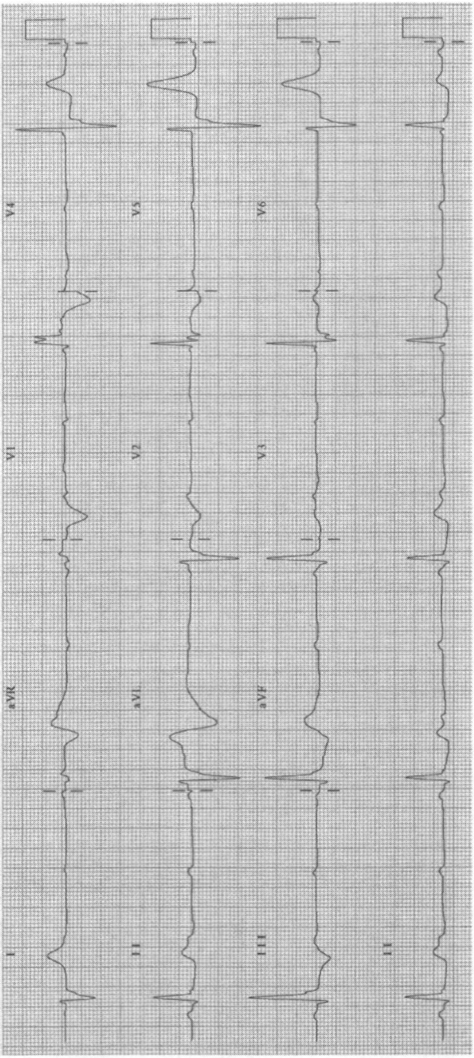

Fig. 24.27 There are regular non-conducted P waves with a broad complex QRS escape rhythm. There is no association between the atrial and the ventricular rates. For management see p.139.

Atrial fibrillation

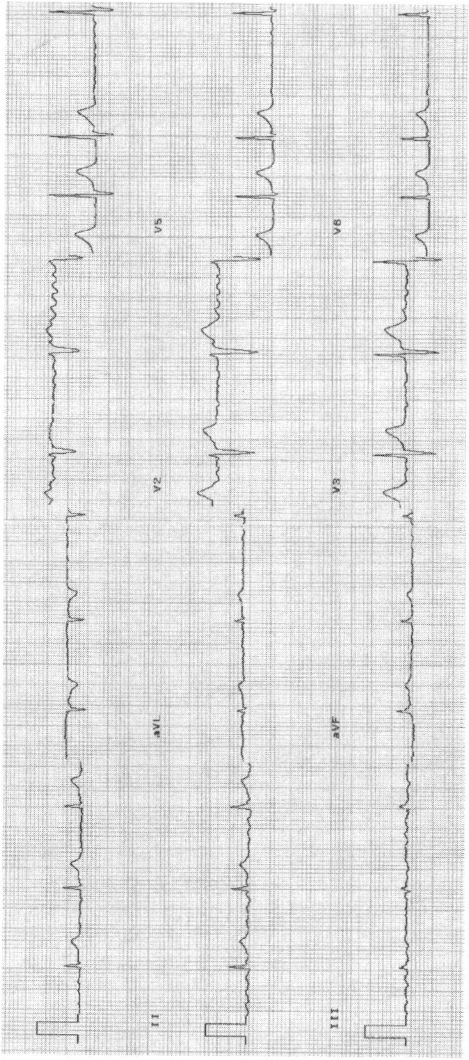

Fig. 24.28 Irregularly irregular ventricular rhythm with no discernible P waves. For management see p.151.

Pre-excited atrial fibrillation

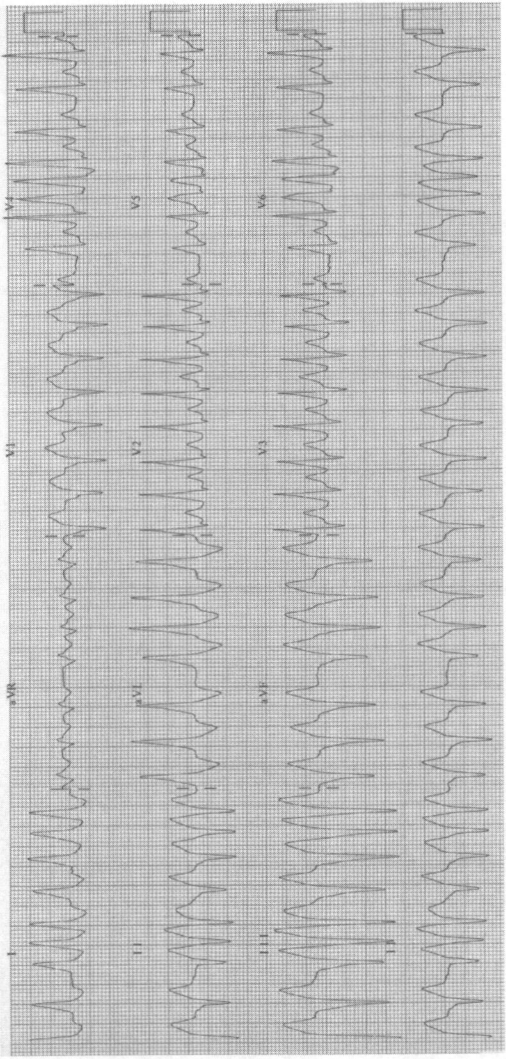

Fig. 24.29 An irregular broad complex tachycardia with very rapid ventricular activation and conduction. For management see p.165.

Atrial Flutter

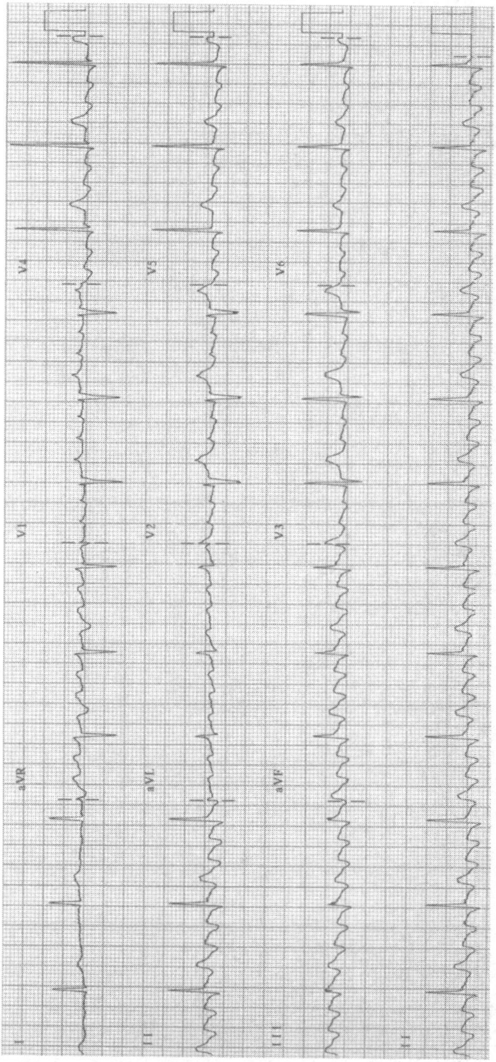

Fig. 24.30 The baseline is irregular with a 'saw-tooth' pattern. The flutter waves are conducted with a 4:1 pattern to the ventricle. For management see p.157.

Atrial Tachycardia

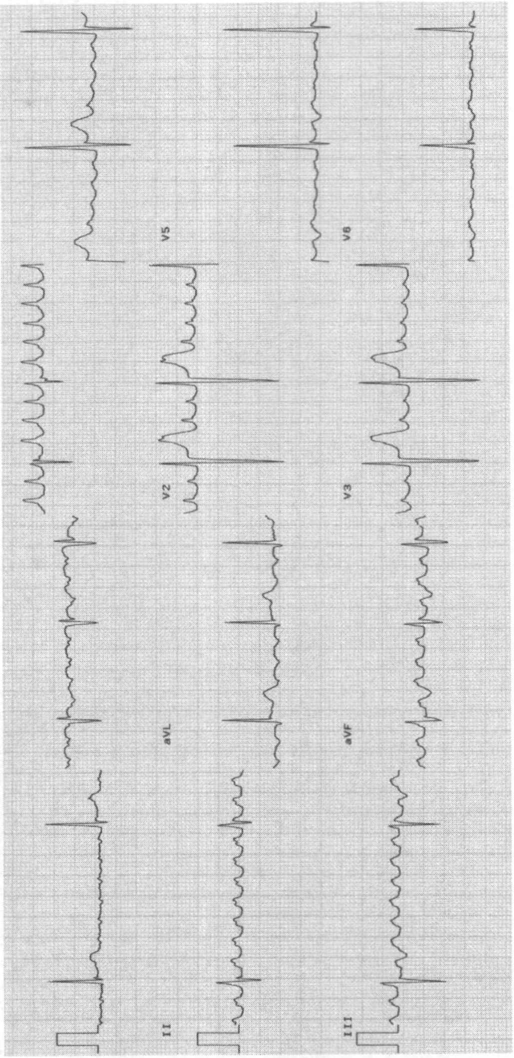

Fig. 24.31 The baseline is irregular with very rapid atrial activation (300 bpm) and a positive P wave in V1 suggesting a focal atrial tachycardia. The baseline returns to normal between each atrial beat.

Supraventricular tachycardia (AVNRT)

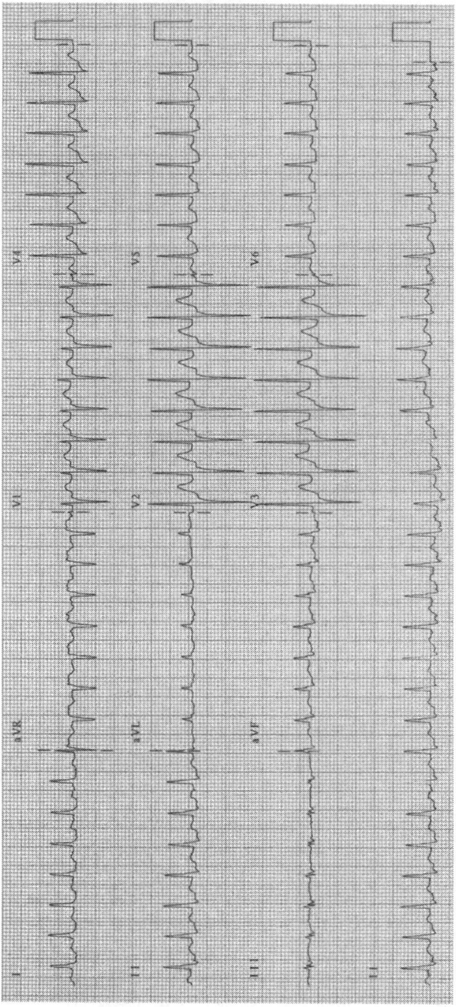

Fig. 24.32 A narrow complex tachycardia (SVT). Differentiation from AVRT on the ECG is difficult but can be suggested: the terminal deflection on the R wave in V1 is likely to represent the R-prime (R') sign which suggests a terminal portion of P wave is visible there (the rest is hidden 'behind' the QRS). With a ventricular-to-atrial conduction time so short, AVNRT is the most likely diagnosis. For management see p.163.

Supraventricular tachycardia (AVRT)

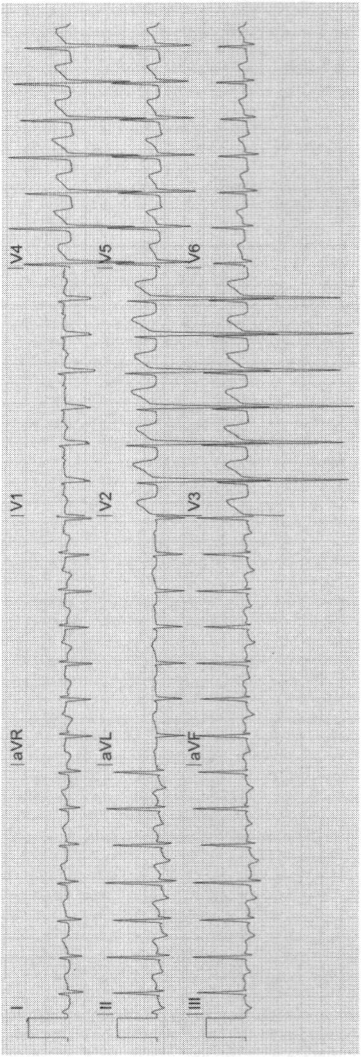

Fig. 24.33 A narrow complex tachycardia. There is retrograde P wave activation (clearly seen in V1 before the QRS complex).

Pre-excitation

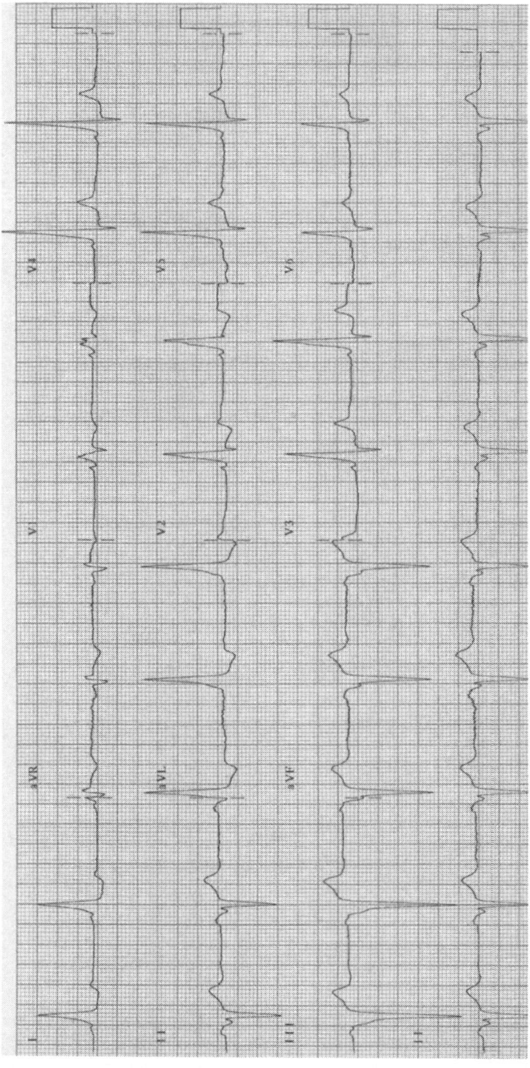

Fig. 24.34 Short PR interval due to the presence of a delta wave. There is a RBBB-type pattern present, suggesting the accessory pathway is left sided. The negative delta waves inferiorly suggest that the accessory pathway is posteroseptal. For management see p.385.

Ventricular tachycardia

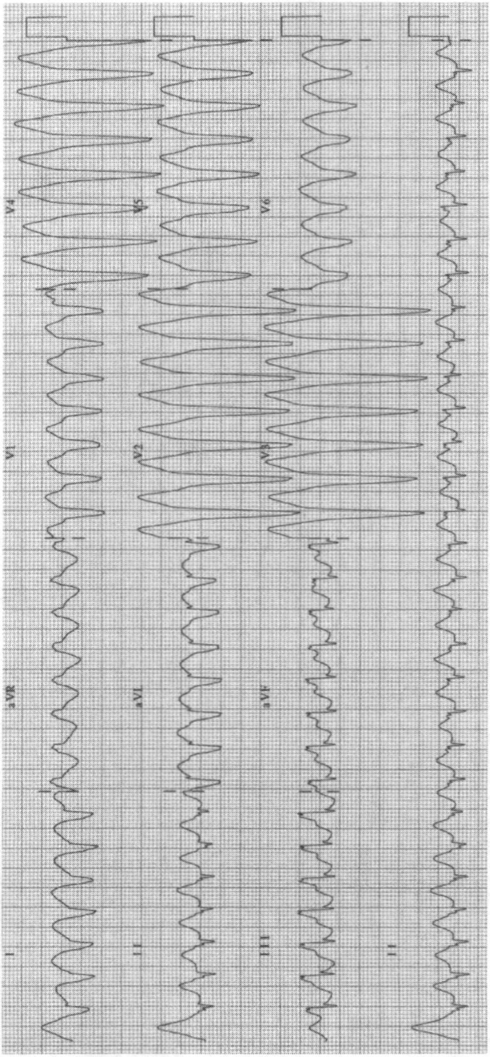

Fig. 24.35 A broad complex tachycardia with a ventricular rate of 180 bpm. AV dissociation is seen with buried P waves in V6. There is concordance across the chest leads. For management see p.169.

Fascicular ventricular tachycardia

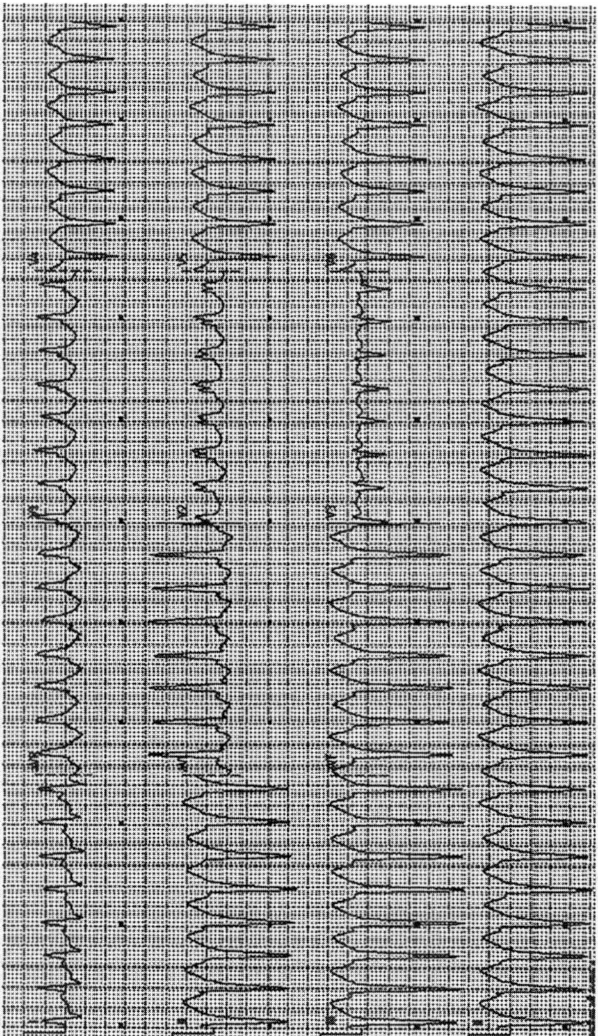

Fig. 24.36 A broad complex tachycardia with a ventricular rate of 182 bpm. Note the vertical 'straight up' axis (strongly negative in II/III/AVF) and relatively narrow QRS duration, suggesting fascicular VT.

Ventricular fibrillation

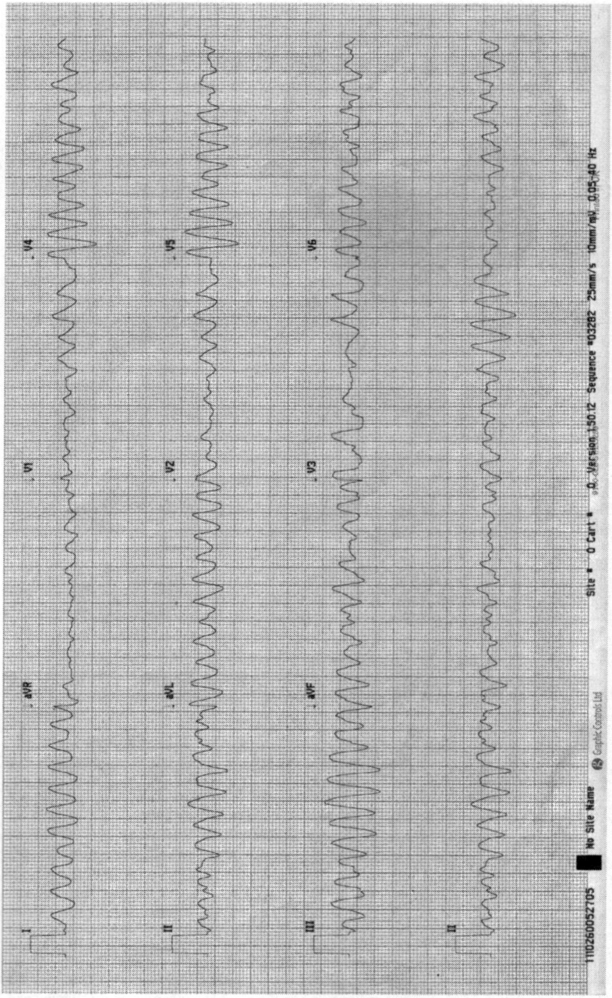

Fig. 24.37 Broad complex ventricular rhythm without cardiac output consistent with fine polymorphic VT/VF. Immediate DCCV is required.

Accelerated idioventricular rhythm

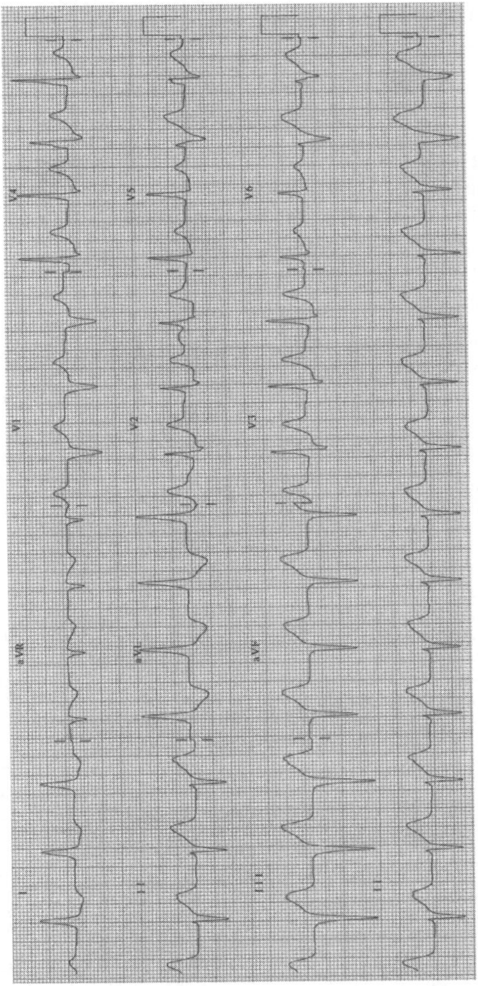

Fig. 24.38 An automatic ventricular rhythm with a rate < 100 bpm. Usually seen in the context of myocardial ischaemia or MI.

Long QT

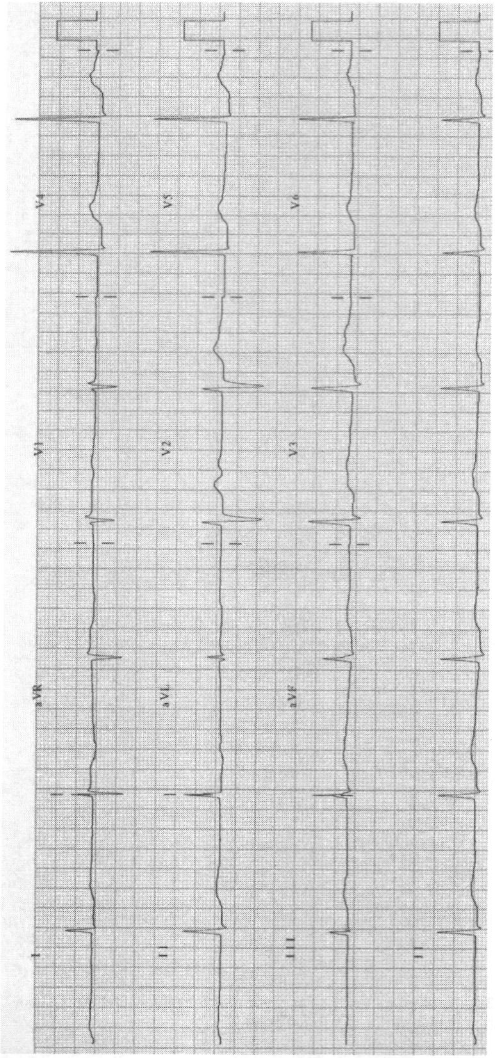

Fig. 24.39 The QT interval (start of the Q wave to the end of the T wave) is prolonged (> 600 ms). See Inherited long QT syndrome p.349; Drug-induced long QT p.313.

Brugada syndrome

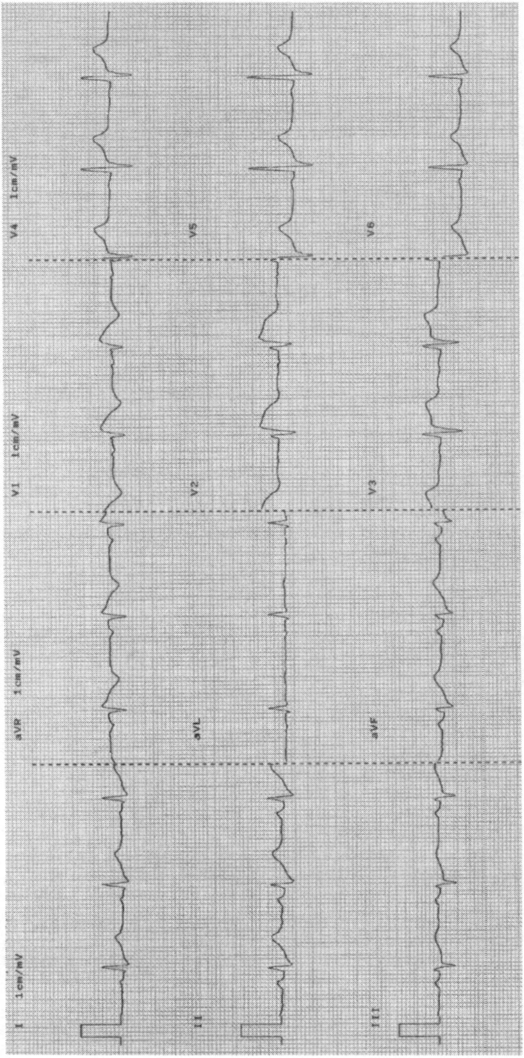

Fig. 24.40 Right precordial ST elevation with T-wave inversion in V1–V3. Association with SCD. See p.351.

Hypertrophic cardiomyopathy

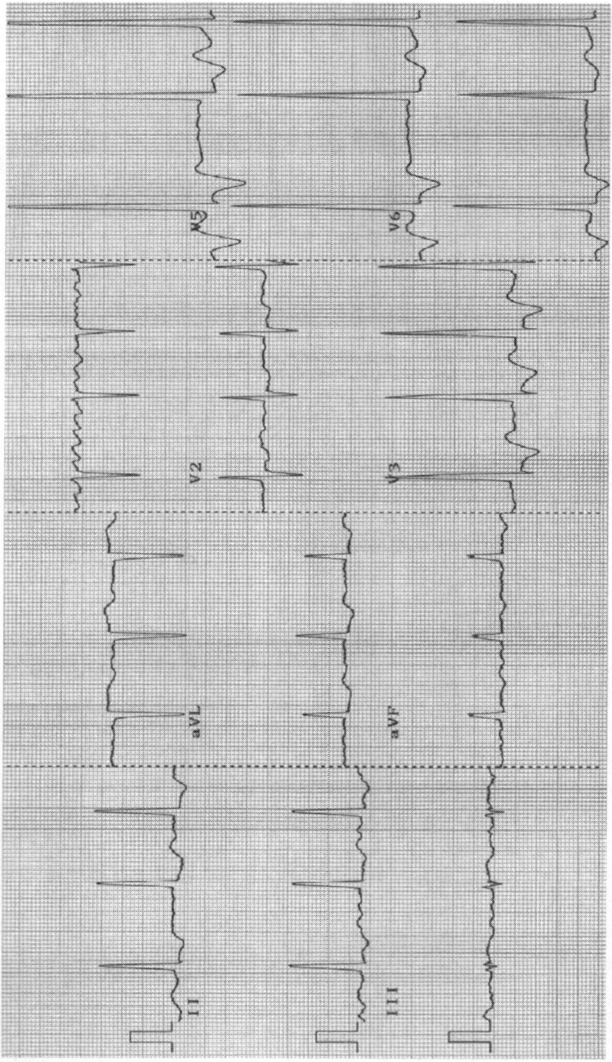

Fig. 24.41 The underlying rhythm is AF. Tall R waves are seen along with repolarization changes in V3–V6, in keeping with LV hypertrophy. See p.343.

Arrhythmogenic right ventricular cardiomyopathy

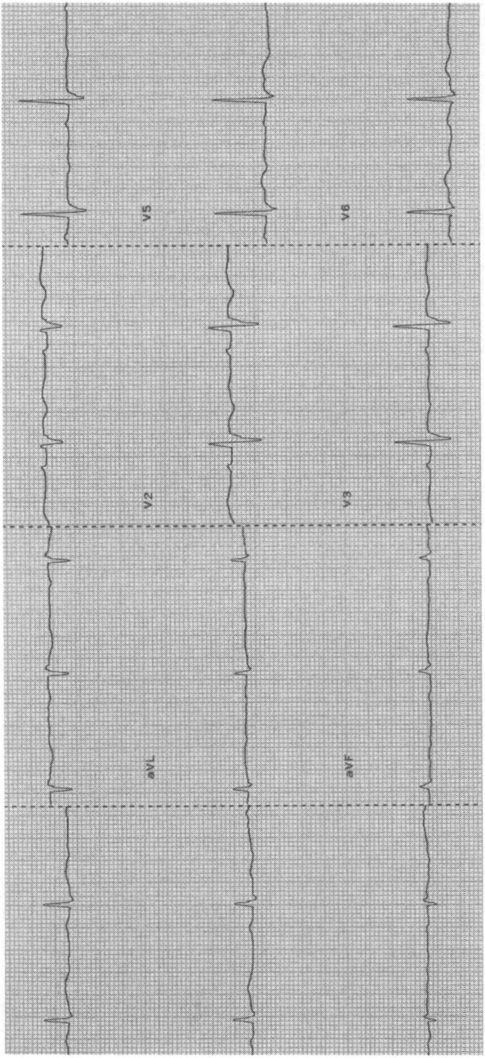

Fig. 24.42 T-wave inversion is seen in the right precordial leads (V1–V3). There is an epsilon wave (a small spike representing a late RV potential) seen in V1 and V2 in the upstroke of the ST segment. Associated with VT. See p.345.

Single chamber pacemaker

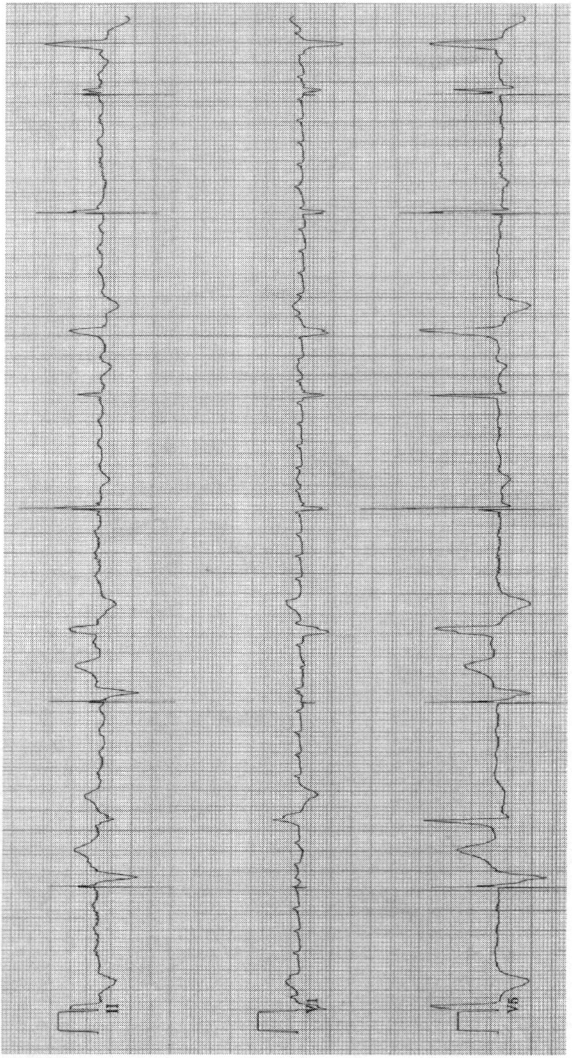

Fig. 24.43 The underlying rhythm is atrial flutter with intermittent ventricular conduction and bigeminy. Pacing spikes precede widened (captured) ventricular complexes and narrow (fusion) ventricular beats.

Dual chamber pacemaker

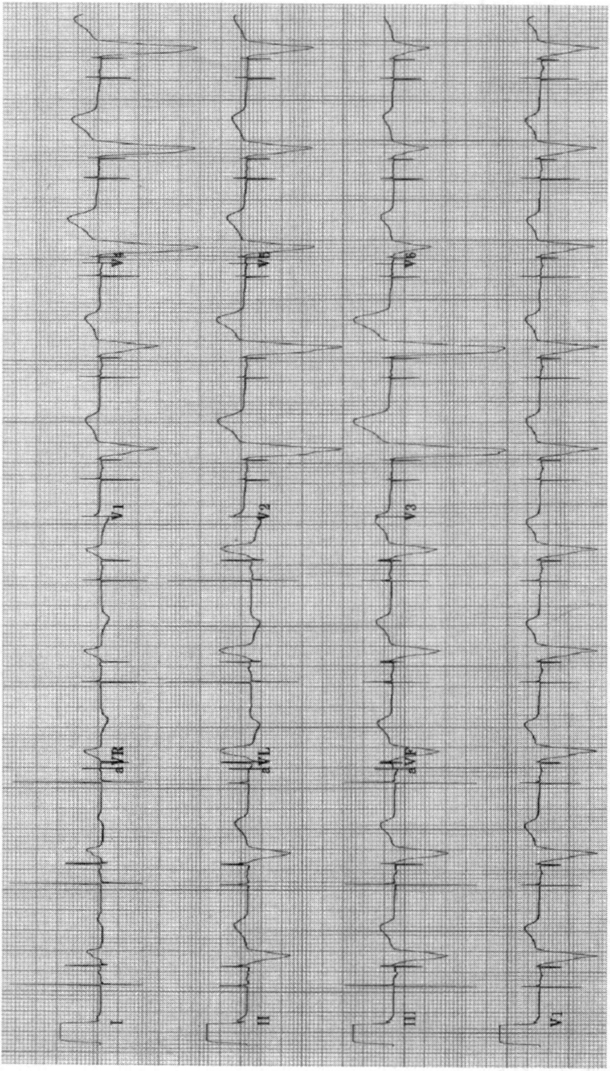

Fig. 24.44 There are pacing spikes preceding each atrial and ventricular complex.

Pacemaker lead failure

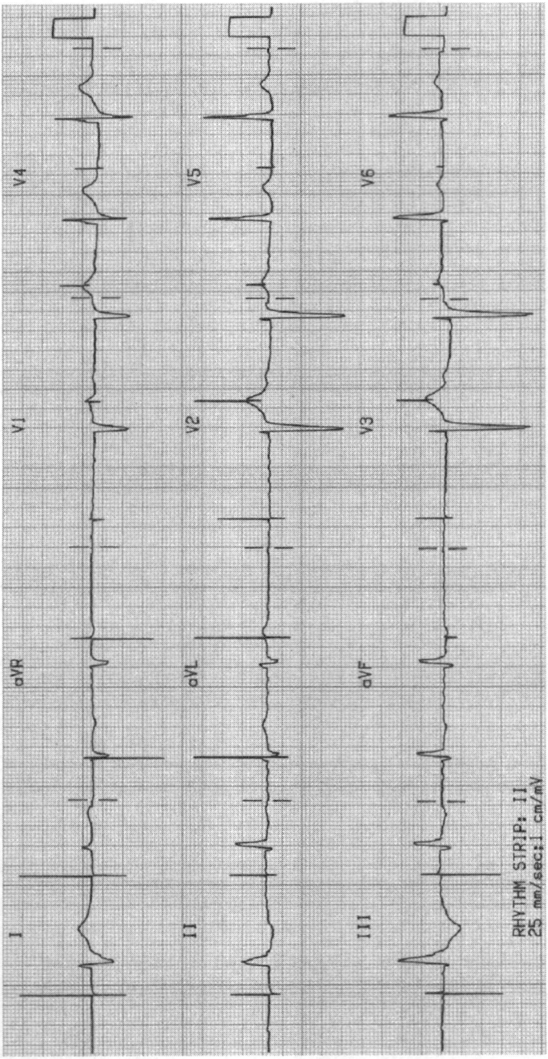

Fig. 24.45 Pacemaker spikes can be seen with no ventricular capture. The ventricular lead had displaced.

Chapter 25

Emergency imaging

Introduction

Patients presenting with unstable cardiovascular disease require rapid and comprehensive assessment integrating clinical findings with appropriate emergency imaging.

Echocardiography remains the most versatile and cost-effective imaging modality for the assessment of critically unwell patients, with alternative modalities used in selected cases. Understanding the advantages and limitations of imaging modalities is important in ensuring the correct assessment and diagnosis is made.

Cardiac CT can be safely undertaken in many patients given the proximity of CT services to emergency departments and rapid protocols.

MRI is not feasible in unstable patients but can be useful in the sub-acute phase to clarify diagnoses.

Unstable cardiovascular disease requiring emergency imaging can include the following clinical scenarios:

- Acute coronary syndrome ➲ p.47
- Cardiogenic shock ➲ p.11
- Mechanical complications of acute coronary syndromes
- Acute aortic pathology ➲ p.179
- Acute pulmonary embolism ➲ p.208
- Cardiac tamponade ➲ p.201
- Acute valvar regurgitation ➲ p.97
- Takotsubo cardiomyopathy ➲ p.50
- Hypertrophic cardiomyopathy ➲ p.343
- Pericarditis ➲ p.198

The majority of these conditions will include symptoms of chest pain and/or breathlessness along with haemodynamic disturbance such as hypotension and/or tachycardia.

Emergency transthoracic echocardiography

Transthoracic echocardiography (TTE) at the patient bedside can rapidly augment the clinical assessment and provide diagnostic information and guide treatment.

It is appropriate to use TTE in the following scenarios:

- Haemodynamic instability with suspected cardiac aetiology
- Suspected myocardial ischaemia with non-diagnostic ECG or biomarkers
- Suspected complication of myocardial ischaemia
- Respiratory failure with suspected cardiac aetiology
- Suspected acute pulmonary embolism

The focus of emergency TTE is to assess ventricular function, the pericardium and the aortic valve, and proximal ascending aorta.

Emergency TTE protocol during cardiopulmonary resuscitation

A protocol for a rapid, focused echo in cardiac arrest includes:

- Parasternal long axis
- Parasternal short axis
- Apical 4 chamber
- Subcostal and IVC

With these four views utilizing 2D imaging only, rapid interpretation and subjective assessment of the following should occur:

- Myocardial insufficiency—pump failure ➲ p.73
- Pericardial collection—tamponade ➲ p.201
- Pulmonary embolism—right heart dysfunction ➲ p.208
- Hypovolaemia—right heart size and filling

Emergency transoesophogeal echocardiography

Transoesophogeal echocardiography can be performed at the bedside although it usually requires sedation and care with airway and oxygenation, so may not be safely achievable in all patients. In emergency departments emergency CT is likely to be more practical, but in patients with cardiovascular emergencies on intensive and critical care units prompt CT may be less feasible and TOE more appropriate.

TOE provides superior assessment of the aortic valve, ascending aorta, mitral valve, left atrium, and posterior pericardium than TTE.

Emergency cardiac CT

Cardiac CT can rapidly evaluate the coronary arteries, aorta, and pulmonary vasculature in most patients. While patients with confirmed or high-risk acute coronary syndrome should undergo invasive diagnostic angiography with follow-on revascularization, patients with low to moderate risk of acute coronary syndrome can be considered for emergency CT coronary angiography.

Acute coronary syndromes

(See ➲ p.47.)

Patients presenting with chest pain and ECG evidence of pathological ST elevation fulfilling criteria for STEMI should undergo assessment with invasive coronary angiography with immediate PCI if an occluded culprit vessel is identified. There is no role for CT or MRI, and uncomplicated cases should not have invasive angiography delayed by assessment with echocardiography.

Patients presenting with chest pain and ischaemia on ECG but without ST elevation should also undergo prompt invasive angiography without further imaging assessment.

Patients presenting with chest pain and elevated or borderline cardiac biomarkers but without ECG evidence of ischaemia should be assessed with urgent imaging to either identify ischaemia or confirm coronary artery pathology. Cardiac CT angiography is appropriate in these patients to evaluate coronary artery anatomy. Dynamic assessment with stress echocardiography or stress/rest CMR can also be considered but is less widely available.

Mechanical complications of acute coronary syndromes

Infarction or ischaemia of myocardium can lead to acute rupture of ventricular walls leading to either ventricular septal defects or free wall rupture and tamponade. The latter is usually fatal although rarely can be contained and treatable. If ischaemia affects a papillary muscle, then rupture will lead to acute severe mitral regurgitation.

Emergency assessment of patients with confirmed infarction or ischaemia who go on to develop acute heart failure and shock includes bedside transthoracic echocardiography to identify the aetiology.

Potential findings at echocardiography include:

- Dilated and impaired right ventricle with abnormal flow across a ventricular septal rupture
- Pericardial collection with evidence of free wall rupture
- Torrential mitral regurgitation with flail portion of mitral valve

If suspected but not confirmed on transthoracic echocardiography then a TOE can be considered once the patient is haemodynamically stabilized which would usually require intubation, ventilation, and intra-aortic balloon pump support.

Cardiogenic shock

(See ➲ p.11.)

Patients with chest pain and hypotension (< 90 mmHg) with evidence of impaired perfusion and end-organ damage need emergency evaluation with bedside transthoracic echocardiography while initial resuscitation and assessment is undertaken. Identification of pump failure with impaired ventricular systolic function should prompt consideration of invasive angiography and vasopressor or mechanical circulatory support.

Acute aortic pathology

(See ➲ p.179.)

Suspected acute aortic dissection or intramural haematoma is best evaluated with emergency CT. Transthoracic echocardiography may be required if there is hypotension and concern over possible progression to aortic root involvement and pericardial effusion.

Transoesophogeal echocardiography is excellent at assessing the ascending aorta and upper descending aorta and can be considered if CT is not readily available, or if immediate surgery to relieve tamponade is required where assessment of the dissection anatomy can guide the surgical approach.

MRI can evaluate the whole aorta and assess for dissection but is not practical or safe in a potentially unstable patient.

Acute pulmonary embolisms

(See ➲ p.208.)

Echocardiography can be normal in up to half of patients with acute pulmonary embolism, for this reason a CT pulmonary angiogram is preferable to echocardiography for diagnosis of suspected pulmonary embolism. Echocardiography can help to guide management in patients with confirmed pulmonary embolism and inform the likely outcome, particularly in patients with significant right ventricular dysfunction.

Cardiac tamponade

(See ➲ p.201.)

Tamponade is a clinical diagnosis, but bedside transthoracic echocardiography is the ideal imaging assessment in patients with suspected tamponade physiology. Evidence of a pericardial collection with reduced cardiac output and increased ventricular interdependence confirms the diagnosis and can also be used to simultaneously guide therapeutic aspiration.

CT can identify pericardial fluid although it often overestimates the amount of fluid present and cannot assess the haemodynamic impact of a pericardial collection.

MRI is accurate for the diagnosis of pericardial effusion and can evaluate cardiac output and respiratory impact on filling but is not relevant in emergency pathology.

Acute valvular regurgitation

(See ➲ p.92.)

Acute severe aortic or mitral regurgitation can present with cardiogenic shock and/or pulmonary oedema. Bedside transthoracic echocardiography is appropriate to rapidly evaluate valve and ventricular function and exclude addition or alternate pathology.

The identification of acute valvar regurgitation should prompt consideration of infective endocarditis and exclusion of aortic pathology in aortic regurgitation, and myocardial infarction with papillary muscle rupture in mitral regurgitation.

Takotsubo cardiomyopathy

(See ➲ p.50.)

Acute left ventricular dysfunction in a pattern not typical for coronary occlusion leading to myocardial dysfunction can be identified with transthoracic echocardiography and is appropriate in patients with chest pain and/or ST elevation where Takotsubo cardiomyopathy may be suspected. Frequently invasive angiography is also required to confidently exclude coronary artery disease, although a CT coronary angiogram may also be considered if the patient is well enough to comfortably undergo this.

Hypertrophic cardiomyopathy

(See ➲ p.343.)

The potential for hypertrophic cardiomyopathy to influence left ventricular outflow tract haemodynamics and mitral valve function make transthoracic echocardiography the preferred modality to assess patients with known or suspected hypertrophic cardiomyopathy presenting with chest pain or breathing difficulties. Careful evaluation of anterior mitral valve leaflet motion, outflow tract gradients, and the timing and direction of mitral regurgitation are important for the full assessment of a patient with ventricular hypertrophy and symptoms.

Pericarditis

(See ➲ p.198.)

Pericarditis is a clinical diagnosis based on a typical history of pain worsening with inspiration and a supine position, supported by ECG changes. Echocardiography is normal in most cases, which can help to exclude alternative diagnoses but is not routinely recommended. Patients with suspected pericarditis and additional symptoms such as breathlessness or hypotension should be assessed with echocardiography to exclude a significant pericardial effusion or wall motion abnormalities that might suggest coronary ischaemia or myocarditis.

Chapter 26

Digital technologies

Introduction

Digital technologies are becoming increasingly used in all aspects of medicine. This includes artificial intelligence (AI) and large language models, virtual reality, wearables and devices, telemedicine, and mobile apps. These technologies enhance early detection, improve patient monitoring, support rapid and informed decision-making, and provide advanced training.

Artificial Intelligence

AI-based image and ECG interpretation

AI in echocardiography

- Automated reporting can help provide key parameters of cardiac structure and function instantly
- Application of complex diagnostic algorithms to detect conditions such as heart failure with preserved ejection faction (HFpEF)
- AI-guided image acquisition software can guide non-experienced operators to acquire diagnostic-quality images
- Automated image interpretation to identify regional wall motion abnormalities

AI in cross-sectional imaging

- Rapid CT coronary angiogram with AI-assisted detection of severe stenosis may identify candidates who need emergency revascularization
- AI in plaque analysis, perivascular inflammation, and fractional flow reserve may also detect those at the highest risk
- Automated segmentation in cardiovascular magnetic resonance (CMR) imaging can provide accurate measurements rapidly
- New AI technologies promise to identify patterns of late gadolinium enhancement without using gadolinium contrast, a process known as virtual native enhancement

AI in ECG

- AI-powered ECG interpretation apps are available and provide rapid advice on likelihood of significant events such as an occlusive myocardial infarction

AI-based decision support tools

AI large language model interfaces

- Can be used to triage patients in the emergency department or referrals based on history, risk factors, and clinical parameters
- Can offer real-time, evidence-based guidance to healthcare providers during cardiac emergencies (Fig 26.1)

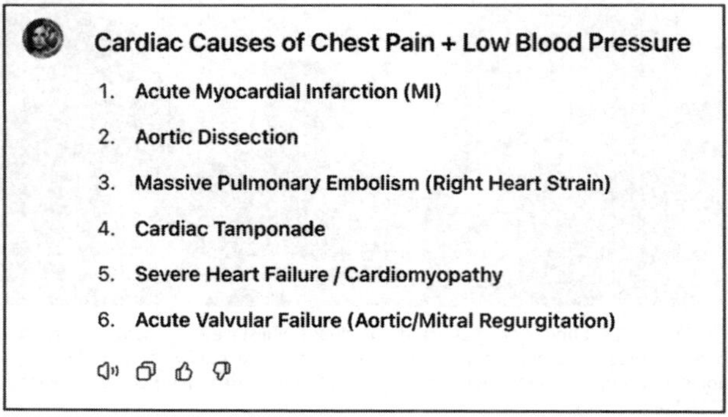

Fig. 26.1 HollieAI using ChatGPT and prompt 'Cardiac causes of chest pain presenting with low blood pressure'.

Virtual reality

Anxiolytic during procedures

- VR immerses patients in calming virtual environments, reducing anxiety during procedures like pericardiocentesis or vas-cular access
- VR can serve as a distraction technique, minimizing the perception of pain and discomfort (Fig. 26.2)
- Patients can use VR headsets to engage in guided relaxation exercises, enhancing their overall procedural experience

Procedural training

- VR simulations provide realistic, hands-on training for medical professionals, allowing them to practise complex procedures in a controlled environment
- Detailed anatomy visualization and interactive scenarios help trainees understand spatial relationships and procedural steps
- Repetitive practice in VR improves proficiency, confidence, and procedural accuracy, leading to better patient outcomes

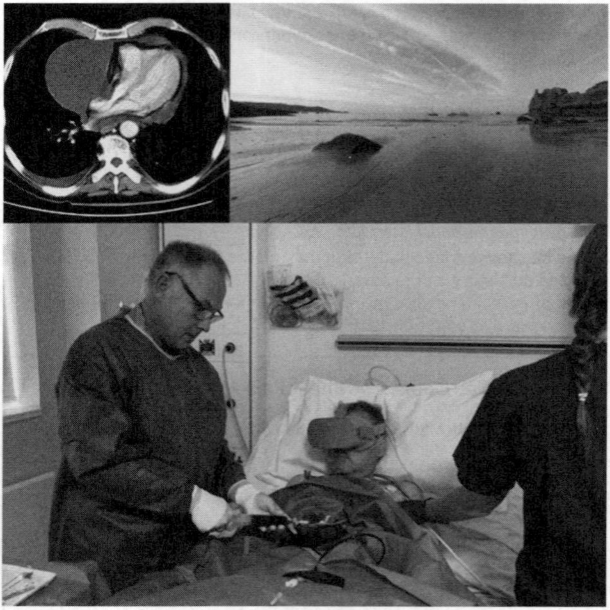

Fig. 26.2 Patient undergoing pericardial drainage whilst viewing images of a calm beach in Jersey. Reproduced with permission from Virtual reality as a therapy adjunct during emergency pericardiocentesis. *European Heart Journal Case Reports* 2020 May 19; 4(4): 1.

Wearables

Monitoring devices

Smart watches and smart phones

- Can monitor heart rhythm and perform single-lead ECGs
- Can track physical activity levels and sleep patterns
- Newer systems can record cuffless blood pressure
- Data can be downloaded from smart phones for review by healthcare provider
- Similar technology is now being applied to other devices such as glasses, rings, and shoes

Newer technologies

- Technology integrated into shirts and vests has shown promise in detecting changes in intrathoracic impendence which may precede heart failure decompensation
- Patch-based ultrasound devices are being developed to non-invasively measure haemodynamics and can detect changes in stroke volume

Real-time monitoring

- Continuous data collection from wearables allows for the immediate detection of cardiac abnormalities, enabling prompt intervention
- Wearables empower patients to take an active role in managing their heart health, increasing adherence to treatment plans and lifestyle modifications

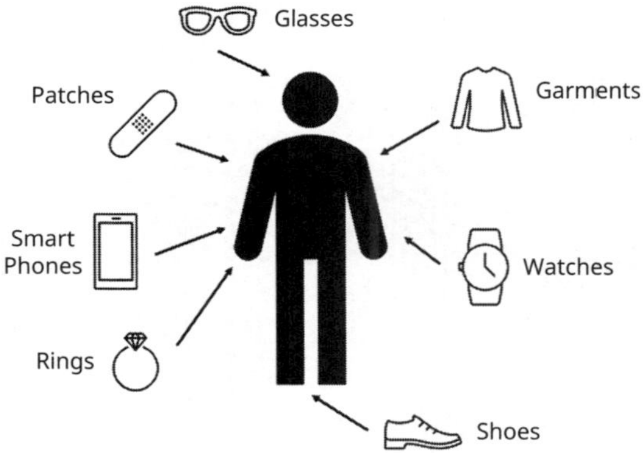

Fig. 26.3 Examples of wearable technology in detecting cardiac disease.

Devices

Cardiac-implanted electronic devices

- Include pacemakers, implantable cardioverter defibrillators (ICDs), and cardiac resynchronization therapy (CRT) devices
- These devices continuously monitor and regulate heart rhythms, providing life-saving interventions when necessary
- Remote monitoring capabilities allow healthcare providers to track device performance and patient status in real time

Portable ECGs

- Portable ECG devices including watches that connect to smart phones, enabling patients to record and share ECGs with their healthcare providers instantly
- Provides a convenient way for patients to monitor their heart health and detect arrhythmias early

Automated external defibrillators

- Can analyse heart rhythms and deliver shocks to restore normal rhythm in cases of sudden cardiac arrest
- Modern AEDs use AI to enhance rhythm analysis accuracy, ensuring appropriate and timely defibrillation

Telemedicine

Remote consultations

- Telemedicine platforms enable cardiologists to provide consultations and follow-ups for patients in remote or under-served areas
- Facilitates real-time communication between emergency medical services and cardiologists, improving patient triage and initial management

Guiding practical procedures

- Telemedicine can guide less experienced healthcare providers through complex procedures, such as thrombolysis or pericardiocentesis, in real time
- Can enhance the quality of care delivered in pre-hospital settings and during transport to medical facilities

Mobile Health Applications

Patient management apps

- Medication reminders and adherence tracking help patients follow prescribed treatment plans
- Integration with wearable devices and other health data sources provides a comprehensive view of patient health, aiding in proactive management
- Automated alerts based on critical health data can notify patients to seek emergency medical attention

Clinician management apps

- Can provide tools to track patient status during emergencies, monitor vital signs, and manage drug administration
- Interactive management algorithms to follow during emergencies

Chapter 27

Palliative care

Recognizing dying

Recognizing that a patient is at risk of dying in the next few days or hours is an essential skill. Recognition of dying allows the patient and their families to be informed and included in individualized decision making about end-of-life care. It shifts the approach from active, interventional medicine to providing clear information about dying and delivering best supportive care. Caring for a dying patient necessitates regular reviews as their condition changes, with cessation of futile, often burdensome, treatments and tests.

Patient at risk of dying

- Several hospital admissions, with decreasing time between each one
- Functional decline with an increasing burden of symptoms
- Weight loss and poor appetite
- No single biochemical marker or scan result is indicative of dying but collectively the following suggest poor chance of recovery:
  - Persistently low Hgb, albumin, or sodium
  - Worsening liver or renal failure
  - Progressive disease on diagnostic testing
  - Cognitive decline, which is often rapid
- Increasing dependence on others
- Increasing frailty: enquire about the 4 Fs (forgetfulness, falls, functional decline, and fatigue)

Young patients (< 60 years), those who have been fit and active, and/or those with rapid progression of their illness, may compensate well and then deteriorate quickly. Dying can go undetected in these patients until it is too late to have important conversations.

Recognizing active dying

The following indicate that a patient is actively dying (hours to days):

- Excessive drowsiness (not medication-related)
- Bedbound and/or profoundly weak
- New-onset or worsening confusion or delirium
- Minimal or no oral intake or fluids (coughing on fluids)
- Unable to take oral medications

Reassure patients and their families that these findings are expected and a normal part of dying. Speech and language therapy and dietetic input is rarely indicated. Some patients may aspirate on oral fluids, risk feeding is often acceptable. See below for advice on IV fluids and non-oral delivery of medications. Good mouth care is essential.

Managing dying

The patient (or their family) has often already thought that they could be dying. Traditionally, medicine is about sustaining life and, to give hope, we offer more treatments. Talking openly and honestly about dying often brings relief. Discussions about the futility of cardiopulmonary resuscitation and other treatments will follow relatively easily.

Discussing patient wishes

- Where does patient want to be when they die?
- How do we ensure that they don't receive futile treatment?
- What symptoms might be expected and how will we manage them?
- Do they have a will or other instructions to share before they die? Some people like to write letters (particularly for children)
- Can they be an organ or tissue donor?
- What happens after death?

Many hospitals will have a booklet that can support these discussions.

Transitioning to end-of-life care

- Document that the patient is dying, and all decisions/discussions
- Complete the DNACPR form (and/or ReSPECT form, if used)
- Stop all tests including blood tests, unless they direct symptom management
- Stop venous cannulation
- Stop observations
- Request regular mouth care, pressure-relieving mattresses, and repositioning (to avoid pressure sores)
- Request regular reviews by the nursing team even if observations are not being recorded
- Consider referral to the palliative care—for support, advice on symptom management, and logistics or transfer of the patient to a hospice or home

Prognostication

- This is challenging: explain to patients that they may live longer, or shorter, than doctors predict
- The rate of change in symptoms can help predict the time to death—deterioration every day suggests the patient is entering the last days of life

Drugs

A patient's medications should be reviewed and rationalized when dying is recognized: don't wait until the patient cannot swallow to stop drugs. Stop all medications that do not control symptoms and/or are futile or unpleasant for a dying patient.

Drugs and devices

- Antibiotics—stop unless doing so will result in poor symptom control (e.g. painful infected wound, fevers/rigors). Don't re-cannulate dying patients for IV drugs unless essential for symptom control
- Antiepileptics—patient may need subcutaneously (seek advice)
- Antidepressants—stop
- Antihypertensives—usually stop
- Anticoagulation—usually stop (even in those with thromboemboli and metallic heart valves); patient will die before harm arises
- Antiplatelets—usually stop; patient will die before harm arises
- Diuretics—usually stop; continuing diuretics as this stage can cause excessive dryness and thirst. Try without but prescribe furosemide subcutaneously PRN (see Table 27.1)
- ICD—deactivate, if present
- Rate-controlling drugs—stop unless recent decompensation or symptomatic tachycardia
- Statins—stop
- Steroid may help with pain and nausea, but cause hyperglycaemia, heighten appetite (unwelcome when dying), and can cause agitation. Reduce or stop depending on the indication
- Vitamins, minerals, nutritional supplements—stop

Diabetes management

- Stop dietary restrictions
- Type 1 diabetes
  - Accept capillary blood glucose (CBG) of 10–20 mmol/L
  - Reduce basal insulin to achieve target CBG (usually by 25–50%)
  - Stop regular short-acting insulin (prescribe PRN)
  - Do not test for ketones (usually elevated in dying patients)
  - Stop insulin when patient is completely unresponsive
  - Seek input from diabetes/palliative care teams on continuous monitoring devices and insulin pumps
- Type 2 diabetes
  - Stop all medications including insulin
  - Stop checking CBGs

Fluids and blood products

Patients at the end of life rarely require parenteral fluids, but a trial of fluids is sometimes indicated (e.g. for thirst). Blood products are rarely useful and can cause harm. Tranexamic acid may be indicated if patients are persistently bleeding. Stop checking and chasing FBC.

Symptom management

The preferred route of medication delivery at end of life (in the UK) is subcutaneous. This route can be used for 'as required' medications or as a continuous subcutaneous infusion (CSCI).

A CSCI device allows medications to be delivered via subcutaneous line connected to a portable syringe driver. The CSCI bypasses the need for the oral and IV routes, and issues with drug elimination. Lines can remain *in situ* for 3–7 days.

Most common drug combinations are compatible and can be delivered via one CSCI, namely analgesia (morphine or alternative opioid), anxiolytic/sedative (midazolam), anticholinergic (hyoscine butylbromide) for secretions, and antiemetic (metoclopramide or haloperidol). Other drugs must be delivered individually due to incompatibility or volume (e.g. furosemide).

Palliative care input is advised for patients who have required multiple PRN doses and/or who have persistent symptoms. Also seek advice about conversion of medications to the subcutaneous route (e.g. antiepileptic drugs).

Table 27.1 Common symptoms and subcutaneous medications for management at end of life.

Symptom	Key issues	Drugs (via SC route unless otherwise stated)
Breathlessness	Use opioid and/or benzodiazepines Morphine is usually first line unless established on an alternative opioid	**Midazolam** 2.5 mg 1 hrly PRN **Morphine** 2.5 mg 1 hrly PRN
Restlessness or anxiety	Assess for reversible causes. Is patient in pain, urinary retention or constipated?	**Midazolam** 2.5–5 mg 1 hrly PRN 10–30 mg/24 h CSCI
Agitation	As above: address reversible causes	**Haloperidol** 0.5–1.5 mg bd (2–5 mg/24 h CSCI)
Respiratory secretions	Start medications as soon as secretions appear Counsel family: it may not be possible to stop secretions; patient will not be distressed if they have reduced conscious level	**Hyoscine butylbromide** (not *hyoscine hydrobromide*) 20 mg 1 hrly PRN (60–120 mg/24 h CSCI) **Furosemide (if pulmonary oedema)** 20 mg PRN (up to 200 mg/24 h CSCI)
Pain	Morphine is usually first line unless established on an alternative opioid	**Morphine in opioid naïve** 2.5 mg 1hrly PRN (5–10 mg/24 h CSCI)

(*Continued*)

Table 27.1 (*Contd.*)

Symptom	Key issues	Drugs (via SC route unless otherwise stated)
Seizures	For new or worsening seizures, use midazolam	**Midazolam** 10 mg SC or IM PRN (30–60 mg/24 h CSCI)
Nausea and vomiting	Gastric stasis/general antiemetic	**Metoclopramide** 10 mg qds (30–60 mg/24 h via CSCI)
Nausea and vomiting	Opioid-related/renal failure/ hypercalcaemia	**Haloperidol** 0.5–1 mg bd (1–2 mg/24 h CSCI)
Nausea and vomiting	Brain metastases/raised ICP/Parkinson's disease	**Cyclizine** 25 mg tds (75–150 mg/24 h via CSCI)
Bleeding (including haematemesis, haemoptysis, epistaxis, haematuria, bleeds from tumours)	Consider tranexamic acid (oral, IV, topical, SC) to control persistent mild–moderate bleeds Risk of large-volume bleeds: prepare the family (but not always the patient) Put brown/green towels in patient's room or nearby STOP anticoagulants and antiplatelet drugs Prescribe midazolam as PRN. Make team aware.	**Tranexamic acid** Soak gauze with solution for injection and apply to low volume, superficial bleeds. If persistent: 2000 mg/24 h via CSCI **Midazolam—for large-volume (likely terminal) bleeding** **IM/IV** 10 mg stat and repeat after 5 minutes if needed. IM/IV onset quicker than SC DON'T BE AFRAID TO GIVE, if the patient survives the bleed, they will not be harmed by midazolam given in this manner.

After death

Give relatives the opportunity to see or remain with the patient after death.

Patients who die in hospital will usually be moved to a hospital mortuary within hours. Direct families to your bereavement office who will guide them through the next steps.

From 2024: all deaths in UK are reviewed by medical examiner. This process includes a call to the bereaved families to ask if they understand the cause of death and have any concerns or questions. It is good practice to tell families about this.

When to refer to the coroner

- Cause of death is not known
- Death during surgery, under anaesthesia, or in the early post-operative period
- Death related to poisoning, use of a controlled drug, or medicinal product
- Death related to neglect or failure of care
- Mesothelioma (or industrial disease)
- Death was violent, suspicious, or unnatural (accidents, suicide)

Tissue donation

- Many patients with chronic conditions cannot donate organs but may be able to donate tissue (eyes, bones, skin, heart valves, or tendons)
- Patients with blood-borne viruses, haematological malignancies, or dementia cannot donate tissue
- In the UK, the process of tissue donation is usually coordinated by the National Referral Centre (NHS Blood and Transplant)
- Retrieval of tissue after death needs to occur within 24 hours for eye donation and 48 hours for other tissues

Box 27.1 Resources

- End of life care: One chance to get it right. Improving people's experience of care in the last few days and hours of life, the Leadership Alliance for the Care of Dying People (2014)
- Talking about DNACPR: http://talkcpr.wales/
- What to do when someone dies: step by step www.gov.uk/when-someone-dies
- Tissue Donation: www.organdonation.nhs.uk/helping-you-to-decide/about-organ-donation/tissue-donation/

Index

For the benefit of digital users, indexed terms that span two pages (e.g., 52–53) may, on occasion, appear on only one of those pages.

Tables, figures, and boxes are indicated by an italic *t* , *f* , and *b* following the page number.

A

F

G

H

Q

R

S